Formulation tools for pharmaceutical development

Published by Woodhead Publishing Limited, 2013

Woodhead Publishing Series in Biomedicine

1 Practical leadership for biopharmaceutical executives
J. Y. Chin
2 Outsourcing biopharma R&D to India
P. R. Chowdhury
3 Matlab® in bioscience and biotechnology
L. Burstein
4 Allergens and respiratory pollutants
Edited by M. A. Williams
5 Concepts and techniques in genomics and proteomics
N. Saraswathy and P. Ramalingam
6 An introduction to pharmaceutical sciences
J. Roy
7 Patently innovative: How pharmaceutical firms use emerging patent law to extend monopolies on blockbuster drugs
R. A. Bouchard
8 Therapeutic protein drug products: Practical approaches to formulation in the laboratory, manufacturing and the clinic
Edited by B. K. Meyer
9 A biotech manager's handbook: A practical guide
Edited by M. O'Neill and M. H. Hopkins
10 Clinical research in Asia: Opportunities and challenges
U. Sahoo
11 Therapeutic antibody engineering: Current and future advances driving the strongest growth area in the pharma industry
W. R. Strohl and L. M. Strohl
12 Commercialising the stem cell sciences
O. Harvey
13 Biobanks: Patents or open science?
A. De Robbio
14 Human papillomavirus infections: From the laboratory to clinical practice
F. Cobo
15 Annotating new genes: From *in silico* screening to experimental validation
S. Uchida
16 Open-source software in life science research: Practical solutions in the pharmaceutical industry and beyond
Edited by L. Harland and M. Forster

Published by Woodhead Publishing Limited, 2013

17 Nanoparticulate drug delivery: A perspective on the transition from laboratory to market
V. Patravale, P. Dandekar and R. Jain

18 Bacterial cellular metabolic systems: Metabolic regulation of a cell system with ^{13}C-metabolic flux analysis
K. Shimizu

19 Contract research and manufacturing services (CRAMS) in India: The business, legal, regulatory and tax environment
M. Antani and G. Gokhale

20 Bioinformatics for biomedical science and clinical applications
K-H. Liang

21 Deterministic versus stochastic modelling in biochemistry and systems biology
P. Lecca, I. Laurenzi and F. Jordan

22 Protein folding *in silico* : Protein folding versus protein structure prediction
I. Roterman

23 Computer-aided vaccine design
J. C. Tong and S. Ranganathan

24 An introduction to biotechnology
W. T. Godbey

25 RNA interference: Therapeutic developments
T. Novobrantseva, P. Ge and G. Hinkle

26 Patent litigation in the pharmaceutical and biotechnology industries
G. Morgan

27 Clinical research in paediatric psychopharmacology: A practical guide
P. Auby

28 The application of SPC in the pharmaceutical and biotechnology industries
T. Cochrane

29 Ultrafiltration for bioprocessing
H. Lutz

30 Therapeutic risk management of medicines
A. K. Banerjee and S. Mayall

31 21st century quality management and good management practices: Value added compliance for the pharmaceutical and biotechnology industry
S. Williams

32 Sterility, sterilisation and sterility assurance for pharmaceuticals
T. Sandle

33 CAPA in the pharmaceutical and biotech industries: How to implement an effective nine step programme
J. Rodriguez

34 Process validation for the production of biopharmaceuticals: Principles and best practice.
A. R. Newcombe and P. Thillaivinayagalingam

35 Clinical trial management: An overview
U. Sahoo and D. Sawant

36 Impact of regulation on drug development
H. Guenter Hennings

37 Lean biomanufacturing
N. J. Smart

38 Marine enzymes for biocatalysis
Edited by A. Trincone

Published by Woodhead Publishing Limited, 2013

39 Ocular transporters and receptors in the eye: Their role in drug delivery
A. K. Mitra
40 Stem cell bioprocessing: For cellular therapy, diagnostics and drug development
T. G. Fernandes, M. M. Diogo and J. M. S. Cabral
41 Oral Delivery of Insulin
T.A Sonia and Chandra P. Sharma
42 Fed-batch fermentation: A practical guide to scalable recombinant protein production in *Escherichia coli*
G. G. Moulton and T. Vedvick
43 The funding of biopharmaceutical research and development
D. R. Williams
44 Formulation tools for pharmaceutical development
Edited by J. E. Aguilar
45 Drug-biomembrane interaction studies: The application of calorimetric techniques
Edited by R. Pignatello
46 Orphan drugs: Understanding the rare drugs market
E. Hernberg-Ståhl
47 Nanoparticle-based approaches to targeting drugs for severe diseases
J. L. Arias
48 Successful biopharmaceutical operations: Driving change
C. Driscoll
49 Electroporation-based therapies for cancer: From basics to clinical applications
Edited by R. Sundararajan
50 Transporters in drug discovery and development: Detailed concepts and best practice
Y. Lai
51 The life-cycle of pharmaceuticals in the environment
R. Braund and B. Peake
52 Computer-aided applications in pharmaceutical technology
Edited by J. Djuris
53 From plant genomics to plant biotechnology
Edited by P. Poltronieri, N. Burbulis and C. Fogher
54 Bioprocess engineering: An introductory engineering and life science approach
K. G. Clarke
55 Quality assurance problem solving and training strategies for success in the pharmaceutical and life science industries
G. Welty
56 TBC
57 Gene therapy: Potential applications of nanotechnology
S. Nimesh
58 Controlled drug delivery: The role of self-assembling multi-task excipients
M. Mateescu
59 *In silico* protein design
C. M. Frenz
60 Bioinformatics for computer science: Foundations in modern biology
K. Revett
61 Gene expression analysis in the RNA world
J. Q. Clement

Published by Woodhead Publishing Limited, 2013

62 Computational methods for finding inferential bases in molecular genetics
Q-N. Tran

63 NMR metabolomics in cancer research
M. Čuperlović-Culf

64 Virtual worlds for medical education, training and care delivery
K. Kahol

Published by Woodhead Publishing Limited, 2013

Woodhead Publishing Series in Biomedicine: Number 44

Formulation tools for pharmaceutical development

EDITED BY
J. E. AGUILAR

WP
WOODHEAD
PUBLISHING

Oxford Cambridge Philadelphia New Delhi

Published by Woodhead Publishing Limited, 2013

Woodhead Publishing Limited, 80 High Street, Sawston, Cambridge, CB22 3HJ, UK
www.woodheadpublishing.com
www.woodheadpublishingonline.com

Woodhead Publishing, 1518 Walnut Street, Suite 1100, Philadelphia, PA 19102-3406, USA

Woodhead Publishing India Private Limited, G-2, Vardaan House, 7/28 Ansari Road, Daryaganj, New Delhi – 110002, India
www.woodheadpublishingindia.com

First published in 2013 by Woodhead Publishing Limited
ISBN: 978–1–907568–99–2 (print); ISBN: 978–1–908818–50–8 (online)
Woodhead Publishing Series in Biomedicine ISSN 2050-0289 (print); ISSN 2050-0297 (online)

British Library Cataloguing-in-Publication Data: A catalogue record for this book is available from the British Library.

Library of Congress Control Number: 2013932368

Typeset by RefineCatch Limited, Bungay, Suffolk

The innovation point is the pivotal moment when talented and motivated people seek the opportunity to act on their ideas and dreams

W. Arthur Porter

To my son Pablo, who changed my life and is my inspiration to want to be better and better.

J. E. Aguilar

Published by Woodhead Publishing Limited, 2013

Contents

Published by Woodhead Publishing Limited, 2013

List of figures

Published by Woodhead Publishing Limited, 2013

Published by Woodhead Publishing Limited, 2013

List of tables

Published by Woodhead Publishing Limited, 2013

Foreword

Formulation Tools for Pharmaceutical Development describes the application of selected computer based tools for pharmaceutical development with the aim to improve its efficiency. Broadly, these tools aid developers to leverage prior knowledge more effectively. It is my privilege to provide a context for this book and I hope readers will find this useful.

Like many of the authors of chapters in this book, I also trained as a pharmacist – pharmaceutical engineer – and I too aspire to improve how high-quality pharmaceutical products are developed and manufactured. Early in my academic career I studied the application of Artificial Neural Networks for this purpose and progressed the idea of 'Computer Aided Formulation Design'.[1,2] As a regulator (at the US FDA) one of my interests was to improve the utility of prior knowledge and scientific development reports in regulatory review and inspection decisions – this interest, in part, culminated in the development of a framework for Quality by Design of pharmaceutical products.

The ability to leverage prior knowledge for decision making poses several challenges. Overcoming these challenges provides a means to improve the development process as it helps to: (a) prevent repeating past mistakes, (b) understand patterns in formulation-process variables and variance in product performance, and (c) identify a set of optimal conditions, without having to conduct a large number of trial-and-error experiments, to achieve a desired product quality and performance.

Chapters in this book describe useful practical applications of neural networks, expert systems and mathematical modeling to a range of problems in pharmaceutical development. As you read these chapters, take a moment to consider how you can apply these tools in your work. Keep in mind that your ability to generate 'testable predictions', which can be validated empirically, will improve the process of product development and facilitate regulatory communication. Please do also reflect on the importance collecting the 'right information'. This exercise should help to inform improvements in your approach for collecting, organizing, modeling and analyzing data. An important goal is to generate knowledge that improves understanding of underlying patterns and mechanism. Doing so will, I believe, help make you and your organizations more effective in completing your future projects in less time and at lower cost.

As an ex-regulator and as a champion of Quality by Design I see significant value (e.g., competitive advantage) to be gained by companies that effectively leverage prior knowledge in product development and related regulatory submissions. In closing I share with you the following words of wisdom from Deming: 'Experience by itself teaches nothing ... Without theory, experience has no meaning. Without theory, one has no questions to ask. Hence, without theory, there is no learning.'[3]

Ajaz S. Hussain, Ph.D., Frederick, MD, USA.
a2zpharmsci@msn.com

References

1. Hussain, A.S., Yu, X., and Johnson, R.A.: Application of Neural Computing in Pharmaceutical Product Development. *Pharm. Res.* 8: 1248–1252 (1991).
2. Hussain, A.S., Shivanand, P., and Johnson, R.A.: Application of Neural Computing in Pharmaceutical Product Development: Computer Aided Formulation Design. *Drug. Dev. Ind. Pharm.* 20: 1739–175 (1994).
3. Deming, W.E. *The New Economics for Industry, Government, Education.* M.I.T. Press (1991).

Dr. Hussain currently serves as the Chief Scientific Officer and the President Biotechnology at Wockhardt Ltd. Prior to this appointment in 2012 he held position of CSO and Vice President at Philip Morris International (PMI) and Vice President Biopharmaceutical Development at Sandoz. At PMI he contributed towards development of a platform for manufacturing vaccines in tobacco plant and on tobacco harm reduction thru assessment of modified risk tobacco products. At Sandoz he led the development and registration of several of biosimilar products and established a 'quality by design' framework for biosimilar development. Prior to his industrial experience Dr. Hussain served as Deputy Director, Office of Pharmaceutical Science at the US FDA. There he championed

Published by Woodhead Publishing Limited, 2013

the FDA's initiatives on Process Analytical Technology and Quality by Design. He started his professional career in academia (University of Cincinnati and the Ohio Northern University). His major scientific contributions have been in the areas of application of Artificial Neural Networks, Computer-Aided Formulation Design, Biopharmaceutics Classification System, In vitro In Vivo Correlations, Process Analytical Technology and Quality by Design. He is the recipient of several prestigious awards such as the FIP's Industrial Pharmacy Medal and the Scientific Achievement Award of AAPS. He is a Fellow of American Association of Pharmaceutical Scientists and the Swiss Society for Pharmaceutical Sciences.

About the authors

Johnny E. Aguilar Ph.D.

Dr. Johnny Aguilar has over 12 years of experience in the pharmaceutical industry in different areas such as quality control, quality assurance, highly potent compound management, launching, quality operation, vaccines and diagnostics management and manufacturing science and technology departments; this experience was gained working in major international pharmaceutical companies in Spain, Australia and Switzerland. He was also Professor on a master's programme in Business Management of the Pharmaceutical Industry and of the Programme for Specialists in Industrial Pharmacy by the Spanish Government at the department of Pharmaceutical Technology at the University of Barcelona, Spain. He studied pharmacy at the National University of Trujillo (Peru) and holds a Master in Management of the Pharmaceutical Industry and a Ph.D. in Pharmacy and Pharmaceutical Technology from the University of Barcelona. He has participated in many scientific congresses about pharmaceutical technology, both national and international. He is the author or co-author of more than 20 international scientific papers and one book on pharmaceutical technology. He holds two awards, one from ISPE-Spain and one Accesit Dr Esteve award of the Royal Academy of Pharmacy of Catalonia. He was also invited in 2010 to be an associate member of the Peruvian Academy of Health in Lima and his Ph.D. thesis received the Extraordinary Doctoral Award (2010–2011) from the University of Barcelona. Dr. Aguilar can be contacted at aguiljo9f@hotmail.com.

Aleš Belič

Aleš Belič is an associate professor at the Faculty of Electrical Engineering, University of Ljubljana where he is involved in modelling and analysis of biological and pharmaceutical systems with major stress on the analysis of EEG signals, system biology, pharmacokinetics, and modelling in pharmaceutical technology. He received his B.Sc. and Ph.D. degrees from the Faculty of Electrical Engineering, University of Ljubljana in 1994 and 2000, respectively, for the modelling in pharmacokinetics and pharmacodynamics. He collaborates with many people and groups at:

Faculty of Pharmacy at the University of Ljubljana, Centre for Functional Genomics and Biochips at Medical Faculty (University of Ljubljana), Institute for Clinical Neurophysiology at University Clinical Centre Ljubljana, Krka Pharmaceuticals d.d., Sandoz Research Centre Mengeš, Institute for Analysis and Technical Computing at the Technical University of Vienna, Chemical Research Centre at the Hungarian Academy of Sciences in Budapest. He has been involved in several industrial projects as well as national and international research activities (6th and 7th European Framework Projects).
He may be contacted at ales.belic@fe.uni-lj.si.

Roser Fuster García
Roser Fuster García graduated as a Technical Engineer specialising in Industrial Chemistry from the Industrial School of Barcelona of the UPC (Spain) in 1978. She worked as a laboratory technician in Quality Control and then as a technician in development of new products in Galenical Development until 1990 in the Pharmaceutical Industry: Dr. Andreu. Then she worked as a laboratory technician in Laboratorios Hosbon (in quality control and pharmaceutical development), Laboratorios Salvat (pharmaceutical development) and Parke-Davis (quality control). She joined the Service of Development of Medicines (SDM) at the Faculty of Pharmacy at the University of Barcelona in 2004, where she is working on the investigation and development of new medicines and implementation of new methodologies used in characterization and quality control of solid dosage forms, which have been published in a significant number of scientific papers.

Dra. Encarna García Montoya
Dra. García Montoya studied pharmacy at the University of Barcelona (Spain). She started her career working as a quality assurance technician at Laboratorios Hosbon (Group Roussel Uclaf-Hoescht) and then worked as a quality control technician at Laboratorios Uriach (Spain). She then joined the Department of Pharmacy and Pharmaceutical Technology at the University of Barcelona, where she was appointed to Quality Assurance, responsible for the Service of Development of Medicines (SDM) of the Faculty of Pharmacy. She holds a Ph.D. in Pharmacy and Pharmaceutical Technology from the same University (2001), and became Titular Professor in 2003. Dr. García Montoya has been recognized as a Specialist in Industrial Pharmacy by the Spanish Government in 2005 and Specialist in Quality and Control of Medicines in 2006. She has also participated in a substantial number of basic and applied research projects

developed in the SDM. She is the author or co-author of several international scientific papers and co-author of six books on *Pharmaceutical Technology and Pharmaceutical Quality*, edited by Dr. Ramon Salazar. In addition, she has been Coordinator of the Master in Business Management of the Pharmaceutical Industry (UB) since 1996. She has participated in a significant number of scientific congresses about pharmaceutical technology, both national and international. Her research interests have focused on the area of pharmaceutical quality, multimedia tools applied to the pharmaceutical industry and direct compression technology.
Dra. García Montoya can be contacted at encarnagarcia@ub.edu, egarciamontoya@gmail.com.

Dr. M. Landin
Mariana Landin studied pharmacy at the University of Santiago de Compostela (Spain) and holds a doctorate from the same University (1991). After a three-year postdoctoral stage in the UK, she again joined the Department of Pharmacy and Pharmaceutical Technology at the University of Santiago, becoming a professor in 1998. Dr. Landin was recognized as a Specialist in Industrial Pharmacy by the Spanish Government in 2005. She has participated in a substantial number of basic and applied research projects, both national and international. She has supervised more than 10 Ms.D. and Ph.D. students and collaborated in the organization of international and national symposia. She is the author or co-author of more than 50 international papers, some of them included as main references in the *Handbook of Pharmaceutical Excipients*. She has a background and broad experience in the areas of pharmaceutical material science and processing, such as raw materials characterization and variability or scale-up process. She also has extensive experience in the design and evaluation of immediate and controlled drug delivery systems. Over recent years her research interests have been focused on the applicability of artificial intelligence tools (artificial neural networks, neuro-fuzzy logic and genetic programming) for modelling biological and technological process in order to aid better understanding and rational design of new and/or better dosage forms.
Dr. Landin can be contacted at m.landin@usc.es.

Dr. Hans Leuenberger
Dr. Hans Leuenberger is Professor Emeritus in Pharmaceutical Technology at the University of Basel in Switzerland. He is also CEO of the Intitute for Innovation in Industrial Pharmacy and CSO of Cincap. He holds an M.Sc. in Physics, a Ph.D. in Nuclear Physics and Private Docent in

Pharmaceutics, all obtained from the University of Basel. He was Private Docent in Pharmaceutics, full Professor and Head of the Institute of Pharmaceutical Technology, Head of the Department of Pharmaceutical Sciences and Dean of the Faculty of Science at the University of Basel. He holds different awards related to pharmaceutical sciences from different universities and, in 2007, he received a Ph.D honoris causa in Pharmaceutics from the Mahidol University in Bangkok, Thailand, and another in 2008 from the Mendeleyev University of Chemical Technology of Russia. Since 1990, he has been a Fellow of the American Association of Pharmaceutical Sciences, Corresponding Member of the Royal Academy of Pharmacy in Spain, foreign member of the Russian Academy of Engineering and Honorary member of the Swiss Academy of Engineering Sciences. His major fields include: Quality by Design, Process Analytical technology, Right First Time concept and workflows, solid dosage form design, percolation theory, Formulation Computer Aided Design, Fractal geometry and New Process Technologies.

Aleksander Mendyk Ph.D.

Aleksander Mendyk studied pharmacy at the Jagiellonian University Medical College Cracow (graduated 1997) and in 2004 got his Ph.D. with distinction. He is now Assistant Professor at the Dept. of Pharmaceutical Technology and Biopharmaceutics at the Jagiellonian University Medical College in Cracow. He has supervised numerous M.Sc. students and co-supervised Ph.Ds. He has participated in several grants, among them as the Principal Investigator and member of steering committee of European projects. He is the author and co-author of over 47 publications and a reviewer for the *European Journal of Pharmaceutical Sciences*. He was also scientific consultant for several pharmaceutical companies. His scientific interests are mainly in the computational pharmacy area, namely computational intelligence systems such as artificial neural networks, neuro-fuzzy systems but also drug dissolution description and pharmaceutical equivalence, bioequivalence and in vitro–in vivo correlation (IVIVC). Dr Mendyk is also an Open Source software developer, focused on pharmaceutical data processing – his project KinetDS has gained a lot of international attention.

Dr. Mendyk can be contacted at mfmendyk@cyf-kr.edu.pl or at aleksander.mendyk@uj.edu.pl.

Dra. Montserrat Miñarro Carmona

Dra. Miñarro Carmona studied pharmacy at the University of Barcelona (Spain). She started her career working as a Deputy Pharmacist in the

Published by Woodhead Publishing Limited, 2013

Pharmacy Department of National Paraplegic Hospital 'GUTTMAN' (1989) in Barcelona, then as a researcher in Pharmaceutical Development Lab ESTEVE-FBG (1990–1991), then Pharmaceutical Technical Manager Lab TAMARANG (1991–1992), Technician of Regulatory Affairs in Lab SALVAT (1992–1995), Manager of Regulatory Affairs in Lab SALVAT (1995–2001) and Pharmaceutical Technical Manager Ind. Quimica SALVAT (2000–2001). She joined the Department of Pharmacy and Pharmaceutical Technology at the University of Barcelona and became Technical Manager of Regulatory Affairs of the Service of Development of Medicines (SDM) in the Faculty of Pharmacy. She received her doctorate from the same University in 1995, becoming Titular Professor in 2001. Dra Miñarro Carmona has been recognized as a Specialist in Industrial Pharmacy by the Spanish Government in 2001 and specialist in the Analysis and Testing of Medicines and Drugs in 2003. She has participated in a significant number of basic and applied research projects developed in the SDM, and a significant number of scientific congresses about pharmaceutical technology, both national and international. She is the author or co-author of several international papers and she is co-author of 10 chapters in five books about Pharmaceutical Technology or Pharmaceutical Quality.

Dr. Nopphadol Chalortham

Dr. Nopphadol Chalortham received his B.S. in Pharmacy and M.S. in Management and Information Technology from Chiangmai University in 1996 and 2004, respectively. He also received the Ph.D. degree in Pharmaceutical Science from Chiangmai University in 2010. He is now with the Faculty of Pharmacy there. His research interests centre on ontology development, expert system and drug formulation, which includes herbal and generic drugs.

Dr. Nopphadol Chalortham can be contacted at nopphadolc@gmail.com

Dr. Pilar Pérez Lozano

Dr. Pérez Lozano studied pharmacy at the University of Barcelona (Spain). She started her career working as a collaborator in the Service of Development of Medicines (SDM) located in the Faculty of Pharmacy of the University of Barcelona (1995–1997) and she was also researcher at the Department of Pharmacy and Pharmaceutical Technology in the same University. Later she led the quality assurance projects carried out in the Service of Development of Medicines (SDM) at the Faculty of Pharmacy. She holds a Master in Liquid Chromatography and obtained a doctorate from the same University in 2002, becoming

'Lector' Professor in 2008. She has participated in a significant number of basic and applied research projects developed in the SDM, and she participated in a significant number of scientific congresses about pharmaceutical technology both national and international. She is the author or co-author of several international papers and co-author of four books about Pharmaceutical Technology or Pharmaceutical Quality.

Dr. Phuriwat Leesawat

Dr. Phuriwat Leesawat received his M.S. degree in Industrial Pharmacy from Chulalongkorn University in 1991 and his Ph.D. degree in Industrial and Physical Pharmacy from Purdue University, USA in 1999. From 1999 to the present, he has been with the pharmaceutical science department, Pharmacy faculty, Chiangmai University in Thailand.

Dr. Maxim Puchkov

Dr. Maxim Puchkiv graduated from Mendeleyev University of Chemical Technology of Russia (MUCTR), in Moscow in 2000. He obtained his Ph.D. in chemical engineering at MUCTR in 2002, and in the same year he joined the group of Prof. Dr. H. Leuenberger (Pharmaceutical Technology, University of Basel) as postdoctoral fellow. In 2007 he became the CEO of the Center for Innovation in Computer-Aided Pharmaceutics (CINCAP GmbH) and in 2010 he joined the group of Prof. Dr. Jörg Huwyler as scientific collaborator. His scientific interests are focused on massively-parallel computational models for design of pharmaceutical formulations; discrete element models for design, understanding, and optimization of pharmaceutical processes and unit operations; interactive and process-oriented computer tools and simulators for advanced teaching and training of industrial unit operations.

Manuel Roig Carreras

Manuel Roig Carreras studied pharmacy at the University of Barcelona (Spain), graduating in 1962. He has been recognized as a Specialist in Industrial Pharmacy by the Spanish Government and holds a Postgraduate Degree in Bioavailability and Bioequivalence from the University of Santiago de Compostela in Spain and qualifications in Pharmaceutical Development for veterinary specialities carried out by Doxa Group. He worked in Laboratorios PEVYA (Molins de Rey-Barcelona) as a laboratory technician in the Department of Biochemistry until 1964. From 1964 until 1991 he was Head of the Department of Pharmaceutical Development

Published by Woodhead Publishing Limited, 2013

in Laboratorios Dr. Andreu and Technical Director of Farminter, then from 1991 until 1999 in Laboratorios S.A.V.A.T. (Barcelona) and from 1999 to 2004 he was technical assessor of Laboratorios Rubió (Barcelona). He has collaborated in the Service of Development of Medicines (SDM) located in the Faculty of Pharmacy of the University of Barcelona since it was founded. He has contributed to a significant number of basic and applied research papers related to the design of pharmaceutical dosage forms and in the implementation of new methodologies used in the characterization and quality control of solid dosage forms developed in the SDM, which were also used in some patents in Laboratorios Dr. Andreu, Laboratorios S.A.L.V.A.T. and the SDM.

Raymond C. Rowe B.Pharm., Ph.D., D.Sc., F.R.Pharm.S., C.Chem., F.R.S.C., C.Phys., MInst.P.
Ray Rowe is currently Chief Scientist at Intelligensys Ltd (a UK company dedicated to the development of intelligent and simulation software for product formulation). Until 2009 he was also a part-time professor of Industrial Pharmaceutics at the University of Bradford, where he was director of the PROFITS (PROduct Formulation using InTelligent Software) Special Interest Group with the aim of helping companies apply the technology of artificial intelligence to improve the formulation and processing of their products. Formerly he was a Senior Principal Scientist at AstraZeneca, UK, where he advised senior management in pharmaceutical and analytical research and development on the science and technology in the formulation and development of new medicines. He joined AstraZeneca (formerly ICI Pharmaceuticals and then Zeneca Pharmaceuticals) in 1973 having received his B.Pharm. from the University of Nottingham in 1969 and his Ph.D. from the University of Manchester in1973. Ray Rowe's research interests lie in the areas of polymer film coating, powder technology including compaction and granulation, the structural characterization of complex colloid systems and the application of knowledge engineering and advanced computational techniques in formulation. He has published over 350 research papers and reviews including eight patents, a book entitled *Intelligent Software for Product Formulation* and is currently co-editor of the *Handbook of Pharmaceutical Excipients*. In 1992 he was designated Fellow of the Royal Pharmaceutical Society for distinction in the Science of Pharmacy, and in 1993 he was awarded a D.Sc .from the University of Manchester. In 1998 he was awarded the Chiroscience Industrial Achievement award, and in 1999 he was elected Chairman of the British Pharmaceutical Conference. He has been an adjunct professor at the University of Illinois at Chicago and a visiting professor at the Universities

of Santiago de Compostela and Strathclyde. He is also a Chartered Chemist and Fellow of the Royal Society of Chemistry and a Chartered Physicist and Member of the Institute of Physics.

Dr. Rowe can be contacted at rowe@intelligensys.co.uk.

Igor Škrjanc

Igor Škrjanc received B.Sc., M.Sc. and Ph.D. degrees in electrical engineering, from the Faculty of Electrical and Computer Engineering, University of Ljubljana, Slovenia, in 1988, 1991 and 1996, respectively. His main research interests are intelligent, predictive control systems and autonomous mobile systems. In 2007, he received the highest research award of the University of Ljubljana, Faculty of Electrical Engineering, and, in 2008, the highest award of the Republic of Slovenia for Scientific and Research Achievements, Zois award for outstanding research results in the field of intelligent control. He also received the Humboldt Research Fellowship for Experienced Researchers for the period between 2009 and 2011. Currently, he is a Professor of Automatic Control at the Faculty of Electrical Engineering and the head of the research programme in Modelling, Simulation and Control.

Dr. Josep M. Suñé Negre

Dr. Suñé Negre studied pharmacy at the University of Barcelona (Spain). He started his career working as a Deputy Pharmacist in the Pharmacy Department of University Hospital General 'Vall d'Hebrón' Barcelona (1984–1986). He was also investigator in the department of Galenic Pharmacy and Pharmaceutical Technology in the Research Center of the Pharmaceutical Industry: 'Ferrer Internacional', and worked as Head of Manufacturing of the Pharmaceutical Industry: Dr. Andreu (1986). He joined the Department of Pharmacy and Pharmaceutical Technology at the University of Barcelona, where he was appointed manager of the Service of Development of Medicines (SDM) located in the Faculty of Pharmacy. He holds a doctorate in Pharmacy and Pharmaceutical Technology in the same University. He became Titular Professor in 1988. Dr. Suñé Negre has been recognized as a Specialist in Industrial Pharmacy by the Spanish Government in 2001 and specialist in Analysis and Testing of Medicines and Drugs in 2003. He has participated in a significant number of basic and applied research projects developed in the SDM, and also a significant number of scientific congresses about pharmaceutical technology, both national and international. He is the author or co-author of several international scientific papers and he is co-author of 10 books about Pharmaceutical Technology or Pharmaceutical Quality. He is Director of the Masters in

Business Management for the Pharmaceutical and Similar Industries at the Universidad de Barcelona, and he is Numerary Academic of the Royal Pharmacy Academy of Catalonia.

Taneth Ruangrajitpakorn

Taneth Ruangrajitpakorn is at the Human Language Technology Lab at NECTEC in Thailand. His expertise covers Natural Language Processing, Parsing, Ontology and digital language resources.

Dr. Thepchai Supnithi

Dr. Thepchai Supnithi received his B.S. degree in Mathematics from Chulalongkorn University in 1992. He received M.S. and Ph.D. degrees in Computer Engineering from Osaka University in 1997 and 2001, respectively. Since 2001, he has been with the Human Language Technology Lab at NECTEC in Thailand. He has researched in several fields including Knowledge Engineering, Natural Language Processing and E-learning.

Dr. Josep Ramón Ticó Grau

Dr. Ticó Grau studied pharmacy at the University of Barcelona (Spain). He started his career working as a Deputy Pharmacist in the Pharmacy Department of National Paraplegic Hospital 'GUTTMAN' in Barcelona. He was also Research and Deputy Manager in the Department of Pharmaceutical Technology at the Research Centre of the Pharmaceutical Industry 'ALMIRALL Ltd'. He joined the Department of Pharmacy and Pharmaceutical Technology at the University of Barcelona and became the Deputy Manager of Service of Development of Medicines (SDM) of the Faculty of Pharmacy. He received his doctorate from the same University in 1987, becoming Titular Professor in 1989. Dr. Ticó Grau has been recognized as a Specialist in Industrial Pharmacy by the Spanish Government in 2001 and specialist in the Analysis and Testing of Medicines and Drugs in 2003. He has participated in a significant number of basic and applied research projects developed in the SDM, and also a significant number of scientific congresses about pharmaceutical technology, both national and international. He is the author or co-author of several international scientific papers and he is co-author of seven books about Pharmaceutical Technology or Pharmaceutical Quality. At the moment he is Head of the Pharmacy and Pharmaceutical Technology Department at the University of Barcelona, and Academic of the Royal Pharmacy Academy of Catalonia.

David Tschirky

David Tschirky obtained his master's degree in Pharmacy from the University of Basel. In his work for the degree he contributed to the assessment of computer-based calculation models used in the development of software for the design and development of pharmaceutical formulations.

Franc Vrečer

Franc Vrečer is an associate professor at the Faculty of Pharmacy, University of Ljubljana, where he is involved in preformulation and formulation research, process and formulation optimization and quality assurance. As well as his scientific activities at the university he works full time in the pharmaceutical industry, where he is assistant director of R&D in KRKA, d.d., Novo Mesto and is involved in development activities of new pharmaceutical products. He received his B.Sc., M.Sc. and Ph.D. degrees from the Faculty of Pharmacy, University of Ljubljana in 1983, 1988 and 1992, respectively, for pharmaceutical technology. He is author and co-author of several scientific publications and patents.

Dr. Wei-san Pan

Dr. Wei-san Pan studied pharmacy at Shenyang Pharmaceutical University (China) and got his Ph.D. He started his career working as a lecturer in the school of Pharmacy of Shenyang Pharmaceutical University in 1989. He became Titular Professor in 1999. Dr. Wei-san Pan has been recognized as Specialist in Pharmaceutics by the Chinese Government in 2002 and specialist in Pharmaceutical Education in 2003. He has participated in and hosted an important number of basic and applied research projects developed in Pharmaceutics. He has published over 300 papers on pharmacy and applied for 40 patents. He is the author or co-author of several international papers and he is co-author of 18 books about Pharmaceutical Technology. At present, he is Head of the School of Pharmacy in Shenyang Pharmaceutical University (China).
Dr. Wei-san Pan can be contacted at ppwwss@163.com.

Dr. Zhi-hong Zhang

Dr. Zhi-hong Zhang studied pharmacy at Shenyang Pharmaceutical University (China). He started his career working in AustarPharma (USA), doing formulation R&D. He joined the CSPC institute of pharmaceutical research (China) for a period. He received his doctorate from the same university in 2009, becoming Titular Engineer in 2010. He

Published by Woodhead Publishing Limited, 2013

has participated in a number of basic and applied research projects developed in oral dosage forms, especially extended release dosage forms. He is the author or co-author of several international papers about Pharmaceutical Technology. He oversees the activities of the R&D, scale up and industrialization of extended release products.
Dr. Zhi-hong Zhang can be contacted at zhangzhihong198210@163.com.

Damjana Zupančič-Božič

Damjana Zupančič-Božič is head of the Technology Operation Center in KRKA, d.d. Novo Mesto, responsible for technology transfer, scale-up procedures and process optimization of pharmaceutical dosage forms in the pharmaceutical industry. She is also actively involved in the implementation of automatization of production documentation and manufacturing execution system (MES) and ERP system SAP. She received B.Sc., M.Sc. and Ph.D. degrees from the Faculty of Pharmacy, University of Ljubljana in 1990, 1995 and 2008, respectively, for the pharmaceutical technology of solid dosage forms.

1

Introduction

Johnny Edward Aguilar

The way in which medicines are developed is changing and the regulatory environment is also changing. Consequently, formulators require full understanding of a product and its process of development. In addition, it is desirable for formulators to detect any gaps in drug formulas which, if not addressed, could be linked to inadequate quality or problems with the product. Different methodologies have been implemented to try to improve the existing pharmaceutical process in the industrial environment, such as lean and six sigma. High variability and continuous problems during manufacturing could be avoided by ensuring that a good product design is used in the initial stages when developing new medicine. This is not an easy step because of complex non-linear relationships between the formulation composition, process conditions, and product properties. In most cases, a formulation consists of a drug, a number of formulation ingredients, and process conditions, interactions between which affect the quality of the final product. Thus, formulation design is based on a multi-dimensional space that is difficult to conceptualize for scientists working in this field (Rowe and Roberts, 1998; Shao et al., 2007).

A good understanding of processes and interactions between different components of formulations is key to understanding the complex relationships in product formulations. This can be attained using appropriate tools that avoid unnecessary trials in the laboratory and optimize this goal in an efficient manner. These kinds of tools also provide information which can be used in the optimization of the formulation, so that the final formulation is obtained by fixing any gaps previously detected by these formulation tools. The tools also assist formulators in avoiding problems related to quality which can occur in the subsequent development phase or during commercial manufacturing.

Understanding of these processes and implementation of continuous improvements are becoming ever more important. Therefore, such tools and their derivate software are highly appreciated for a better understanding of our processes by formulators, scientists, and similar professionals in the pharmaceutical industry or research centers. It is noted that the development of such tools has increased recently, for example they are being used in design or development of formulations such as expert systems, artificial intelligence technologies and tools such as artificial neural networks, etc.

The methodologies termed lean and six sigma are commonly used in routine manufacturing. These apply basic statistics to evaluate the behavior of a process, permitting identification of an advantageous change or detection of a possible trend beforehand. However, there are alternatives that can be used to reach this goal, such as preformulation and formulation tools. In contrast to the traditional statistical approach, these tools allow analysis of complex and non-linear relations and provision of additional information that can be used during the analysis phase. They can help to propose assertive solutions during optimization. For example, SeDeM methodology, detailed in this book, can provide information on differences in rheology properties in a powdered formulation for tablets, which can be used when comparing suppliers used for raw materials. This tool uses routine tests of pharmacopeia to allow identification of variances between two different suppliers of the same component, excipient, or drug substance, and provides information on any gaps that must be corrected before executing the pilot and commercial batches. Analysis using this tool ensures a successful formula and a robust validation.

Factors related to productivity and reduction of cost are also taken into account when developing medicines. The tools described in the subsequent chapters can assist with cost reduction by providing information to lead to a better understanding of formulations under development, and by decreasing the lead time in development and avoiding unnecessary trials because the old (expensive) methodology trial error is not applied. The use of these tools is highly appreciated by pharmaceutical companies and research centers as good product design leads to lean processes and cost improvements.

During the lab phase, the physical and chemical properties of a drug are determined and then the desired dosage form and critical attributes are designed. The design of experiment is performed in the pilot scale, which helps to obtain a detailed understanding of the different steps implemented in the process. The data are generated and used in the

Published by Woodhead Publishing Limited, 2013

scale-up and the subsequent phase corresponding to commercial manufacturing. Preliminary design space and the criteria of final specifications are determined during this phase.

Review of the design space is then initiated. This information related to the manufacturing process is used in improvement studies and for future troubleshooting, which can be necessary in routine manufacturing of commercial batches.

All these phases are strictly linked and require exchange of information in trying to understand the complex non-linear relationships between the formulation composition, process conditions, and product properties. This information is not only useful at the development stage, but also subsequently for identifying root causes and supporting implementation of effective corrective and preventive actions.

The pharmaceutical development phase provides information critical to form the basis of process understanding. This can be used for various new technologies; it facilitates scientists to reach a better understanding of the chemical and physical phenomena of the drug. There are some cases wherein this learning is compiled on paper, in electronic data, books or in the personal experience of pharmacists or professionals working in development of medicines; however, there are also unpublished experiences and knowledge, which are therefore unknown to the scientific community. If that information were treated and compiled using appropriate software or managed with an adequate methodology, it could provide a high probability of a good and effective solution in case of problems with the formulation. The use of an expert system or other artificial intelligence tools is recommended to achieve this. 'Expert system' (ES) is a versatile term, as ES occur in many disciplines such as economics, mathematics, etc; however there are some common definitions:

- 'Computer program that draws upon the knowledge of human experts captured in a knowledge base to solve problems that normally require human expertise' (Partridge and Hussain, 1994).
- 'The label "expert system" is broadly speaking, given to a computer program intended to make reasoned judgements or give assistance on a complex area in which human skills are fallible or scarce' (Lauritzen and Spiegelhalter, 1988).

There is a need to introduce newer methods in mathematical modeling of stochastic phenomena, such as power behavior which could be of a single component or a mixture in a final formulation. However, it is important to have an overview of the main directions of past modeling trends. One of the main objectives in the second half of the twentieth century was to develop artificial intelligence-based modeling methods for aiding design of pharmaceutical dosage forms. Artificial intelligence can capture the knowledge of a formulation expert, document it, and make it available and user-friendly. Turban compared artificial intelligence (AI) with—as he called it—natural intelligence (NI) of experts as follows (Turban, 1995):

- NI depends on persons, which results in a dependency on personnel changes.
- NI is difficult to transfer, whereas AI can be moved from one computer to another.
- AI can reduce costs.
- AI is consistent, decisions are traceable and can easily be documented.
- AI is not creative.
- NI uses a wider context of experience to solve problems.

These methods are restricted to sequential processing of knowledge; however, a different approach is to use neural networks. As the name implies, artificial neural networks are inspired by the functionality of the human brain. The artificial neuron takes one or more inputs, each multiplied with a weight factor, and potentially creates an output which is forwarded to another neuron. Whether an output is generated or not depends on the inputs, which must exceed a defined threshold. The threshold activation is computed by transformation functions, which can be linear or non-linear. Compared with expert systems, neural networks need short development time, but need to be trained. The training consists of linking inputs and outputs and adapting weight-values until inputs give a result that is close to the experimentally determined result.

A classic algorithmic overview of pharmaceutical development indicates that it requires a recompilation of knowledge with a foundation in many disciplines that could assist with understanding drug substances and the different interactions with excipients. It is important to consider the variables used during the process which could potentially impact the quality of the medicines, and to avoid those considered unnecessary. However, as previously mentioned, this is not an easy task because they are not universal theories or principles. Mechanisms can be identified by those with professional experience; however, innovative preformulation and formulation tools are under development which could help reach better understanding of these complex relations. These tools could suggest a model for use to define the final formulation and the appropriate process to apply, therefore having a high impact on the final formulation.

Published by Woodhead Publishing Limited, 2013

Finally it is concluded that the life sciences industry is changing rapidly and the historical rules, regulations, and government oversight are under pressure to modernize. The recent introduction of Quality Systems and Quality by Design (QbD) concepts has challenged the traditional view that simple compliance with the basic Good Management Practices (GxP) rules is enough to satisfy stakeholders, regulators, and patients. A better understanding of processes is required. The strategies used for development of new medicines are also changing and they are being carried out based on a strategy of quality by design and not quality by evidence. There are tools described in this book which could help to design a robust formulation and to understand the interaction between components, and could provide some argument towards the final decision required by a formulator, scientist or process expert without requiring execution of many experiments, therefore reducing lead time. The tools also reduce the resources required in development as unnecessary trials are avoided.

1.1 References

Partridge, D and Hussain, K, 1994 *Knowledge-Based Information System.* s.l.:McGraw Hill.

Lauritzen, S and Spiegelhalter, D, 1988 Local Computations with Probabilities on Graphical Structures and their Application to Expert Systems. *J R Statist Soc*, 2, 157–224.

Shao Q, Rowe RC and York P, 2007 Investigation of an artificial intelligence technology—Model trees Novel applications for an immediate release tablet formulation database. *EurJP*, 3, 137–44.

Rowe, RC and Roberts, RJ, 1998 *Intelligent Software for Product Formulation.* Taylor and Francis Ltd., London.

Turban, E., 1995. *Decision Support Systems and Expert Systems.* 4. ed. s.l.:Englewood Cliffs.

2

Artificial neural networks technology to model, understand, and optimize drug formulations

Mariana Landin, University of Santiago, Spain, and Raymond C. Rowe, Intelligensys Ltd, Stokesley, UK

DOI: 10.1533/9781908818508.7

Abstract: This chapter presents the fundamentals of different artificial intelligence methods, artificial neural networks (ANN), genetic algorithms and fuzzy logic, as useful tools to model the effect of different variables (continuous and nominal) and their interactions on the properties of pharmaceutical formulations. ANN allow for generation of complex multidimensional models of easy and quick numerical solutions. The strength of AI methods lies in their ability to detect and quantify complex non-linear relationships between inputs and outputs as well as their capability to generalize distorted or partially occluded patterns. AI methods can be used to study the knowledge space and establish the design space within the framework of Quality by Design.

Key words: artificial intelligence, optimization, design space, artificial neural networks, genetic algorithms, fuzzy logic.

2.1 Introduction

Development or improvement of pharmaceutical formulations involves many raw materials and process variables that interact in a complex way, making control and optimization a complex task. For decades, pharmaceutical development has been attempted via trial and error supplemented by the previous experience and knowledge of the formulator. Formulation quality was assured by final testing. As a result 'acceptable formulations' were delivered to the market and some remain commercially available. But companies often report problems associated with changes in suppliers of raw materials or batches or in the manufacturing process that affect the quality of the formulations, making them unacceptable. Such problems can arise because, although the formulations meet standard requirements, the complex relationships between all the variables involved and the responses are not well understood and their effects are not really under control.

Optimization approaches, employing systematic Design of Experiments and statistical analysis, came to partially substitute such trial and error procedures. The use of experimental designs, especially factorial designs in the development of solid dosage forms became common practice in the 1980s, and appropriate statistical treatments allowed determination of critical parameters of complex processes, comparison between materials, or the improvement or optimization of formulations (Wehrlé and Stamm, 1994; Lewis et al., 1999). Some of these works were published but most remain part of the in-house material of pharmaceutical companies.

In 2002, the FDA announced a new initiative (cGMPs for the 21st century: A risk-based approach) intending to modernize its regulations of pharmaceutical quality for human drugs and to establish a new regulatory framework focused on Quality by Design (QbD), risk management, and quality systems (Jiang and Yu, 2009).

The International Conference on Harmonization guideline (ICH Q8, 2009) states that QbD is a systemic approach to development that starts by predefining objectives and emphasizes product and process understanding and process control, based on sound science and quality risk management. QbD requires an understanding of how formulation and process variables influence product quality (knowledge space) and a definition of the design space inside the knowledge space (García et al., 2008).

ICH Q8 defines the design space as 'the multidimensional combination and interaction of input variables (e.g. material attributes) and process parameters that have been demonstrated to provide assurance of quality' (ICH Q8, 2009).

When developing a new formulation the formulator should identify and distinguish critical from non-critical variables, establish the design space and define a control strategy to assure process performance and product quality (Figure 2.1).

For the pharmaceutical industry, adoption of QbD represents both an opportunity and a challenge. This approach should reduce cost and time

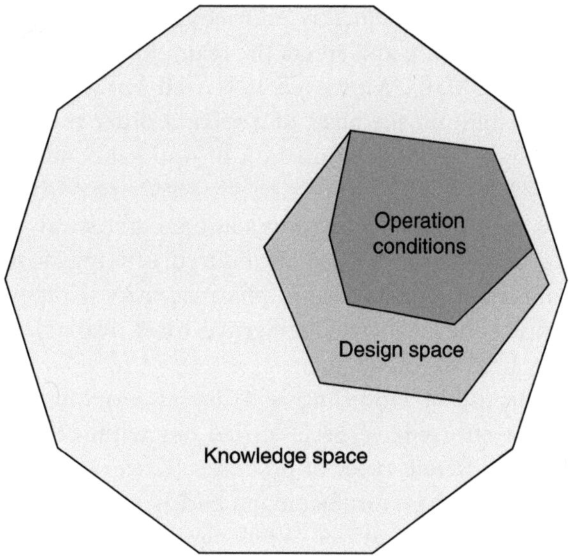

Figure 2.1 Relation between the knowledge space, the design space and the normal operation conditions

and improve process efficiency and quality of the formulations (Zomer et al., 2010). Moreover, from a regulatory standpoint, operating within the design space is not considered as a change in a formulation and does not require regulatory oversight, but movements outwith the design space are considered changes and need regulatory approvals (Jiang and Yu, 2009).

Recent and significant technological advances applied to pharmaceutical development mean that researchers face an unprecedented influx of large data sets from different types of variables (binomial, discrete and continuous) and nominal factors, which hinder the utility of traditional methodologies such as response surface methodology (RSM). RSM, including statistical experimental designs and multiple linear regression analysis under a set of constrained equations, is a recommended method for establishing 'the design space' with the inconvenience that nominal factors cannot be included in those designs (Lunney et al., 2008). In those cases, a valid alternative strategy would be to repeat the response surface design for each level of the discrete factors.

The usual recommendation and procedure is that response surface designs should be considered after a thorough screening using factorials of fractional factorial experiments which are useful in modelling the relationships between variables and results, but as the number of variables in those processes is frequently enormous, their numerical solution is highly time consuming and enters the realm of complex statistics (Singh et al., 2005a, 2005b). Moreover, it is well known that prediction of response variables on the basis of a second order polynomial equation sometimes results in poor estimation of optimal conditions (Takayama et al., 1999b).

In recent years, together with traditional statistical techniques, soft computing methods have been introduced offering novel solutions to improve modelling and control in pharmaceutics (Colbourn and Rowe, 2009). Among the artificial intelligence tools available, ANN are the most widely used for modelling.

As the purpose of modelling is to increase our understanding of a process, great efforts have been carried out within the pharmaceutical field to model different types of processes (Kremer and Hancock, 2006) and formulation behaviour (Siepmann and Siepmann, 2008).

Mechanistic, empirical or semiempirical mathematical models, continuum or discrete models have been employed to understand the behaviour of formulations or process, to allow comparisons between them, to predict their properties or find the best procedure to formulate a dosage form (Gibson, 2009).

For development of any mathematical model it is necessary to follow certain steps: a) identification of the problem or process to be simulated, understood, controlled and/or optimized; b) selection of data, variables (input and outputs) and the most important aspect, what is the model for, what is the question to be answered; c) introduction of accurate and precise data according to each variable and selection of the type of modelling procedure. In white box models the selection of equations (mainly algorithms) is often required; in black box models this a priori information is not available. If the black box model is chosen, some parameters should be determined to fit the model to the system (in neural networks the selection of those parameters is called training); and d) model evaluation to check the gaps between the observed and predicted data (which should be as low as possible).

The validity of the model is not only about if it fits well or not with empirical observations, but also about its ability to generalize and predict in the range of the study and/or provide new insight which is partially occluded in the data, and which cannot be known from direct observation or from statistical data analysis of the process. If this is not achieved, the model is likely to be unnecessary, time consuming and useless.

One important issue to consider when modelling is the quality of data. The model will be excellent and useful if data are excellent. Models do not produce miracles. Bad quality data (non-accurate, dispersed or non-precise) are not the best option to fit good models, especially if they are selected for a black box model, as neural networks are.

2.2 Artificial neural networks fundamentals

Artificial neural networks (ANN) are mathematical models generated by computational systems that simulate biological neural networks. A few decades ago, computers able to learn from experience were science fiction but they have progressed to be a distinct and tangible reality with applications in disciplines as diverse as engineering design, the detection of mobile phone fraud (Krenker et al., 2011) and scientific research in pharmacy or medicine (Hartnell and Mackinnon, 2003).

ANN technology has been widely described in recent literature (Ichikawa, 2003; Russell and Norvig, 2003; Rowe and Roberts, 2005; Krenker et al., 2011), but to better understand its applications it is pertinent to briefly review their design and function.

ANN are biologically inspired systems, having a strong similitude to biological neural systems. The main elements of biological neural networks are the neurons, electrochemical excitable cells that can receive signals or stimuli from other neurons via synapse connections (Figure 2.2). The cell body of a neuron can have multiple dendrites, but never more than one axon. Stimuli, received through the dendrites, are transmitted to the cell body. If a stimulus is intense enough, the neuron generates another stimulus that is transmitted along the axon to the next neuron via synapses. In this way biological neurons establish millions of connections making a three-dimensional neural network.

In an artificial neural system the main element is the artificial neuron also called a 'perceptron' or node (Figure 2.2). Nodes are organized into groups called layers. The ANN architecture is an interconnected assembly of those individual processing elements. As for biological neurons, artificial neurons receive one or more inputs from neighbouring neurons, process the information and produce an output to be transmitted to the next perceptron. The strengths of connections between the artificial neurons are called 'weights' (Takayama et al., 1999a). While computing the output, the input information (X_i) is weighed either positively or negatively. To solve or interpret a given problem, the computational approach should define those weights and assign an internal threshold

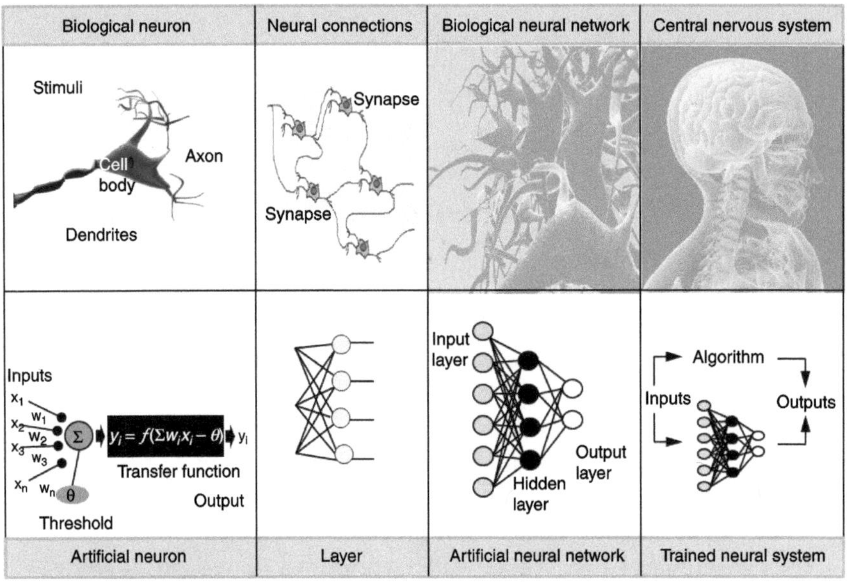

Figure 2.2 **Basic comparison between a biological neuronal system and an artificial neural system. x = input variable; w = weight of input; θ = internal threshold value; f = transfer function.**

value (θ). At each node, the input values (X_n) are multiplied by their associate weight (W_n) to give a result, which is adjusted by its threshold value. The output is then determined using a function 'f', 'transfer function' or 'activation function' (Figure 2.2; Eq. 2.1).

$$y_i = f\ (\Sigma W_n.X_n - \theta_i) \tag{2.1}$$

The transfer function can be linear or non-linear. Among the non-linear functions that can be applied, hyperbolic, tangent or radial basis form, etc., the sigmoid function (Eq. 2.2) is the most commonly used (Figure 2.3). Sigmoid function, $f(y_i)$, is conducted to the following layer as an output value. Alpha is a parameter relating to the shape of the sigmoid function. Non-linearity of the sigmoid function is strengthened with an increase in α.

$$f(y_i) = 1/[1 + \exp(-\alpha y_i)] \tag{2.2}$$

By connecting artificial neurons (many hundreds of thousands), complex ANN can be obtained. Figure 2.2 illustrates the topology of one

Published by Woodhead Publishing Limited, 2013

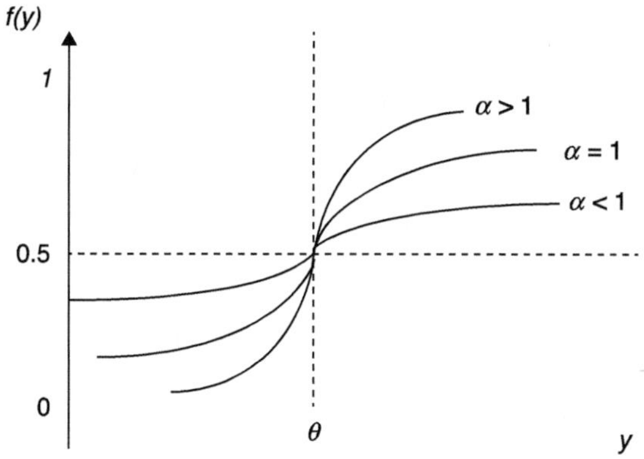

Figure 2.3 Representation of the sigmoid function (modified from Ichikawa, 2003)

of the most popular and successful network architectures, a multilayer perceptron (MLP) network, consisting of three simple layers: one input layer, one output layer and one hidden layer. A neural network can have multiple layers between the input and the output layer but, in practice, this simple hierarchy-type network with just three layers has been successfully applied to many pharmaceutical problems (Erb, 1993; Ichikawa, 2003; Rafienia et al., 2010).

ANN must be trained for them to 'learn'. This learning process is done in a manner similar to how children learn not to touch the oven after being burned a few times. Unlike conventional computer programs, which are explicitly programmed, the ANN are trained with a number of examples or facts (a set of empirical data), the number of which should lie between three and ten times the number of connections (Erb, 1993; Sun et al., 2003). Additionally, 10–20% of the facts should be randomly set aside to be used for testing the fitted network.

During the 'training process' the system is able to establish the relationship between inputs and outputs using algorithms designed to alter the strength (weights) of the connections in the network to produce a desired signal flow. The back-propagation method has been the most frequently used for adjusting the weights, being called back-propagation because the size of the error is fed back into the calculation for the weight changes (Erb, 1993).

The ability of the network to memorize and process the information lies in the weights assigned to the inter-node connections, which determines the conductivity through the network. When the computed output is acceptable, compared with experimental output, the network has attained a good generalization of the problem domain. Once the multidimensional model has been established, it is able to quickly estimate the corresponding output for any other untested combination of inputs (Colbourn and Rowe, 2009). The difference between experimental and predicted outputs is usually quantified by means of an error function similar to those used in statistics.

In different research fields, it has been proposed that the performance of a well-designed MLP network is comparable with that achieved using classical statistical techniques (Rowe and Roberts, 1998), and therefore is suitable for a wide range of applications including the selection of raw materials and process variables in the development and optimization of formulations as tablets (Takagaki et al., 2010), microspheres (Labouta et al., 2009), microparticles (Leonardi et al., 2009), nanoparticles (Ali et al., 2009), emulsions (Agatonovic-Kustrin et al., 2003; Glass et al., 2005; Wei et al., 2008; Gasperlin et al., 2008), hard capsules (Guo et al., 2002) and gels (Lee et al., 2008); the development of analytical procedures and/or interpretation of analytical data (Agatonovic-Kustrin et al., 1998; 2000); establishment of in vivo–in vitro correlations (De Matas 2007; 2008; Fatouros et al., 2008); establishment of a quantitative structure–property relationship (Andrea and Kalayeh, 1991); and establishment of the relationship between a complex formulation and its efficiency (Qiao et al., 2010; Zhou et al., 2010).

2.2.1 Strengths of artificial neural networks

The strength of ANN lies in their ability to detect and quantify complex non-linear relationships between inputs and outputs as well as their capability to generalize distorted or partially occluded patterns (Taylor, 1996; Ichikawa, 2003; Shao et al., 2006).

From a formal point of view, ANN have several advantages over statistics and traditional methods: a) they can process different types of data together (continuous, binomial, discrete); b) they can be used to produce complex models without applying specific mathematical functions or the prior assumption of the nature of the relationships between input and output parameters, so they can discover subtle relationships in the data; c) they do not require specific experimental design, being able to use incomplete data, data acquired during a series of trial and error experiments or even historical data (Colbourn, 2003; Colbourn and Rowe, 2005); d) a significant advantage of ANN is that input variables can be cross-correlated, which facilitates their ability to recognize patterns (Erb, 1993).

ANN allow a design space inside the knowledge space to be defined through the use of a relative small amount of data (Woolfson et al., 2010) and to generate complex multidimensional models of easy and quick numerical solutions.

2.2.2 Limitations of artificial neural networks

This powerful technology has limitations that must be identified. Most classical neural networks involve a trial and error approach to find the optimal architecture, transfer function and learning paradigm (Takagaki et al., 2010). The network architecture is an aspect to study. Although MLP have proved efficient in solving an important number of pharmaceutical development problems, the formulator must consider that no single software or modelling algorithm can solve 'all' problems (Labouta et al., 2009; Rafienia et al., 2010).

No analytical methods are available to determine the optimum number of neurons required for a specific problem (Su and Khorasani, 2001; Lawrence et al., 1996). The number of hidden neurons depends on factors such as the number and the distribution of data training. There is no general rule, despite some authors (Wei et al., 2008) having applied the principle that number of weights must be smaller than number of training data constitution pairs as described by the function:

$$N_{\text{hidden}} \times N_{\text{inputs}} + N_{\text{hidden}} \times N_{\text{outputs}} \leq N_{\text{training data}}$$

Models can involve undertraining or overtraining. The number of hidden neurons must be kept to a minimum to avoid overtraining (Labouta et al., 2009). If overtraining occurs, the network learns the noise within the data and loses the ability to accurately predict properties of records out of the training set (Takagaki et al., 2010). Differences between software mainly rely on the back-propagation algorithm used for network training, the activation functions applied at network nodes and the mechanism of limiting network overtraining.

ANN technology has also limitations related to the difficulties of interpreting the results in simple form or to elaboration of formal reasoning or extraction of general rules (Colbourn, 2003). If the number of variables is important, the complex multivariate 'black box' models derived from ANN can be really difficult to analyse using 2D or 3D plots (Figure 2.4). One can stand in front of a wonderful non-linear model and an excellent collection of graphs showing the effects of inputs on outputs and still maintain the great question: 'And, what should I do now?'

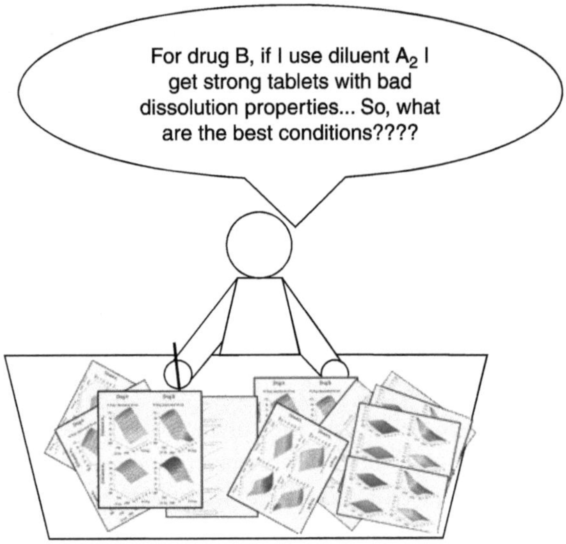
For drug B, if I use diluent A_2 I get strong tablets with bad dissolution properties... So, what are the best conditions????

Figure 2.4 Example of how much information cannot solve practical problems

In order to avoid such limitations, ANN can be coupled with other AI techniques such as fuzzy logic technology or genetic algorithms (Agatonovic-Kustrin and Beresford, 2000; Agatonovic-Kustrin and Alani, 2001), to give hybrid systems, the results of which are easier to interpret and generalize, allowing the formulator to acquire real knowledge on the process and/or find the combination of inputs to give the requested outputs (Plumb et al., 2005; Shao et al., 2006; Shao et al., 2007; Gago et al., 2010b).

2.3 Genetic algorithms

Genetic algorithms (GA) are also bio-inspired artificial intelligence tools. They are based on the biological principles of genetic variation and natural selection, mimicking the basic ideas of evolution over generations (Cartwright, 1993). As evolution selects the 'best adapted individuals', genetic algorithms are designed to select the best solution for a specific problem, or, in other words, the optimization of the process studied (Rowe and Roberts, 1998).

When combining ANN and genetic algorithms (Figure 2.5), the 'search' for the best solution starts by randomly generating a set of candidate

Published by Woodhead Publishing Limited, 2013

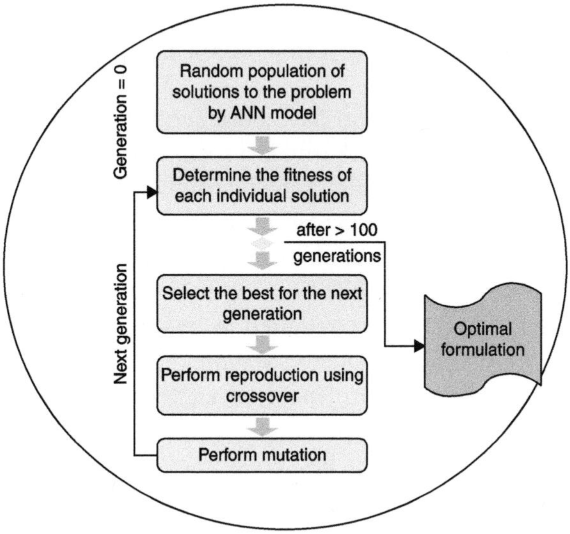

Figure 2.5 Steps in the search process for the optimal formulation when artificial neural networks and genetic algorithms are coupled

solutions to the problem (a set of inputs and their corresponding predicted outputs from the ANN model). Candidate solutions are then selected according to their fit to previous established criteria; the best are used for evolving new solution populations to the problem using crossover and mutation. This is repeated until the criteria are satisfied. After several generations (>100) an optimum must be achieved, because the most suitable solutions are most likely to be reproduced.

For a genetic algorithm to function it must possess several features. Firstly, a numerical description of how good a solution is to the problem (desirability function). Secondly, a logical method of selecting individual solutions to become parents of the next generation, and, finally, a logical method of mixing the different elements to produce new solutions (Mitchell, 1998; Glezakos et al., 2010).

Pharmaceutical product development is a multivariate optimization problem. It involves finding the best combination of ingredients and process variables to obtain various optimal characteristics simultaneously. It is well known by the formulator that a desirable formulation for one property is frequently undesirable for other characteristics. Therefore, finding an 'optimal' solution means finding the best compromise solution (Agatonovic-Kustrin and Beresford, 2000). ANN coupled with GA have been shown to be useful in achieving the compromise solutions required in dosage forms development (Leane et al., 2003; Díaz-Rodríguez and Landín, 2011).

ANN coupled with GA also have been successfully proposed to deal with different pharmaceutical problems such as the rational selection or production of raw materials (Godavarthy et al., 2009; Valizadeh et al., 2009), quantitative structure–property relationship design (Neely et al., 2009) and variable selection in analytical procedures (Xiaobo et al., 2010).

When several responses are required to be optimized simultaneously, the desirability function is a function of more than one response (Leonardi et al., 2009). The procedure involves creating a function for each individual response (di), and obtaining a global function D that should be maximized by choosing the best conditions of the designed variables. The function D ranges from 0 (value totally undesirable) to 100 (all the responses lie in the desirable range simultaneously).

Recently, some commercial computer program developers such as Intelligensys (Stokesley, UK), NeuralWare (Carnegie, USA) and Neuro Dimension (Gainesville, USA), have developed software packages for prediction/optimization applications combining ANN and GA software.

2.4 Quality by Design case study: an integrated multivariate approach to direct compressed tablet development

To illustrate the use of ANN technology, we have selected the pharmaceutical development of a direct compression tablet formulation. This type of formulation is complicated enough to be a good example when explaining the use of this technology, but simple enough to easily describe the aspects that can affect formulation quality. At a minimum, those aspects should include active product ingredients (APIs), excipients (EXP), manufacturing process and packaging system. The formulator should establish which are the critical aspects for product quality and define the control strategy for the product.

Following the ICH Q8 guideline, an Ishikawa diagram can be established to identify potential variables affecting the quality of direct compression tablets (Figure 2.6). Within the raw materials (API and excipients), product specifications such as physical chemical properties (e.g. solubility, water content, particle size, crystal properties. . .) and

Published by Woodhead Publishing Limited, 2013

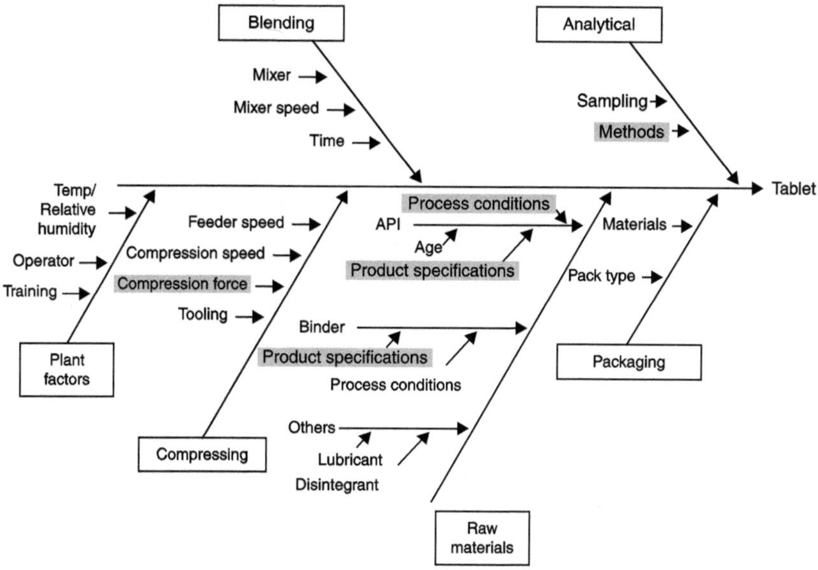

Figure 2.6 Ishikawa diagram identifying the potential variables that can have an impact on the quality of direct compression tablets

biological characteristics (biological activity, permeability. . .) can be considered and interrelated (e.g. compatibility of API with excipients). Additionally, process conditions related to the use of raw materials (e.g. percentage in the formulation) must be defined.

The process development program should also define the appropriateness of the equipment used (e.g. compression or blending tools) and identify any critical process parameters that should be monitored and/or controlled (e.g. mixing time, compression force. . .).

As can be seen, despite direct compression being a 'simple' procedure, the number of variables (inputs) involved in the process is enormous.

Another interesting aspect to consider is that some variables are numerical and continuous (e.g. mixing time, compression force) but many others are nominal (type of binder or lubricant, mixer, compression tool. . .).

The process development program also includes establishment of the Critical Quality Attributes (CQA), which are physical, chemical, biological or microbiological properties that should be within an appropriate limit, range or distribution to ensure the desired product quality. CQA are generally associated with the API, excipients, intermediate and final products. For direct compression tablets, the CQA are related to purity, mechanical properties (crushing strength, weight loss by friability. . .), drug release properties and stability. CQA (outputs) should be prioritized and/or increased as product knowledge and process understanding increase.

Once the significant parameters (inputs and outputs) are identified, they can be further studied (e.g. appropriate design of experiments and modelling) to achieve a high level of process understanding.

To start with our hypothetical example, we can fix some of the parameters such as the plant factors, compression and mixing tools, mixing operation conditions, etc., and select the ones we are going to study (Figure 2.6, variables in the grey areas). The tablets will be produced by direct compression of the mixtures prepared in a Turbula T2C mixer at 30 rpm for 15 min. In all cases, 0.5% w/w magnesium stearate as lubricant will be added. For the tabletting process, an eccentric tablet machine (Korsch EKO) will be used. The machine will be equipped with 9 mm flat punches and piezoelectric transducers to measure the upper punch compression force. Lower punch will be adjusted to produce 200 mg tablets. The production rate will be 33 tablets/min.

As study variables, we have selected the type of drug (drug A and drug B), the percentage of drug in the formulation (from 0% to 10%), the type of binder (binder A_1 and binder A_2 with different nominal particle size) and the compression force.

Following the characteristic steps in modelling processes suggested earlier, the process to be simulated, understood, controlled and/or optimized is the development of direct compression tablets of drug A or drug B at specific conditions of plant factor, compression and mixing tools, mixing operation conditions, lubricant type and conditions, etc.

Within this process we have selected four inputs (drug type, drug percentage, binder type and compression force) and five outputs (CQAs) (weight variation coefficient (%), crushing strength (kg), weight lost by friability (%), disintegration time (s) and drug dissolved at 60 min (%)). The questions to be answered in this example could be: is this process of direct tabletting robust enough to produce pharmacopoeia acceptable tablets for the two selected drugs? To what extent does the use of either binder affect the results?

The third step in the modelling process proposed is the introduction of the accurate and precise data according to each variable and the selection of the type of model. In our in-house material we had data from different experiments that fulfil an experimental design for four variables (although ANN technology does not require a specific experimental design); drug

Published by Woodhead Publishing Limited, 2013

and binder types at two levels (drug A and drug B; binder A_1 and A_2) and drug percentage (0%, 5%, 10%) and compression force (900, 1700 and 2500 N) at three levels, the limits of which will constitute our knowledge space.

Outputs were tested and recorded following USP specifications.

The network structure chosen was a multilayer perceptron (MLP) network, consisting of three simple layers: one input layer including four inputs, one output layer including five outputs or CQAs and one hidden layer with five nodes. Selected training parameters are shown in Table 2.1.

Data (36 facts in Table 2.2) were divided in two groups, 33 facts for training the network and three randomly selected for testing the error and avoiding overtraining.

ANOVA parameters and correlation coefficients were used to perform the model evaluation and check the gaps between the observed and predicted data. Training and test data ANOVA correlation coefficients greater than 75% together with f-ratios higher than critical f values for the corresponding degrees of freedom are indicative of good performance

Table 2.1 **Training parameters used for ANN modelling**

	Network structure	
	No. hidden layers	1
	No. nodes in hidden layer	5
Back propagation type:		RPROP
Transfer function in:		
	Output transfer type	Linear
	Hidden layer	Symmetric sigmoid
Targets:		
	Target epochs	1000
	Target MS error	0.0001
	Random seed	10 000
Test data:		
	Screen update set	5
	Smart stop enabled	Toggled on
	Minimum interactions	20
	Test error weighting	0.2
	Autoweight	Toggled on

Table 2.2 **Differential characteristics of the formulations studied and mean values of the parameters used to characterize them**

Binder	Drug	% drug	CF (N)	WVC (%)	TS (kg)	F (%)	DT (s)	%D (30 min)
A_1	A	0	900	0.48	3.18	0.19	12	0
A_1	A	0	1700	1.40	6.50	0	16	0
A_1	A	0	2500	0.97	9.17	0	17	0
A_1	A	5	900	0.35	3.25	0.53	16	96.97
A_1	A	5	1700	0.43	6.17	0.16	21	85.91
A_1	A	5	2500	1.15	10.00	0.02	28	75.45
A_1	A	10	900	0.48	2.67	0.74	9	93.71
A_1	A	10	1700	0.48	6.50	0.18	16	92.50
A_1	A	10	2500	0.58	9.83	0.04	20	78.48
A_2	A	5	900	1.29	4.58	0.45	14	98.18
A_2	A	5	1700	1.09	8.08	0.38	29	69.98
A_2	A	5	2500	1.14	10.67	0.24	55	33.18
A_2	A	10	900	0.43	5.75	0.33	21	96.89
A_2	A	10	1700	0.37	9.17	0.29	35	51.29
A_2	A	10	2500	0.29	11.00	0.27	62	25.76
A_1	B	0	900	0.48	3.18	0.19	12	0
A_1	**B**	**0**	**1700**	**1.40**	**6.50**	**0.00**	**16**	**0**
A_1	B	0	2500	0.97	9.17	0.00	17	0
A_1	B	5	900	1.35	2.67	1.60	4	100.0
A_1	B	5	1700	1.41	5.42	0.44	11	77.92
A_1	B	5	2500	1.99	8.58	0.23	16	37.66
A_1	B	10	900	0.49	2.33	2.88	10	100.0
A_1	B	10	1700	0.77	5.83	0.51	13	99.62
A_1	B	10	2500	0.78	8.42	0.25	12	69.57
A_2	B	0	900	0.67	4.50	0.45	16	0
A_2	**B**	**0**	**1700**	**0.77**	**9.00**	**0.19**	**37**	**0**
A_2	B	0	2500	0.67	11.42	0.1	85	0
A_2	**B**	**5**	**900**	**0.32**	**3.08**	**0.81**	**14**	**92.75**
A_2	B	5	1700	0.32	6.78	0.54	23	43.83
A_2	B	5	2500	0.22	9.00	0.49	32	13.30
A_2	B	10	900	0.63	3.33	1.03	9	98.03
A_2	B	10	1700	0.48	6.33	0.67	17	72.72
A_2	B	10	2500	0.63	7.42	0.37	21	52.27

Facts used for test data set are highlighted.

Published by Woodhead Publishing Limited, 2013

of the models (Shao et al., 2006). Good models were successfully developed simultaneously for the five parameters.

Figure 2.7 shows the correlation between experimental and predicted values for the five outputs studied. Slopes close to 1 are indications of the agreement between them. Even for parameters such as friability which have been reported, in some cases, difficult in making predictions (Plumb et al., 2005; Shao et al., 2006), ANN performed well.

As we have pointed out previously, the validity of the model is not only about whether or not it fits well to empirical observations, but also about

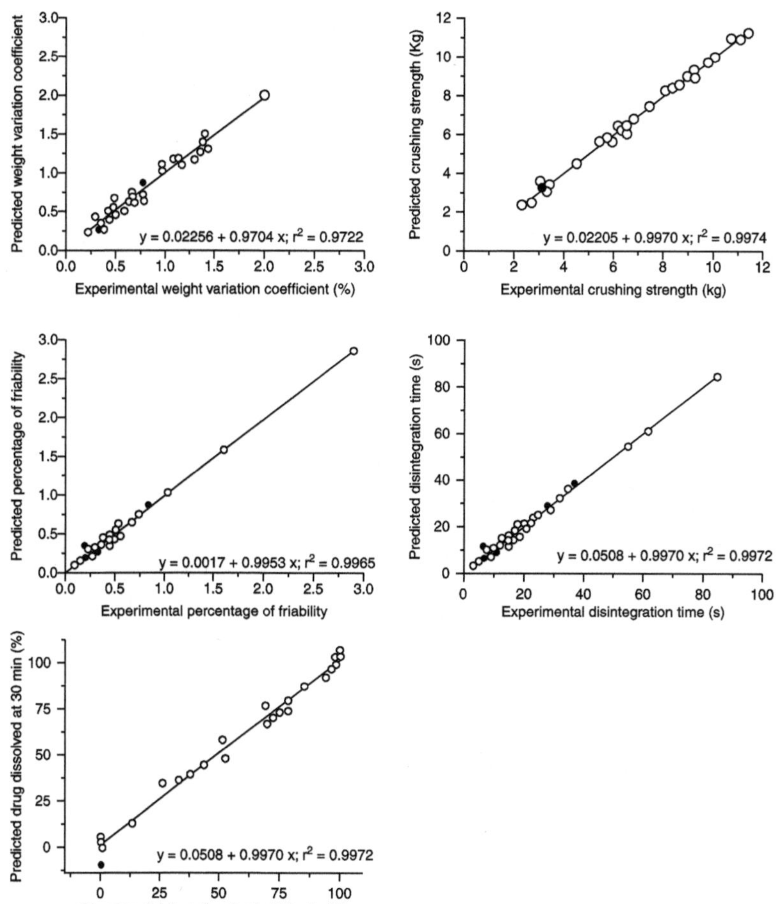

Figure 2.7 **Correlation between experimental values and those predicted by the ANN model for the five outputs studied (open symbols = training data, closed symbols = test data)**

its ability to generalize and predict in the range of the study. In order to test it, the model should be validated using a set of extra unseen data and the fit between experimental and predicted results analyzed.

Once the network has been trained and validated, the black box model allows prediction of the outputs for a specific set of inputs and, for instance, construction of the predicted response surfaces for each parameter.

As examples of response surfaces we have selected one parameter related to tablet mechanical properties, the friability (Figure 2.8) and one parameter related to tablet release properties, the drug released at 30 min (Figure 2.9). As variables, type of drug and binder are categorical, four surfaces can be represented for each parameter.

Important qualitative and quantitative information can be derived from Figures 2.8 and 2.9. Drug A-based tablets are always within the pharmacopoeia limits for friability (friability lower than 1%) whichever binder is used (Figure 2.8). On the contrary, drug B affects tablet mechanical properties negatively, that is for high percentages of drug B

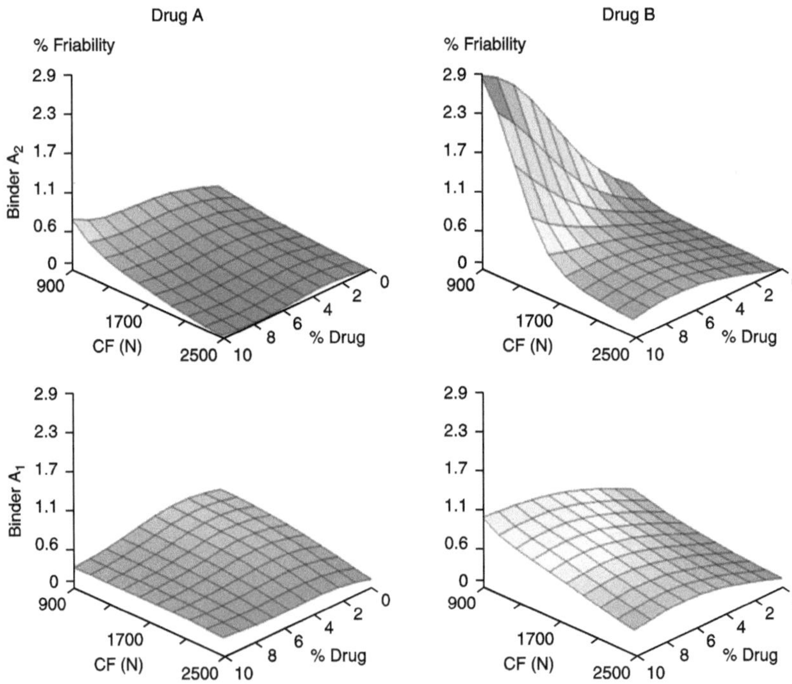

Figure 2.8 3-D plot of percentage of weight lost by friability

Published by Woodhead Publishing Limited, 2013

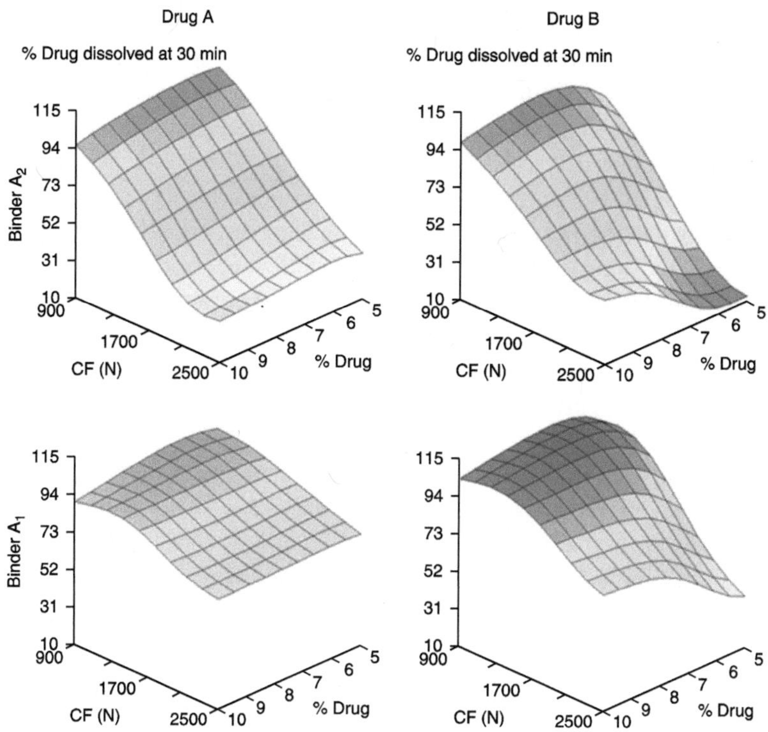

Figure 2.9 **3-D plot of percentage of drug dissolved at 30 min predicted by the model**

the compression force should be high to avoid being out of limits, especially when binder A_2 is used.

Controversial conclusions can be derived when drug release properties are analyzed (Figure 2.9). Whichever drug is used when binder A_1 is incorporated into the formulation, the amount of drug released at 30 min is within the limits (taking as the limits those established by the USP for drug A-based tablets $D_{30min} > 60\%$, and drug B-based tablets $D_{30min} > 80\%$). When binder A_2 is used, the deterioration of the release properties makes tablets compressed at high compression force unacceptable.

Having studied only two of the five outputs, controversial conclusions have already risen. If the five outputs, or more, need to be simultaneously considered, a large collection of graphs should be analyzed. As we have pointed out before, this is a complex task. In such a situation it is appropriate to couple ANN with GA in order to find the best combination or perform formulation optimization.

Let us find the best conditions to produce drug A-based tablets including a therapeutic dose of 12.5 mg. In this case two of the four inputs are fixed type of drug and percentage of drug (6.25%).

Tablets need to fulfil the pharmacopoeia requirements for mechanical and release properties. As has been pointed out before, when several responses need to be optimized simultaneously, a desirability function must be established which is a function of more than one response. The procedure involves establishing the constraints for each individual response. Table 2.3 presents the selection of desirable conditions for the outputs in our example. Weights indicate the priorities for the results fitting the selected variables; firstly, the percentage of drug dissolved at 30 min, followed by the percentage of loss of weight by friability, both pharmacopoeian parameters that must be within the limits (lower than 1% of friability and $D_{30\,min} > 60\%$ for drug A). But we can also introduce constraints for weight variation coefficient (e.g. <2%), crushing strength (e.g. >5 kg) and disintegration time (e.g. < 1.5 min) of that particular formulation.

As an example we have plotted the desirability function for the percentage of drug dissolved in Table 2.3 (Figure 2.10). For drug A-based tablets the pharmacopoeia establishes that the percentage of drug dissolved at 30 min should be higher than 60%, therefore up to a Min (minimum) of 60% is requested. Parameters Mid_1, Mid_2 and Max (maximum) help to establish the shape of the desirability function.

Following the steps in Figure 2.5, GA coupled with ANN selected the conditions in Table 2.4 as the best combination to achieve the results within the constraints established in Table 2.3. For this particular example, all the responses lay in the desirable range simultaneously and with the maximum desirability (100%).

Table 2.3 **Output constraints selected for the optimization process of drug A-based tablets**

Output	Weight	Min	Mid_1	Mid_2	Max	Desirability function
WVC	7	0.22	0.99	1.00	1.99	Down
CS	8	5	6.00	6.50	11.42	Up
F	9	0.8	0.90	0.91	1	Down
DT	6	60	70	85	90	Down
$D_{30\,min}$	10	60	65	70	100	Up

WVC, weight variation coefficient; CS, crushing strength; F, friability; DT, disintegration time; $D_{30\,min}$, percentage of drug dissolved at 30 min

Published by Woodhead Publishing Limited, 2013

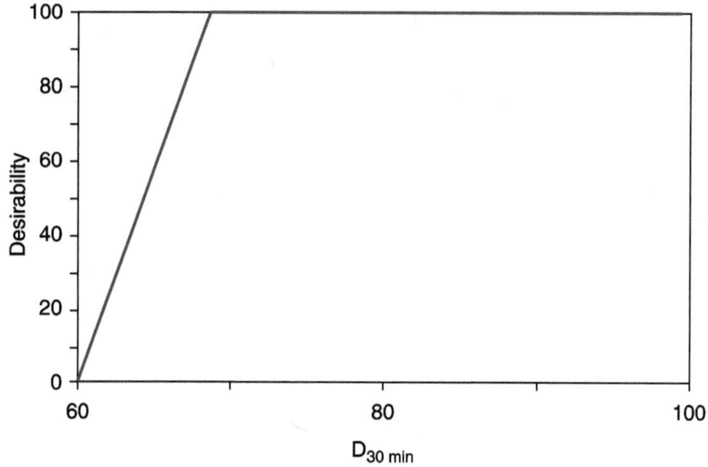

Figure 2.10 Desirability function for percentage of drug dissolved at 30 min following pharmacopoeia requirements for drug A-based tablets

Table 2.4 Selected inputs and predicted outputs for the optimum formulation selected by ANN coupled with GA

Inputs	Value	Fixed	Max	Predicted output		Desirability
Binder	A_2		1.99	WVC (%)	0.98	100
Drug	A	X	11.42	CS (Kg)	10.12	100
Drug percentage	6.25	X	1	F (%)	0.29	100
CF (N)	2122		90	DT (s)	38	100
			100	$D_{30\ min}$(%)	92	100

2.5 Fuzzy logic

Fuzzy logic is an AI tool, especially useful in problem solving, that can be also coupled with ANN to get knowledge from a database and to help understand formulations and processes.

Fuzzy set theory was introduced by Zadeh (1965) as an extension of the classical set theory, which enables processing of imprecise information using the membership concept (Adriaenssens et al., 2004). Prof. Zadeh illustrated the concept of the fuzzy set and the degree of membership with the classical 'tall man' example (Figure 2.11). The conventional characteristic mapping of a classical logic set determines that a man is tall

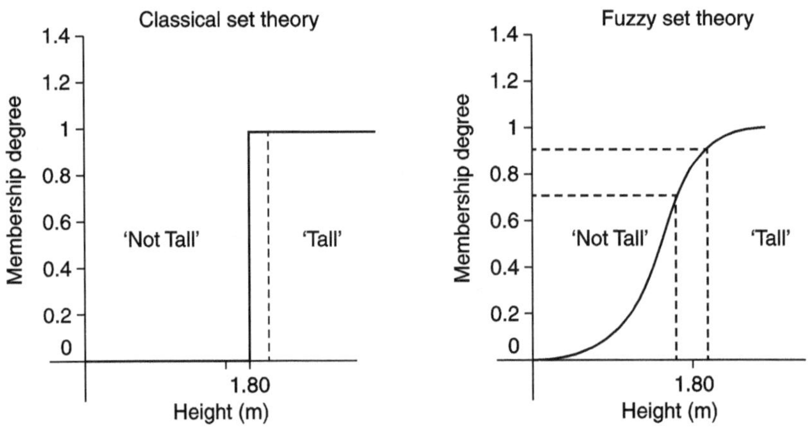

Figure 2.11 **Comparison between classical set theory and fuzzy set theory to illustrate Zadeh's example of the 'tall man' (modified from Zadeh, 1965)**

when his height is over 1.80 m. Therefore, a man of height 1.81 m should be included in the 'tall men' category and a man of height 1.79 m should be included in the 'not tall' man category. With just 2 cm difference in height, the classification of the men into different categories does not seem logical and can have some impractical consequences in the real life (imagine you need two tall men to do a job!).

Zadeh extended the traditional definition of a logic premise from having just two extremes (tall or not tall) to one in which there is a range in degree of truth from 0 to 1. New sets can be described qualitatively by terms as very low, low, average, tall or very tall. Using the fuzzy set theory, an element of those sets can be assigned to a fuzzy set with its membership degree ranging from 0 to 1, so two men of heights 1.79 m and 1.81 m belong to fuzzy set 'tall man' with membership degrees of 0.70 and 0.90, respectively (Figure 2.11). The 1.79 m man is smaller than the 1.81 m man, but is still tall.

As mentioned in the introduction of this chapter, for decades, pharmaceutical development has been attempted via trial and error, supplemented by the knowledge of the formulator. Formulator knowledge is typically built on linguistic tags, not quantitative mathematical data. Often words have higher significance in the real world of formulators than a collection of numerical data (Figure 2.12), and words constitute the basis to solve problems, make decisions or draw conclusions.

When combining ANN and fuzzy logic, the resulting hybrid system technology, neurofuzzy logic is able to break in this topic. This technology

Published by Woodhead Publishing Limited, 2013

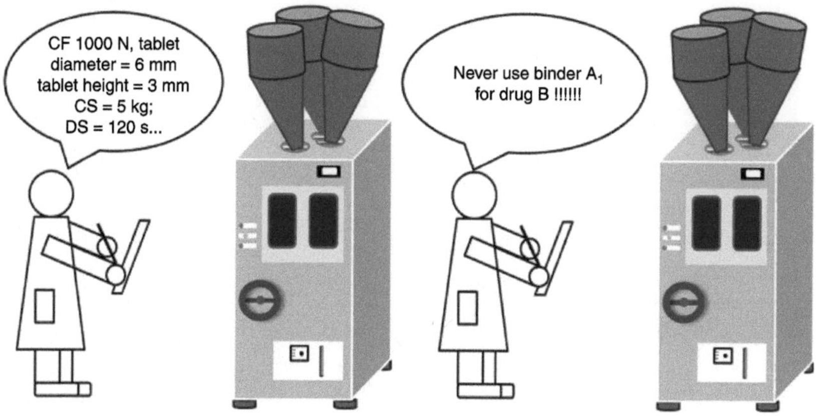
CF 1000 N, tablet
diameter = 6 mm
tablet height = 3 mm
CS = 5 kg;
DS = 120 s...
Never use binder A_1
for drug B !!!!!!

Figure 2.12 The importance of precision and word significance in the real world of the pharmaceutical formulator

combines the adaptive learning capabilities from ANN with the generality and the flexibility of representation from fuzzy logic (Babuska, 1998; Adriaenssens et al., 2004; Shao et al., 2006).

Linguistic tags are fuzzy data or fuzzy variables that can be numerically characterized, but a fuzzyfication process is necessary. For a better understanding of this concept, we will follow the fuzzyfication process of our example on direct compression. Figure 2.13 shows the fuzzyfication process of two variables: a numerical one, the compression force, and a nominal one, the binder type.

The fuzzyfication process of a nominal variable is simple as can be seen in Figure 2.13(a), you use binder A_1 or binder A_2. However, for compression force a more complicated fuzzyfication process is required. In Figure 2.13(b), the x axis is the compression force (N) with ranges for the fuzzy sets in two categories, low and high. The y axis represents the membership function and ranges from 0 to 1 (also could be expressed from 0 to 100%). Any value of compression force can be expressed by a word together with a membership value. For example, 1200 N can be regarded as both low and high compression force but with membership functions of 0.8 and 0.2, respectively. In other words 1200 N is low compression force in a higher degree than it is high compression force.

Therefore, fuzzy logic sets label qualitatively using linguistic terms and also assign varying degrees of membership called membership functions. The membership function then is subjective in nature and is a matter of definition rather than measurement. Chen and Mynett (2003) have

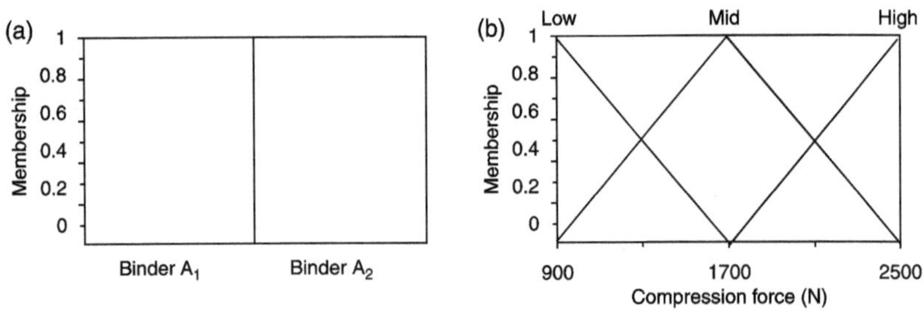

Figure 2.13 **Examples of fuzzy sets for continuous variables (e.g. compression force (N)) and categorical variables (e.g. type of binder) in the direct compression tablet example**

argued that the definition of membership functions and the induction of inference rules is the most difficult part in a fuzzy logic process. This process allows the interaction between linguistic terms (low, high) and the membership functions, making the terms meaningful to a computer. Additionally, it makes expressing the behaviour of a system possible using natural language and enhancing the possibility of concise description of complex tasks or processes.

In fuzzy-rule based systems, after modelling, knowledge is presented by IF–THEN rules. Fuzzy rules are sentences consisting of two parts: an antecedent part stating conditions on the input variable(s), and a consequent part describing the corresponding values of the output variable(s). For a set of the input variables, the degree of fulfilment of each rule is obtained by aggregating the membership degrees of these input values into the respective fuzzy sets. Going back to the example described previously, modelling by neurofuzzy logic allows determination of which inputs have a positive or negative effect on the output study or, in other words, which inputs explain the variations of the outputs. In Figure 2.14 it can be seen that for the parameter crushing strength of our previous example, the most important effect is the compression force (submodel 1 in discontinuous line), followed by the effect of the type of binder used (submodel 2 in continuous line) and the interaction between type and percentage of drug (submodel 3 in continuous line).

By interpreting the IF–THEN rules for the mechanical property, crushing strength, generated by neurofuzzy logic (Table 2.5), it can be easily deduced that:

- The main effect on this mechanical property is the compression force. IF the compression force is low THEN the crushing strength is low.

Published by Woodhead Publishing Limited, 2013

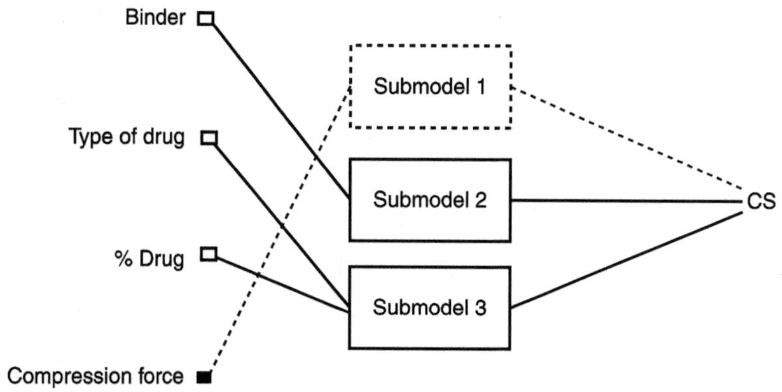

Figure 2.14 Effect of the studied variables on crushing strength parameter (discontinuous lines indicate the more important submodel)

Table 2.5 Examples of a fuzzy output using IF–THEN rules describing the effect of the type of drug and binder, percentage of drug and compression force on the crushing strength of direct compressed tablets

Submodel: 1

IF	CF is LOW	THEN	CS is LOW (1.00)
	CF is HIGH		CS is HIGH (1.00)

Submodel: 2

IF	Binder is A_1	THEN	CS is LOW (0.64)
	Binder is A_2		CS is HIGH (0.80)

Submodel: 3

IF	Drug is A AND %D is LOW	THEN	CS is LOW (0.61)
	Drug is A AND %D is HIGH		CS is HIGH (0.52)
	Drug is B AND %D is LOW		CS is LOW (0.63)
	Drug is B AND %D is HIGH		CS is LOW (1.00)

- Mechanical properties of binder A_2-based tablets are better than mechanical properties of binder A_1-based tablets.
- The incorporation of drug B deteriorates mechanical properties more than incorporation of drug A.

The analysis of the corresponding IF–THEN rules for the different outputs allows us to acquire knowledge on the effect of formulation and process variables on the behaviour of the formulation. The logical structure of rules facilitates comprehension of a semi-qualitative manner, similar to that used by the human brain to analyse the real world (Babuska, 1998).

The major capabilities of fuzzy logic are the flexibility, the tolerance with uncertainty and vagueness and the possibility of modelling non-linear functions, searching for consistent patterns or systemic relationships between variables in a complex data set, data mining and promoting deep understanding of the processes studied by generating comprehensible and reusable knowledge in an explicit format (Setnes et al., 1998; Shao et al., 2006; Yuan et al., 2008; Landín et al., 2009; Gago et al., 2010a).

2.6 Future perspectives

Pharmaceutical systems are complex to understand. Composition and a great number of process variables influence their properties. Nowadays modern technology provides an opportunity to generate a huge amount of data of different types. This storm of information would be useless if at the same time the technology did not solve the associated problems of analysing, integrating and extracting knowledge from the data. If the technology creates a problem, the technology should solve it.

AI technologies, those currently in use and those forthcoming, will help the researchers with those difficult tasks: to integrate variable information, to explain what is going on, to model and finally to predict what will happen in a specific situation.

As described above, neural networks can be used for a wide range of application domains in the field of pharmaceutical research, giving models as least as good as those obtained using statistical techniques and more traditional modelling. Neural networks combined with genetic algorithms can predict the combination of variables that would yield the optimum solution when independent variables are fed into the network, as has been pointed out in this chapter. Also, neural network technologies have spectacular advantages over other systems in their ability to capture non-linear relationships in the data (wherever their origin or type and even from incomplete data sets), without requiring prior knowledge from

Published by Woodhead Publishing Limited, 2013

the user. In fact, the user does not need to have a deep specific background to employ neural systems effectively. Additionally, the knowledge derived from neural networks can be easily increased by adding new data (inputs and/or outputs) to the database, giving new insights to understand and develop formulations.

We think that these new technologies will become the norms for dealing with pharmaceutical formulation development.

2.7 Acknowledgements

The authors thank Drs P.P. Gallego and J. Gago for their critical review of the manuscript and their useful comments.

2.8 References

Adriaenssens V, De Baets B, Goethals PLM and De Pauw N. Fuzzy rule-based methods for decision support in ecosystem management (2004) *Sci Total Environ*, 319, 1–12. ISSN: 0048–9697.

Agatonovic-Kustrin S, Zecevic M, Zivanovic LJ and Tucker IG. Application of artificial neural networks in HPLC method development (1998) *J Pharm Biomed Anal*, 17, 1, 69–76. ISSN: 0731–7085.

Agatonovic-Kustrin S and Beresford R. Basic concepts of artificial neural network (ANN) modeling and its application in pharmaceutical research (2000) *J Pharm Biomed Anal*, 22, 5, 717–27. ISSN: 0731–7085.

Agatonovic-Kustrin S, Wu V, Rades T, Saville D and Tucker IG. Ranitidine hydrochloride X-ray assay using a neural network (2000) *J Pharm Biomed Anal*, 22, 6, 985–992. ISSN: 0731–7085.

Agatonovic-Kustrin S and Alany RG. Role of genetic algorithms and artificial neural networks in predicting the phase behavior of colloidal delivery systems (2001) *Pharm Res*, 18, 7, 1049–55. ISSN: 0724–8741.

Agatonovic-Kustrin S, Glass BD, Wisch MH and Alany RG. Prediction of a Stable Microemulsion Formulation for the Oral Delivery of a Combination of Antitubercular Drugs Using ANN Methodology (2003) *Pharm Res*, 20, 11, 1760–5. ISSN: 0724–8741.

Ali HSM, Blagden N, York P, Amani A and Brook T. Artificial neural networks modeling the prednisolone nanoprecipitation in microfluidic reactors (2009) *Eur J Pharm Sci*, 37, 3–4, 514–22. ISSN: 0928–0987.

Andrea TA and Kalayeh H. Applications of neural networks in quantitative structure-activity relationships of dihydrofolate reductase inhibitors (1991) *J Med Chem*, 34, 9, 2824–36. ISSN: 0022–2623.

Babuska R. Fuzzy modeling for control, In: *International Series in Intelligent Technologies* (1998) Babuska R. (Ed.) Kluwer Academic Publishers, Massachusetts, pp. 1–8.

Cartwright HM. *Applications of Artificial Intelligence in Chemistry* (1993) Oxford University Press, Oxford.

Chen Q and Mynett AE. Integration of data mining techniques and heuristic knowledge in fuzzy logic modeling of eutrophication in Taihu Lake (2003) *Ecol Model* 162, 1–2, 55–67. ISSN: 0304–3800.

Colbourn E and Rowe RC. Neural computing and pharmaceutical formulation. (2005) In: *Encyclopaedia of pharmaceutical technology*, Swarbrick, J. and Boylan, J.C. (Eds), Marcel Dekker, New York.

Colbourn E. (2003) Neural computing: enable intelligent formulations. *Pharmaceutical Technology Supplement*, 16–20.

Colbourn EA and Rowe RC. Novel approaches to neural and evolutionary computing in pharmaceutical formulation: Challenges and new possibilities (2009) *Future Med Chem* 1, 4, 713–26. ISSN: 1756–8919.

De Matas M, Shao Q, Richardson CH and Chrystyn H. Evaluation of *in vitro in vivo* correlations for dry powder inhaler delivery using artificial neural networks (2008) *Eur J Pharm Sci*, 33, 1, 80–90. ISSN: 0928–0987.

De Matas M, Shao Q, Silkstone VL and Chrystyn H. Evaluation of an *in vitro in vivo* correlation for nebulizer delivery using artificial neural networks (2007) *J Pharm Sci* 96, 12, 3293–303. ISSN: 0022–3549.

Díaz-Rodríguez P and Landín M. (2011) Smart design of intratumoral thermosensitive *β*-lapachone hydrogels by Artificial Neural Networks. *Int J Pharm*. In press ISSN: 0378–5173.

Erb RJ Introduction to back propagation Neural Network Compution (1993) *Pharm Res* 10, 165–70. ISSN: 0724–8741.

Fatouros DG, Nielsen FS, Douroumis D, Hadjileontiadis LJ and Mullertz A. *In vitro-in vivo* correlations of self-emulsifying drug delivery systems combining the dynamic lipolysis model and neuro-fuzzy networks (2008) *Eur J Pharm Biopharm*. 69, 3, 887–98. ISSN: 0939–6411.

García T, Cook G and Nosal R. PQLI Ley Topics-Criticality, Design Space, and Control Strategy (2008) *J Pharm Innov* 3, 60–8. ISSN: 1872–5120.

Gago J, Landín M and Gallego PP. A neurofuzzy logic approach for modeling plant processes: a practical case of *in vitro* direct rooting and acclimatization of *Vitis vinifera* L (2010a) *Plant Sci*, 179, 241–9. ISSN: 0168–9452.

Gago J, Landín M and Gallego PP. Artificial neural networks modeling the *in vitro* rhizogenesis and acclimatization of *Vitis vinifera* L (2010b) *J Plant Physiol*, 167, 1226–31. ISSN: 0176–1617.

Gasperlin M, Podlogar F and Sibanc R. Evolutionary artificial neural networks as tools for predicting the internal structure of microemulsions (2008) *J Pharm Pharmaceut Sci* (*www.cspsCanada.org*) 11, 1, 67–76. ISSN: 1482–1826.

Gibson M. Product optimization (2009) In: *Pharmaceutical preformulation and formulation* 2nd Ed. Gibson M (Ed.) Informa Healthcare, New York, pp. 289–324. ISBN–13:878–1–4200–7317–1.

Glass BD, Agatonovic-Kustrin S and Wisch MH. Artificial neural networks to optimize formulation components of a fixed-dose combination of rifampicin, isoniazid and pyrazinamide in a microemulsion (2005) *Current Drug Disc Tech*, 2, 3, 195–201. ISSN: 1570–1638.

Published by Woodhead Publishing Limited, 2013

Glezakos TJ, Moschopoulou G, Tsiligiridis TA, Kintzios S and Yialouris CP. Plant virus identification based on neural networks with evolutionary preprocessing (2010) *Comput Electron Agric* 70, 263–75. ISSN: 0168–1699.

Godavarthy SS, Yerramsetty KM, Rachakonda VK, Neely BJ, Madihally SV, et al. Design of improved permeation enhancers for transdermal drug delivery (2009) *J Pharm Sci*, 98, 11, 4085–99. ISSN: 0022–3549.

Guo M, Kalra G, Wilson W, Peng Y. and Augsburger LL. A prototype intelligent hybrid system for hard gelatin capsule formulation development (2002) *Pharm Technol North America*, 26, 9, 44–60.

Hartnell, N. and MacKinnon N.J. Neural networks: From Science fiction to pharmacy (2003) *Am J Health-Syst Pharm*, 60, 1908–9. ISSN: 1079–2082.

Ichikawa, H. Hierarchy neural networks as applied to pharmaceutical problems (2003) *Adv Drug Deliv Rev*, 55, 1119–47. ISSN: 0169–409X.

ICH Q8. *International Conference On Harmonisation of technical requirements for registration of pharmaceuticals for human use (2009) Pharmaceutical Development Q8 (R2) http://www.ich.org/fileadmin/Public_Web_Site/ICH_Products/Guidelines/Quality/Q8_R1/Step4/Q8_R2_Guideline.pdf.* Last consulted December 2011.

Jiang W and Yu LX. Modern Pharmaceutical Quality Regulations: Question-based Review (2009) In *Developing solid oral dosage forms: pharmaceutical theory and practice.* Qiu, Y, Chen Y, Liu L, Zhang GGZ (Eds) Academic Press, New York, pp. 885–901.

Kremer DM and Hancock BC. Process simulation in the pharmaceutical industry: a review of some basic physical models (2006) *J Pharm Sci*, 95, 3, 517–29. ISSN: 0022–3549.

Krenker A, Bešter J and Kos A. Introduction to the Artificial Neural Networks (2011) In: *Artificial Neural Networks – Methodological Advances and Biomedical Applications*, Suzuki, K (Ed.) 1–18. ISBN 978–953–307–243–2.

Labouta HI, El-Khordagui LK, Molokhia AM and Ghaly GM. Multivariate modeling of encapsulation and release of an ionizable drug from polymer microspheres (2009), *J Pharm Sci*, 98, 12, 4603–15. ISSN: 0022–3549.

Landín M, Rowe RC and York P. Advantages of neurofuzzy logic against conventional experimental design and statistical analysis in studying and developing direct compression formulations (2009) *Eur J Pharm Sci*, 38, 325–31. ISSN: 0928–0987.

Lawrence S, Giles CL and Tsoi AC. *What Size Neural Network Gives Optimal Generalization? Convergence Properties of Backpropagation.* (1996) University of Maryland Technical Report CS-TR–3617 http://clgiles.ist.psu.edu/papers/UMD-CS-TR–3617.what.size.neural.net.to.use.pdf.

Leane MM, Cumming I and Corrigan OI. The use of artificial neural networks for the selection of the most appropriate formulation and processing variables in order to predict the in vitro dissolution of sustained release minitablets (2003) *AAPS PharmSciTech* 4, E26. ISSN: 1530–9932.

Lee Y, Khemka A, Yoo J and Lee CH. Assessment of diffusion coefficient from mucoadhesive barrier devices using artificial neural networks (2008) *Int J Pharm*, 351, 1–2, 119–26. ISSN: 0378–5173.

Leonardi D, Salomón CJ, Lamasa MC and Olivieria AC. Development of novel formulations for Chagas' disease: Optimization of benznidazole chitosan microparticles based on artificial neural networks (2009) *Int J Pharm* 367, 140–7. ISSN: 0378–5173.

Lewis GA, Mathieu D and Phan-Tan-Luu R. *Pharmaceutical and Experimental Design* (1999) Marcel Dekker. New York. ISBN: 0–8247–9860–0.

Lunney PD, Cogdill RP and Drennen III JK. Innovation in Pharmaceutical Experimentation Part 1: Review of experimental designs used in industrial pharmaceutics research and introduction to Bayesian D-optimal Experimental design (2008) *J Pharm Innov* 3, 188–203. ISSN: 1872–5120.

Mitchell M. *An introduction to genetic algorithm* (1998) The MIT Press, Mitchell, E. (Eds) Massachusetts. ISBN–13: 978–0262631853.

Neely BJ, Madihally SV, Robinson RL Jr and Gasem KA. Nonlinear quantitative structure-property relationship modeling of skin permeation coefficient (2009) *J Pharm Sci* 98, 4069–84. ISSN: 0022–3549.

Plumb AP, Rowe RC, York P and Brown M. Optimisation of the predictive ability of artificial neural network (ANN) models: a comparison of three programs and four classes of training algorithm (2005) *Eur J Pharm Sci* 25, 395–405. ISSN: 0928–0987.

Qiao S, Tang C, Jin H, Peng J, Davis D and Han N. KISTCM: Knowledge discovery system for traditional Chinese medicine (2010) *Appl Intell*, 32, 3, 346–63. ISSN: 0924–669X.

Rafienia M, Amiri M, Janmaleki M. and Sadeghian A. Application of artificial neural networks in controlled drug delivery systems (2010) *Appl Artif Intell*, 24, 8, 807–20. ISSN: 0883–9514.

Rowe RC and Roberts RJ. Artificial intelligence in pharmaceutical product formulation: neural computing and emerging technologies (1998) *Pharmaceutical Science and Technology Today*, 1, 5, 200–5. ISSN: 0975–5772.

Rowe RC and Roberts RJ (2005) *Intelligent Software for Product Formulation*, Taylor and Francis, London. ISBN: 0–7484–0732–4.

Russell SJ and Norvig P. *Artificial Intelligence: A Modern Approach* (2nd ed.) (2003), Upper Saddle River, NJ: Prentice Hall, USA. ISBN–13: 978–0131038059.

Setnes M, Babuska R and Verbruggen HB. (1998) Rule-based modeling: precision and transparency. *IEEE Trans Syst Man Cybern Part C-A Rev*, 28, 1, 165–9. ISSN: 1094–6977.

Shao Q, Rowe RC and York P. Comparison of neurofuzzy logic and neural networks in modeling experimental data of an immediate release tablet formulation (2006) *Eur J Pharm Sci*, 28, 394–404. ISSN: 0928–0987.

Shao Q, Rowe RC and York P. Comparison of neurofuzzy logic and decision trees in discovering knowledge from experimental data of an immediate release tablet formulation (2007) *Eur J Pharm Sci*, 31, 129–36. ISSN: 0928–0987.

Siepmann J and Siepmann F. Mathematical modeling of drug delivery (2008) *Int J Pharm*, 364, 2, 328–43. ISSN: 0378–5173.

Singh B, Kumar R and Ahuja N. Optimizing drug delivery systems using systematic 'design of experiments. Part I: Fundamental aspects (2005a) *Crit Rev Ther Drug Carr Syst* 22, 1, 27–105. ISSN: 0743–4863.

Published by Woodhead Publishing Limited, 2013

Singh B, Dahiya M, Saharan V and Ahuja N. Optimizing drug delivery systems using systematic design of experiments. Part II: Retrospect and prospects (2005b) *Crit Rev Ther Drug Carr Syst* 22, 3, 215–93. ISSN: 0743–4863.

Su Z and Khorasani KA. neural-network-based controller for a single-link flexible manipulator using the inverse dynamic approach (2001) *IEEE Trans Ind Electron* 48, 1074–86. ISSN: 0278–0046.

Sun Y, Peng Y, Chen Y and Shukla AJ. Application of artificial neural networks in the design of controlled release drug delivery systems (2003) *Adv Drug Deliv Rev* 55, 9, 1201–15. ISSN: 0169–409X.

Takagaki K, Arai H and Takayama K. Creation of a tablet database containing several active ingredients and prediction of their pharmaceutical characteristics based on ensemble artificial neural networks (2010) *J Pharm Sci* 99, 4201–14. ISSN: 0022–3549.

Takayama K, Fujikawa M and Nagai T. Artificial neural network as a novel method to optimize pharmaceutical formulations (1999a) *Pharm Res* 16, 1, 1–6. ISSN: 0724–8741.

Takayama K, Takahara J, Fujikawa M, Ichikawa H and Nagai T. Formula optimization based on artificial neural networks in transdermal drug delivery (1999b) *J Control Release* 62, 1–2, 161–70. ISSN: 0168–3659.

Taylor JG. *Neural networks and their applications* (1996) Taylor JG (Eds) John Wiley and Sons Ltd. England. ISBN: 0471962821.

Valizadeh H, Pourmahmood M, Mojarrad JS, Nemati M and Zakeri-Milani P. Application of artificial intelligent tools to modeling of glucosamine preparation from exoskeleton of shrimp (2009) *Drug Dev Ind Pharm* 35, 396–407. ISSN: 0363–9045.

Wehrlé R and Stamm A. Statistical tools for process control and quality improvement in the pharmaceutical industry (1994) *Drug Dev Ind Pharm* 20, 141–6. ISSN: 0363–9045.

Wei H, Zhong F, Ma J and Wang Z. Formula Optimization of Emulsifiers for Preparation of Multiple Emulsions Based on Artificial Neural Networks (2008) *J Dispersion Sci Technol* 29, 319–26. ISSN: 0193–2691.

Woolfson AD, Umrethia ML, Kett VL and Malcolm RK. Freeze-dried, mucoadhesive system for vaginal delivery of the HIV microbicide, dapivirine: Optimisation by an artificial neural network (2010) *Int J Pharm* 388, 136–43. ISSN: 0378–5173.

Xiaobo Z, Jiewen Z, Povey M.J, Holmes M and Hanpin M. Variables selection methods in near-infrared spectroscopy (2010) *Anal Chim Acta* 667, 14–32. ISSN: 0003–2670.

Yuan JS, Galbraith DW, Dai SY, Griffin P and Stewart N Jr. Plant systems biology comes of age (2008) *Trends Plant Sci*, 13, 4, 165–71. ISSN: 1360–1385.

Zadeh L. Fuzzy sets (1965) *Inform Contr*, 8, 338–53. ISSN: 0019–9958.

Zhou X, Chen S, Liu B, Zhang R, Wang Y, et al. Development of traditional Chinese medicine clinical data warehouse for medical knowledge discovery and decision support (2010) *Artif Intell Med*, 48, 2–3, 139–52. ISSN: 0933–3657.

Zomer S, Guptam M and Scott A. Application of Multivariate Tools in Pharmaceutical Product Development to Bridge Risk Assessment to Continuous Verification in a Quality by Design Environment (2010) *J Pharm Innov*, 5, 109–18. ISSN: 1872–5120.

ME_expert 2.0: a heuristic decision support system for microemulsions formulation development

Aleksander Mendyk, Jakub Szlęk and Renata Jachowicz, Jagiellonian University, Poland

DOI: 10.1533/9781908818508.39

Abstract: Artificial neural networks (ANN) and random forest (RF) classifier were employed to model microemulsions (ME) formation. The ME quantitative and qualitative composition was the system input, whereas the decision on ME presence or absence was the output. Molecular descriptors were used to characterize qualitative composition of the ME. A large database of over 300 000 records was gathered and processed to create competent models. Sensitivity analysis of ANN was used for crucial variables selection as a data-mining procedure. Final models with 17 inputs were built both for ANN and RF. In the case of ANN, they were combined into the ensemble systems with total classification rate around 85%. For RF, no ensembles were built as they are collective systems intrinsically – the total classification rate was around 86%. Combination of both ANN and RF did not improve results. The decision support system (DSS) was coded as open source Java-based software (ME_expert 2.0) freely available from *http://sourceforge.net/projects/medss*.

Key words: artificial neural networks, random forest, molecular descriptors, decision support system, ensemble systems, microemulsions.

3.1 Introduction

Efficiency is the major issue when an engineering process is ongoing or projected to be carried out in the future. Efficiency involves such terms as reproducibility of the process, cost-effectiveness, simplicity, etc. It is efficiency of the development process that directly or indirectly determines quality of the final product. The latter is of the utmost importance in the pharmaceutical industry – the drugs are to be effective and safe at the same time, which requires the highest possible precision in the manufacturing process. The above-quoted paradigm has found its way to the pharmaceutical product development strategies in such initiatives as Process Analytical Technology (PAT) or Quality by Design (QbD). A major assumption, being the foundation of these approaches, is that complete, mechanistic understanding of the manufacturing process is the guarantee of its ultimate control, thus resulting in the appropriate quality of the product. This approach has proven valid in a growing number of examples and is recognized today as obligatory for the pharmaceutical industry. However, there are still areas where a mechanistic approach is ineffective or at least difficult to employ. A profound example is the development of a pharmaceutical formulation, where the number of possible relationships between excipients, drug substances and/or preparation technologies is almost infinite. It is very difficult to approach pharmaceutical formulation development using classical engineering procedures. That is why heuristic methodology is being applied and has warranted more attention recently. An example of such an approach will be presented for a microemulsions (ME) formulation process, where no clear and universal physical theory is available of how and under what conditions microemulsions are formed.

ME are thermodynamically stable, homogenous, transparent or translucent, optically isotropic dispersions, either oil in water (o/w) or water in oil (w/o), which are stabilized by surfactant molecules where oil and water phases are present in domains of 10–140 nm [26, 106]. Hoar and Schulman were the first to describe the ME in 1943 [48]. Size of particles makes ME transparent as opposed to classical emulsions which are opaque and milky. Because of the content of toxic surfactants and oil phase, ME were not initially of interest to the pharmaceutical industry. In the late 1970s and 1980s, ME were used to recover oil in hard to reach reservoirs [92]. For the last 30 years, together with a vast development in biocompatible excipients, ME were noticed because of their potential advantages, namely bioavailability improvement,

Published by Woodhead Publishing Limited, 2013

long-term stability, ease of preparation, low toxicity and irritancy and considerable capacity for solubilization of various active pharmaceutical ingredients (API) [9, 24, 35, 42, 74, 97]. ME were found to be suitable for numerous applications, such as cosmetics and pharmaceutical formulations [88, 100], cell culture technology [3] and agriculture and food technology [105, 109]. ME are a suitable dosage form for parenteral [75, 104], oral [96, 107], transdermal [55, 70, 93–95], ophthalmic [6] and intranasal [54] applications. According to the Winsor classification [112], there are four general types of ME: type I oil-in-water (o/w) ME with excess of water phase, type II water-in-oil (w/o) ME with excess of oil phase, type III which is a three-phase system, water phase–ME–oil phase, and type IV which is a single-phase ME. Stability of ME depends on the facial tension at the oil/water interface. High dispersion of ME droplets leads to high energy accumulation at the interface. So as to lower the interfacial energy, mixtures of surfactant and cosurfactant are used, which allow spontaneous formation of ME. General considerations about the stability of ME are discussed as an important issue in the formulation development procedure [62, 99].

ME have many potential advantages and uses as pharmaceutical formulations. However, their formulation process is usually conducted by trial and error or formulator's experience rather than an algorithmic procedure. Therefore, it would be beneficial to provide a tool aiding ME formulation process and reducing the burden of laboratory trials, thus increasing development efficiency. Such computerized tools aiding technological processes are well known in engineering and science as expert systems or more flexible decision support systems (DSS). Every DSS includes a basic set of elements:

- knowledge base;
- inference machine;
- user interface.

A user interface allows communication with the DSS and benefit to be drawn from the DSS predictions. A knowledge base usually consists of a set of all available information gathered in the strict way suitable for processing by any numerical analysis tools to be employed in the future. The data quality and preprocessing is crucial to the future system accuracy. The inference machine is the knowledge processor containing the set of rules or general model of the analyzed problem in order to provide the advisory function of the DSS. A key point of DSS development is to adjust the inference machine type and data processing abilities to completely exploit the available knowledge base. The DSS for ME formulations would have to integrate various sources of information and types of input variables in order to be flexible, precise and versatile for its efficiency. In order to fulfill this demand, computational intelligence (CI) tools are used: among these, artificial neural networks (ANN) and random forests (RF) were chosen for this chapter as possible inference machines of DSS.

ANN are non-linear, information processing systems, which are inspired by biological neural structures both in structure and functionality. Classical ANN, so-called multilayer perceptrons (MLP), are multilayered structures in which the signal is processed only in one direction from input, layer by layer, to the output (Figure 3.1). In ANN structure there are processing units, so called artificial neurons or nodes, connected hierarchically by 'weights' simulating biological synapses.

Through the automatic self-learning process, ANN create the models for complex problems based only on the experimental data [67]. One of the most common training algorithms for ANN is back-propagation (BP), where the teaching signal is the difference between current output and the desired one. The teaching signal is propagated backwards from the output layer to the input layer in order to modify weight values. Automatic training allows creation of models without prior assumptions, which is a common pitfall of classical, statistical modeling procedures.

The empirical modeling approach represented by ANN allows identification of complex and unknown relationships in the data beyond the capabilities of classical statistical tools. The above is based also on the relative ease of ANN in dealing with large amounts of data in terms of

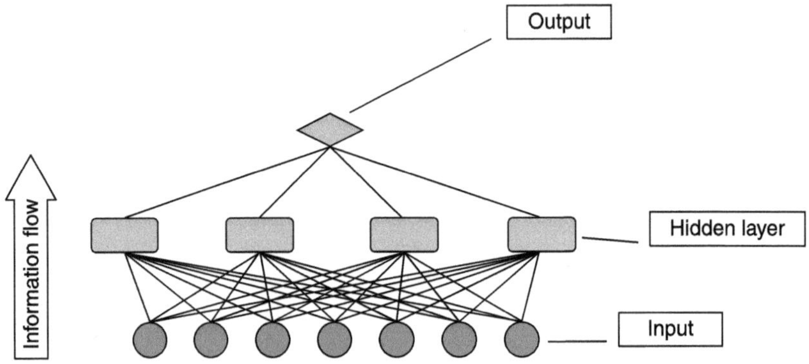

Figure 3.1 Typical layout of a multilayer perceptron-artificial neural network (MLP-ANN)

cases and features. However, the so-called curse of dimensionality is also applicable to the ANN, but is less pronounced than for classical statistical systems. Moreover, ANN are able to decide on input importance by means of sensitivity analysis. This is a way to reduce unnecessary inputs. It improves system performance and also provides knowledge about the analyzed problem. Therefore, ANN are also used as data mining tools allowing for automated knowledge extraction.

Another advantage of ANN is their superior ability to identify non-linear systems, because ANN are usually built on non-linear activation functions – the elements of the artificial neurons. Therefore, ANN are non-linear, data-processing systems themselves. All the above features in a single tool make ANN suitable for dealing with complicated, non-linear and multidimensional problems, where no clear theory exists, thus empirical modeling is the approach of the choice.

ANN have proven to be reliable and flexible tools in many applications in the field of science and technology [63–65, 67, 73, 81, 91]. Their usefulness has been demonstrated in the field of pharmaceutical technology in issues such as granulation [72], solubility assessment [50], powder flow [51], tablet compression [2, 14], dissolution test [10, 17], nanoprecipitate formation [45], formulation of solid dispersions [11, 64] or ME [4, 28, 63, 84] and process validation [13]. Recent studies involving ANN and ME generally focus on prediction of phase boundaries of ME. Richardson et al. [84] developed a simple ANN-based system which had six input neurons, a single hidden layer of 14 neurons with hyperbolic tangent (*tanh*) activation function and one output neuron architecture. The ANN system was able to predict the phase behavior of quaternary systems with acceptable classification error of 83.6–96.5%. The database included ME with lecithin, isopropyl myristate, and water, together with different types of cosurfactants, including short- and medium-chain alcohols, amines, acids, and ethylene glycol monoalkyl ethers.

Djekic et al. [28] used a generalized regression neural network (GRNN) for prediction of solubilization capacity of a water and oil phase for ME containing PEG-8 caprylic/capric glycerides. Satisfactory model performance was obtained where the generalization error expressed as relative root mean squared error (REL RMSE) reached a value of 8.4%. However, the application of the GRNN was very limited because of the narrow range of input data, namely single type of the oil phase, surfactant and cosurfactant as well. A MLP-ANN model with a single hidden layer was applied by Alany et al. [4] to predict formation of ME. Predictions were based on the quantitative composition and hydrophilic-lipophilic balance (HLB) value of surfactants. Classification rate computed on the validation data set was found to be from 85% to 92%, although the base data set was limited to a single type of the oil phase, surfactant and cosurfactant. The most flexible expert system for ME phase boundary prediction based on ANN was developed by Mendyk and Jachowicz [63]. The input data referred to molecular descriptors (CI, connectivity indices, also known as molecular connectivity indices), HLB values, and quantitative composition of ME. The database contained over 65 000 records derived from 118 formulations and the overall performance of the expert system was estimated on 77% correctly classified instances.

Random forest (RF) is an ensemble data mining technique used for classification, prediction, outlier detection and variable selection. The algorithm was developed by Leo Breiman and Adele Cutler [19], and it combines a random selection of features which is an example of the random subspace method proposed by Ho [47] and bootstrap aggregating (bagging) [18]. The advantages of RF are it is an accurate learning algorithm, efficient on large data bases, estimates importance of variables and detects interactions between them, balances errors in class population of unbalanced data sets, and is effective for estimating missing data [83]. RF has found numerous applications in data exploration and understanding. Since RF was first introduced in 2001, many surveys have been published, especially in the fields of genetics [102], molecular biology [27], chemistry [77], pharmacokinetics [86], medicine [101], and toxicology [113]. Despite diverse applications in pharmaceutical science, the RF technique is just beginning to be used in pharmaceutical technology. For example, Palmer et al. [76] used RF algorithms to predict aqueous solubility of potential drug molecules. Based on experimental data for 988 compounds, the RF regression model predicted aqueous solubility more accurately than those created by partial-least-squares regression, support vector machines or ANN. The prediction of solubility for an external test set resulted in R^2 of 0.89 and RMSE of 0.69, and the values of these parameters suggested good model performance.

3.2 Methodology or description of the tool

A complex approach was applied (Figure 3.2) involving several steps:

- database building;
- search for minimum input vector size;
- building of inference machine for DSS;
- implementation of the models into the software.

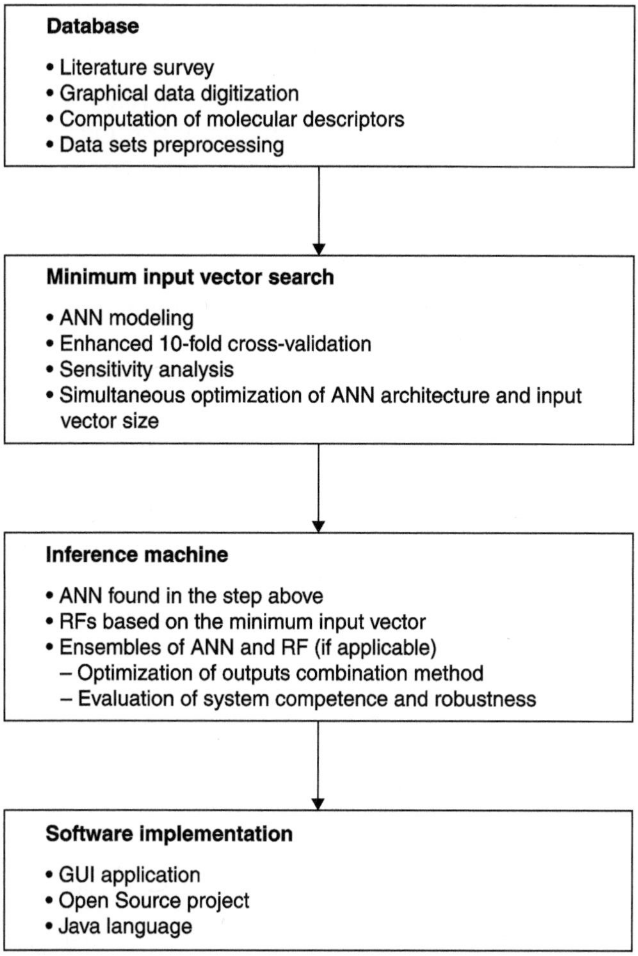

Figure 3.2 Diagram of the work scheme

3.2.1 Database

Literature survey

Data sets were prepared by publication survey of the past 16 years using Scopus® and ScienceDirect® databases. Publication inclusion criteria were as follows:

- clearly defined and illustrated Gibbs phase diagram corresponding to the ME phases boundaries;

- ability to find numerical representation of the component chemical structure and its physicochemical properties.

The formulations were both ternary and pseudo-ternary ME consisting of surfactant (TE), cosurfactant (CO-TE), oil phase (OP), water phase (WP) and miscellaneous surfactant component (MISC) if present. Selected phase diagrams were digitized using Phase_diagr. After the scanning procedure, text files were obtained which consisted of three coordinates (composition of ME) and presence or absence of ME. In cases with more than three components OpenOffice formulas were used to calculate the composition of the mixtures.

Data set

Chemical structures of ME components were drawn in MarvinSketch [61] and 3D-optimized using the Molconvert command-line program included in the Marvin package, which minimized the molecule energy through standard optimization procedure [68]. Resulting *.sdf files were processed further to calculate the chemical descriptors. For each component of ME, 103 physicochemical descriptors were obtained using the Cxcalc Calculator Plugin of Marvin – command-line program with 43 selected plugins (Table 3.1) [21].

Table 3.1 **Molecular descriptors and corresponding Cxcalc plugins used to create the data sets**

Cxcalc plugin	Descriptor group
formula	Elemental Analysis
topologyanalysistable	Charge
composition	
icomposition	
mass	
avgpol	
axxpol	
ayypol	
azzpol	
hasvalidconformer	Conformation
doublebondstereoisomercount	Isomers
resonantcount	

Cxcalc plugin	Descriptor group
enumerationcount	Markush Enumerations
logd	Partitioning
logp	
Pi	Other
Pka	
acceptorcount	
donorcount	
msacc	
msdon	
refractivity	
asa	Geometry
psa	
asymmetricatomcount	
balabanindex	
bondcount	
chiralcentercount	
connectedgraph	
cyclomaticnumber	
dreidingenergy	
fragmentcount	
hararyindex	
hyperwienerindex	
maximalprojectionarea	
maximalprojectionradius	
minimalprojectionarea	
minimalprojectionradius	
molecularsurfacearea	
plattindex	
randicindex	
szegedindex	
wienerindex	
wienerpolarity	

The plugins that produced null or non-numeric output were omitted except the cases which resulted in logical values, where 'true' values were represented by 1 and 'false' by 0. In both cases of Cxcalc and Molconvert, default settings were used. The calculated descriptors from Cxcalc were divided into several groups which included (Table 3.1):

- Elemental Analysis;
- Protonation (pKa Plugin Calculation, Isoelectric Point);
- Partitioning (logP, logD);
- Charge (Polarizability Plugin, Orbital Electronegativity);
- Geometry (Topology Analysis Plugin, Polar Surface Area Plugin (2D), Molecular Surface Area Plugin (3D));
- Markush Enumeration;
- Other (i.e. Hydrogen Bond Donor-Acceptor, Huckel Analysis, Refractivity, Resonance, Structural Frameworks).

Additionally, ionic strength of water phase was calculated according to known qualitative and quantitative composition of water phase. HLB of surfactant and oil phase density were calculated or obtained from the literature. Quantitative composition expressed in compound weight percentages was also included at the input (see Figure 3.3).

Mixtures of compounds were considered as weighted-average according to manufacturer labeling or published data. If a certain ME consisted of a mixture of four or more compounds (i.e. including two surfactants), a particular descriptor was calculated as the weighted-average value of the respective component descriptors according to their individual percentages (Eq. 3.1).

$$Mixt = \sum_{i=1}^{n} R_i * D_i \qquad [3.1]$$

where:

Mixt, weighted average descriptor value;

R, weight ratio (w/w) of the compounds;

D, the value of the descriptor;

n, number of the mixture components;

i, component number.

The assumption that the mixture of compounds like oil or surfactant can be treated as weighted-average of the molecule physicochemical properties is commonly accepted, especially in the field of physical pharmacy [7].

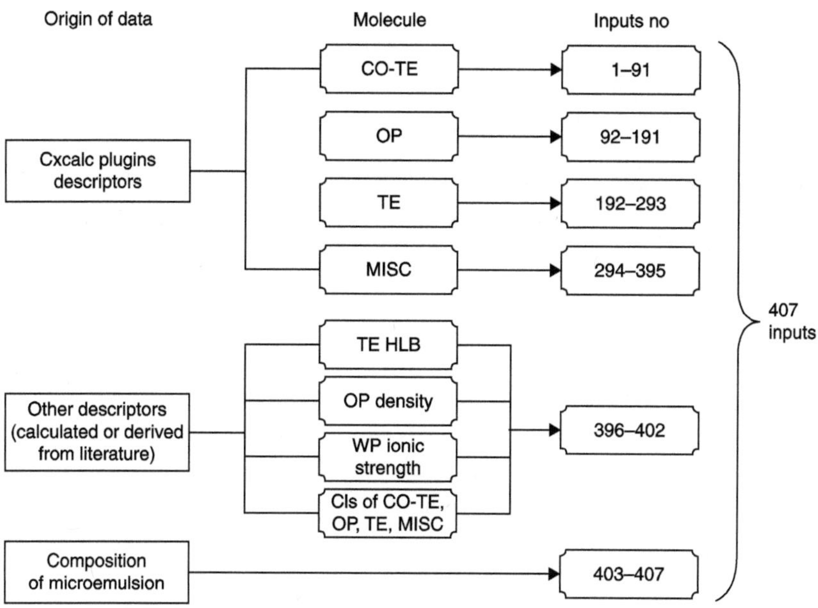

Figure 3.3 **Scheme of the data set processing. CO-TE, cosurfactant; MISC, miscellaneous surfactant component; OP, oil phase; TE, surfactant; WP, water phase**

All components of ME were treated using a unified modeling sequence: sketching 2D chemical structures, 3D optimization, calculation of relevant physicochemical descriptors, and, in cases of a complex mixture, calculation of a single weight-averaged value. The resulting base data set was split randomly according to the enhanced 10-fold cross-validation procedure. The whole formulations were treated as parameters, thus test sets were constructed to include a randomly chosen 10% of formulations but not the data points. The reason for such a modification was to provide ANN with the architecture optimization protocol resembling their future application, namely prediction of unknown formulation behavior. A randomization procedure was carried out without replacement, thus each formulation was included in one of the 10 test data sets. Additionally, in order to match ANN activation functions domains, the data sets were scaled linearly in the range <0.2 ; 0.8> and <–0.8 ; 0.8>, labeled 'orig' or 'scale,' respectively. The noise was added to the data with amplitude ±5% of the original value and double the number of records (ANN labeled as 'rand5x2').

In order to unify the class distribution, a class balancing technique was applied to the data sets. In the 'balance plus' technique, simple multiplication of less represented classes was used. In the 'balance minus' technique, numbers of records of more represented classes were reduced. Both techniques resulted in nearly uniform distribution of classes, but different record numbers.

3.2.2 ANN modeling

ANN modeling was carried out after Mendyk and Jachowicz [65]. MLP with architectures from one to six hidden layers and with two to 200 nodes per layer were applied. Neurofuzzy systems (NFs) with one hidden layer and from five to 100 neurons were trained then tested. Four activation functions were used: linear (*lin*), hyperbolic tangent (*tanh*), logistic (*sigma*) and logarithmic function (*fsr*) presented by Bilski [16]. NFs were simple MISO (multiple inputs – single output) Mamdani systems with *lin* activation function only. Back-propagation (BP) was the learning algorithm with momentum and delta-bar-delta techniques. Jog-of-weights technique (amplitude 1% of each weight value and patience criterion of 100 000 iterations) was also applied to protect ANN from getting stuck in local minima. To avoid ANN overtraining, several training endpoints were used: 1 m (1 000 000), 5 m, 10 m and 20 m iterations. Such a large number of iterations was dictated by the data set size and epoch size equal to 1. The above factors were taken into consideration and number of training iterations (epochs) was adjusted in order to allow for several times of complete presentation of the data set. A total of 198 ANN architectures were used in this study, which for a whole procedure resulted in ca. 50 000 models being trained and tested.

Because of the continuous nature of the ANN activation functions, a binarization procedure was introduced in order to get a simple decision regarding the presence or absence of the ME in a particular case. Simple thresholding was applied, where the output below the threshold was treated as a lack of ME (0) and over the threshold as ME presence predicted (1). In order to determine the best possible generalization abilities of ANN, dynamical thresholding was applied, where the value of the threshold was adjusted empirically. To adjust the decision threshold, *Classif_compute* software was used. The threshold was expressed as a percentage of the minimum–maximum output range. The main criterion for ANN performance assessment was the area

Published by Woodhead Publishing Limited, 2013

under the receiver operating curve (AUROC), which is a common summary statistic for goodness-of-fit in a binary classification task. Its value is equal to the probability that a predictor will rank a randomly chosen positive instance higher than a randomly chosen negative one [15]. It is commonly accepted that AUROC from 1 to 0.9 means very good model fitness, from 0.9 to 0.8 good model fitness, and from 0.8 to 0.7 acceptable model fitness.

Additionally to the AUROC, Good 1 and Good 0 values were calculated as the percentages of correctly predicted formation of ME ('1') and lack of ME ('0'), respectively (Eq. 3.2 and 3.3).

$$Good1 = \frac{x_{Good1}}{n_{pred1}} * 100\% \qquad [3.2]$$

$$Good0 = \frac{x_{Good0}}{n_{pred0}} * 100\% \qquad [3.3]$$

where,

x_{Good1}, x_{Good0} – correctly predicted instances of '1' or '0';

n_{pred1}, n_{pred0} – number of predictions of '1' or '0'.

Efficacy was calculated as the fraction of correctly predicted values, which was the sum of Good 1 and Good 0 predictions divided by the number of all data records (Eq. 3.4).

$$Efficacy = \frac{x_{Good1} + x_{Good0}}{n_{pred}} \qquad [3.4]$$

where,

n_{pred} – number of all predictions.

Performance of ANN models was also expressed as overall classification error (All [%]).

The best ANN architectures were selected to form ensemble systems. These are known to improve classification performance of the system, as different architectures and processing techniques compensate deficiencies of the ensemble members. The results returned by the individual modules were combined in a block of the interpreter in two major ways:

- majority voting technique [34] performed after thresholding of the individual member outputs;

- averaging of the individual member continuous outputs before thresholding.

Thus the ensemble was formed from the ANN independently trained on the available data without any cooperation during the training phase.

A multistart technique was used for the ensemble in order to estimate the system robustness. Coupled with the cross-validation technique, this approach is the most reliable, but also the most computationally expensive [46, 103]. Multistart means that each ANN was trained 10 times, each time from a different, randomly chosen set of weights. Subsequently, the decision threshold was established and performance parameters of each neural net and the decision system were established (AUROC, efficacy, Good '1' and '0'). The robustness was expressed as relative standard deviation (RSD) of the above mentioned parameters.

Sensitivity analysis [66, 87] was used to simplify the model and to investigate factors that mostly contribute to the output variability. The set of best ANN models in terms of the AUROC parameter was chosen. In contrast to the technique proposed by Żurada et al. [115], a set of ANN was used, which met the criterion of AUROC ≥90% of the best result. The final ranking of inputs was the average of all chosen models. Knowledge-based selection of crucial variables was carried out according to Mendyk and Jachowicz [65], where not only the gradient between the values of sensitivity was important but also classification of molecular descriptors.

3.2.3 Random forest modeling

RF modeling was performed after the ANN modeling phase and used a minimum input vector provided by the ANN (Figure 3.3). An extended 10-fold cross-validation procedure was used. In order to allow for a direct comparison of ANN versus RF results, exactly the same pairs of learning/test data sets were chosen as in ANN modeling. Various numbers of trees for RF algorithm were tested: from 10 to 100. Other parameters were kept constant as Weka package defaults such as:

- unlimited depth of the trees;
- random selection of all attributes;
- random seed number set to 1.

Published by Woodhead Publishing Limited, 2013

3.2.4 Software implementation of DSS

Java programming language was chosen in order to provide software independent from the operating system. A Maven project was set up and run with the use of a subversion control system (SVN) providing collaborative work feature. The system was named ME_expert 2.0 as it is the continuation of previously developed Pascal-code-based ME_expert 1.0. The Open Source paradigm of software development allowed consideration of implementation of third-party code developed for the ToxComp system (*www.tox-portal.net*), where Weka interpreter was created as a Java project. ME_expert 2.0 development incorporated the following stages:

- ANN and RF interpreters coding and validation;
- GUI (graphical user interface) development;
- integration of all the above elements;
- documentation writing.

3.2.5 Software and hardware environments

- Nets2010 – own written ANN simulator;
- Weka – Open Source data-mining system for RF simulations;
- Classif_compute – own written software for classification computations;
- Phase_diagr – own written phase diagram digitizer for ME quantitative composition extraction from Gibbs diagrams;
- *dissolve* – own written automatic manager of computational jobs in grid environment;
- MarvinSketch – was used for drawing, displaying, and characterizing chemical structures, Marvin 5.3.0, 2010, ChemAxon (*http://www.chemaxon.com*) [61];
- Cxcalc plugin for Marvin – calculator plugins were used for batch mode of structure property prediction and calculation, Marvin 5.3.0, 2010, ChemAxon (*http://www.chemaxon.com*) [68];
- NetBeans 6.9.1. – Java programming environment;
- OpenOffice 3.1, 2010 (*http://openoffice.org*) [1].

Calculations were performed on seven PCs with Intel/AMD processors under Linux OS environment. PCs with 28 logical processors were connected and formed a local calculation grid-like network. SSH (Secure SHell) protocol was used as a standard communication between workstations.

3.3 Modeling results and tool implementation

3.3.1 The data

After the literature survey, 36 publications matching inclusion criteria were selected. A set of 146 formulations represented by Gibbs phase diagrams was derived and numerically encoded [5, 12, 20, 22, 23, 25, 29–34, 36–41, 43, 44, 52, 53, 57–60, 69, 71, 78, 82, 85, 89, 90, 98, 108, 110, 114]. The base data set consisted of 97 components and over 305 000 records with 424 inputs. A single binary output denoted presence or absence of ME (YES/NO). The initially obtained 424 inputs were reduced during the data set preprocessing procedure. Null or missed inputs were deleted, resulting in 407 inputs. As a result of the enhanced 10-fold cross-validation procedure, test sets counted different numbers of data records. Each set from 1 to 4 consisted of 14 formulations and around 29 000 records, with the remaining test sets consisting of 15 formulations and around 31 000 records.

3.3.2 ANN modeling

The first step of the modeling introduced sensitivity analysis to create possible cut-off points for problem simplification and selection of crucial variables. ANN were trained on the whole available data set with the endpoint of 10 m iterations ensuring good representation of the problem. Assessment of predictive abilities resulted in the ranking of the architectures according to the AUROC values (Table 3.2). It could be noted that the highest ranking positions were associated with ANN based on *fsr* and sigma activation functions. Finally, 32 ANN architectures were selected to the sensitivity analysis based on the 90% of best AUROC criterion (AUROC ≥0.86).

It was found that the minimal number of inputs providing acceptable generalization results was 17. The sensitivity analysis revealed that the most important inputs were: quantitative composition of ME together with the chemical descriptors of surfactant, cosurfactant, and oil phase (Table 3.3, Figure 3.4).

Published by Woodhead Publishing Limited, 2013

Table 3.2 Results of classification analysis for first ten ANN in the ranking based on AUROC

ANN architecture	Activation function	All (%)	Efficacy	AUROC	Good 1	Good 0	Thr (%)
200_100_80_40_20_10	fsr	10.74	0.89	0.95	65.09	95.53	62
200_80_40_20	fsr	10.83	0.89	0.94	71.18	93.84	51
15_7_5	fsr	11.51	0.88	0.93	62.8	95.15	52
20_16_8_4	fsr	11.40	0.89	0.93	70.31	93.34	47
20_16_8_4	sigma	10.80	0.89	0.93	67.61	94.81	53
20	sigma	12.47	0.88	0.93	61.96	94.17	44
40_10_5	fsr	12.00	0.88	0.93	65.71	93.79	43
40_10_5	sigma	11.55	0.88	0.93	66.27	94.21	37
60_20_8	fsr	11.88	0.88	0.93	64.58	94.23	47
60_20_8	sigma	11.61	0.88	0.93	65.58	94.31	37

ANN trained on the whole data set with 407 inputs for sensitivity analysis. All (%), overall classification error. Thr (%), threshold in percentages of the output value range.
ANN, artificial neural network; AUROC, area under the receiver operating curve.

Table 3.3 Ranking of the inputs derived from sensitivity analysis

Rank	Label	Group
1	Water phase (%)	ME composition
2	Oleic phase (%)	ME composition
3	Surfactant (%)	ME composition
4	Fragment count	TE descriptors
5	Cosurfactant (%)	ME composition
6	Pi energy	TE descriptors
7	Surfactant HLB	TE descriptors
8	Connected graph	TE descriptors
9	Balaban index	TE descriptors
10	Miscellaneous surfactant (%)	ME composition
11	pI	TE descriptors
12	Maximal projection area	OL descriptors
13	Ionic strength of water phase	WP descriptors
14	Balaban index	OL descriptors
15	pH=14.00	TE descriptors
16	Dreiding energy	TE descriptors
17	Dreiding energy	CO-TE descriptors

ME, microemulsion; CO-TE, cosurfactant; OP, oil phase; TE, surfactant; WP; water phase.

The factors recognized as the most important inputs determining the presence of ME were as follows:

- Composition of mixture:
  - Water v(w/w %) phase content,
  - Ionic strength of water phase (mol/l),
  - Oleic phase content (w/w %),
  - Surfactant content (w/w %),
  - Cosurfactant content (w/w %),
  - Miscellaneous surfactant content (w/w %).
- Chemical descriptors related to surfactant molecule:
  - Fragment count – the molecule fragment count,

Published by Woodhead Publishing Limited, 2013

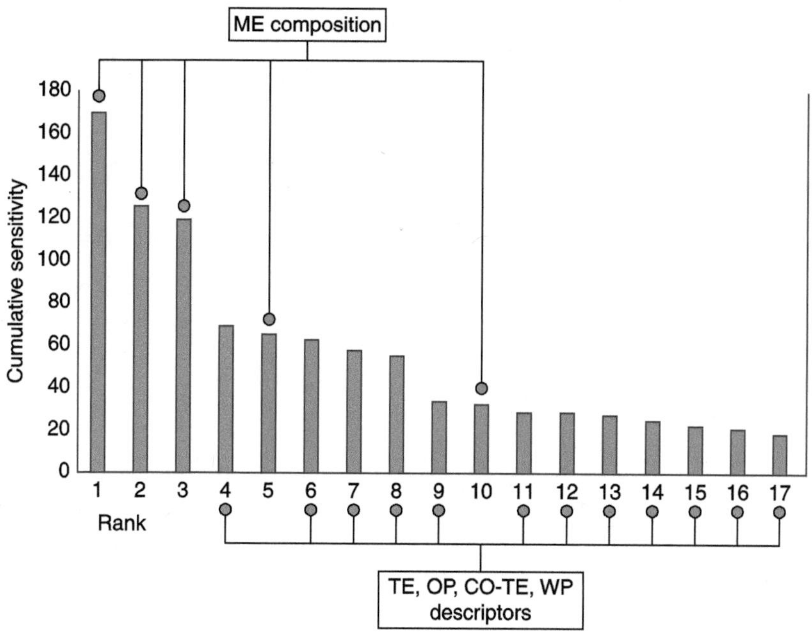

Figure 3.4 **Ranking of inputs obtained after sensitivity analysis, CO-TE, cosurfactant; ME, microemulsion; OP, oil phase; TE, surfactant; WP, water phase**

- Pi energy [dimension β] – value of Pi energy which determines energies of molecular orbitals of Pi electrons in conjugated hydrocarbon systems calculated as Huckle proposed,
- Surfactant HLB – HLB value as published in the literature or an average of HLB values when a mixture of surfactants was present,
- Connected graph – checks whether the molecule graph is connected, returns '1' if the input molecule graph is connected and '0' if it is not,
- Balaban index – the Balaban distance connectivity, or distance connectivity index of the molecule, is the average distance sum connectivity, defined in terms of the vertex distance degrees, which are the row sums of the distance matrix D; calculations are based on the graph theory; the descriptor is related to topostructural properties of molecule [8],
- pI – the isoelectric point,

  - pH=14.00 – the donor atom count at pH 14,
  - Dreiding energy (kJ/mol) – the Dreiding energy of the input molecule is related to the actual 3-D structure (conformer) stability of the molecule.

- Chemical descriptors related to oleic phase:
  - Maximal projection area – which is the radius of the circle surrounding the maximal projection (Angstr.),
  - Balaban index – mentioned above.

- Chemical descriptors related cosurfactant molecule:
  - Dreiding energy (kJ/mol).

The results of sensitivity analysis reveal that specific physicochemical properties involving geometric, energy, and protonation factors of surfactant molecules participate in ME formation, whereas only geometric factors matter in the oil phase. So far, the only molecular descriptors that have been related directly to the formation of ME, as widely described in the literature, are HLB values of the surfactant and the ionic strength of the water phase [56, 84]. Moreover, only the quantity of additional surfactant (MISC) was found to be important for ME formation. However, this might be partially the result of rare occurrences of additional surfactant in the database. The above findings are generally in agreement with Richardson et al. [84], who identified quantitative composition as the crucial factor for ME formation. However, our results show that nearly the same level of importance was assigned for geometric, energy, and protonation descriptors as for composition factors (Figure 3.4).

3.3.3 Ensemble systems of ANN

The ANN ensemble was the result of the ANN optimal architecture search for the smallest input number set, namely 17 inputs. A ranking of architectures was created, where the generalization error obtained during the 10-fold cross-validation was the rank criterion. Top ANN in the ranking were used for the ensemble system (Table 3.4). The initial set of ANN encompassed various training endpoints and pre-processing techniques; however, no clear relationships were found between these parameters and the ANN performance. The only observation was that adding noise to the training data was not beneficial for the system.

Published by Woodhead Publishing Limited, 2013

Table 3.4 **Construction of ensemble systems**

ANN architecture	Activation function	All (%)	Efficacy	AUROC	Good 1	Good 0	Thr (%)
40_10_5 balance_ minus_10m	fsr	16.21	0.84	0.85	50.15	92.51	84
60_20_8 balance_ plus_20m	fsr	16.50	0.84	0.84	53.01	91.44	83
60_20_8 balance_ plus_10m	sigma	17.40	0.83	0.84	57.11	89.24	75
120_50_30_20_10 balance_none_20m	fsr	16.68	0.83	0.84	50.9	91.74	59
7_5 balance_ minus_10m	fsr	17.52	0.82	0.84	55.39	89.48	80
ANN ensemble with voting interpreter (EnV)	–	16.30	0.84	0.77	65.37	88.45	–
ANN ensemble with average interpreter (EnA)	–	15.24	0.85	0.87	52.63	93.1	78

All (%), overall classification error. Thr (%), threshold in percentages of the output value range; balance_{plus,minus,none}, class balancing techniques; {10,20}m, 10 and 20 000 000 training iterations, respectively.

Selection of ANN was strictly empirical and based on the improvement of the whole system performance associated with addition of the following ANN in the ranking. Therefore, initially nine ANN were selected for the ensemble. Two ANN architectures were represented more than once by their training endpoint. By eradicating redundant architectures, the final ensemble system was reduced to five ANN (Table 3.4). It is noticeable that a collective set of ANN surpasses slightly the predicted performance of the best ANN in the ranking. It is expressed in the AUROC and efficacy improvement of the ensemble with average interpreter (EnA) (Table 3.4). However, the system with voting interpreter (EnV) provides substantial improvement in the prediction of ME regions (Good 1) with the price of the Good 0 performance.

Successful prediction of unknown ME composition is presented in Figure 3.5. Although not completely precise, EnV was able to point to the phase diagram region with the largest probability where ME might be

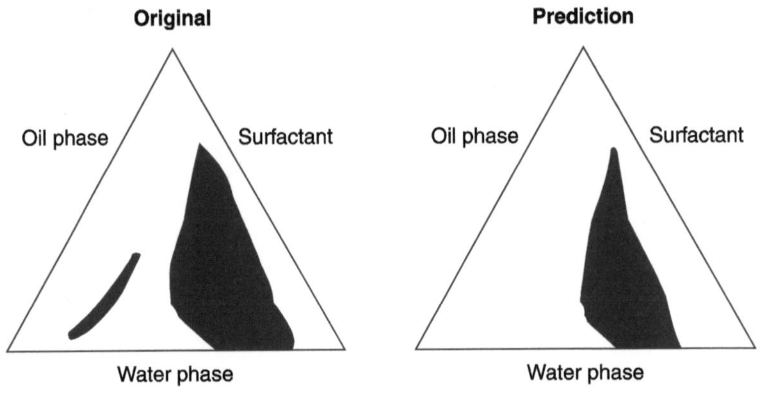

Figure 3.5 Prediction of microemulsion region for unknown to artificial neural network quaternary system: decane (oil phase), sodium dodecyl sulphate (surfactant), hexanol (cosurfactant), water (water phase). Surfactant/cosurfactant ratio = 3:7

found. Thus, it confirmed its function as a DSS – an aid in the formulation of ME.

Stability of the system was confirmed in the multistart procedure, where RSD for most of the diagnostic parameters was below 5%, a commonly used borderline value for variability estimation (Table 3.5). Therefore, it might be concluded that the system is stable and provides good performance for the prospective formulation of ME. In order

Table 3.5 Multistart analysis of ensemble systems

Database	Interpreter	All (%)	Efficacy	Good 1 (%)	Good 0 (%)
10cv	EnA	15.21 (2.12)	0.85 (0.57)	47.41 (7.01)	94.49 (0.59)
	EnV	16.23 (2.81)	0.84 (0.58)	60.72 (1.97)	89.76 (0.83)
BASE	EnA	8.92 (2.70)	0.91 (0.27)	75.83 (1.67)	95.05 (0.52)
	EnV	9.81 (2.41)	0.90 (0.35)	63.37 (9.10)	97.15 (1.70)

10cv, 10-fold cross-validation; EnA, expert committee with average interpreter; EnV, ANN ensemble with vote interpreter; BASE, whole data available. All values are mean (±SD %)

Published by Woodhead Publishing Limited, 2013

to provide the most competent expert system, all the ANN were trained on the whole data set. The latter was also performed in the multistart mode.

3.3.4 RF modeling

The best results were found for a 100 trees-based RF system. Any attempts to extend this number of trees failed to provide better results either because of worse predictive performance of the obtained models or because enormous hardware resources were required for the modeling procedure.

As the RF models are intrinsically ensemble systems, no further ensembles were created, thus the final results were based on the single RF type only, namely the 100 trees-based system (Table 3.6). The results clearly show no substantial advantage of RF models over ANN. This has directed research to find another better generalizing classifier. Several attempts were made among the Weka classifiers with respect to the methodology used in this study, namely the enhanced 10-fold cross-validation scheme.

The results (Table 3.7) show no improvement using any of the 15 Weka classifiers applied. This leads to the conclusion that the modeling results represent the best possible approach due to the nature of the data set itself, not the modeling tool capabilities. An apparent advantage of RF over ANN is the relatively short time of development for RF. Regarding available hardware resources, development of final ANN models required several months of computer work, whereas RF model training required 1 week only. The advantage is apparent as even the actual training of RF is faster than ANN; however, the RF models were based on the reduced input vector provided by ANN. Thus, without the sensitivity analysis provided by ANN no RF model might be created at all.

Table 3.6 Results of 10-fold cross-validation for random forest (RF) system based on 100 trees

RF system	All (%)	Efficacy	AUROC	Good 1	Good 0
100 trees	14.36%	0.86	0.881	55.13	93.44

AUROC, area under the receiver operating curve.

Table 3.7 Other systems for microemulsion modeling [111]

System	All (%)
RotationForest	14.55
J48graft	15.12
J48	15.78
SVM	16.10
SimpleCart	16.24
NBTree	16.54
LTM	16.81
IBk	16.81
REPTree	16.96
Ftree	17.11
LADTree	20.27
DecisionStump	20.57
ADTree	20.92
ADABoost	20.99
VotedPerceptron	27.48

3.3.5 Software development

A software development model was the major issue to start with. Open source paradigm was chosen together with GNU Public license version 3 (GPL v3) [49]. Such a model requires release of the source code of the product software, and allows other users to modify it as long as they also release it under GPL license. It also allows use of other source code released under GNU license. This feature will be exploited in our ongoing project, wherein a Weka interpreter written in Java will be used for in silico toxicity prediction ToxComp (*www.tox-comp.net*) [79, 80].

Java language was chosen for application development, allowing creation of a multiplatform application transparent to the OS. Another reason for choosing Java is its good documentation and the availability of high quality open source Java development environments like NetBeans or Eclipse. Java Swing extensions were chosen for GUI. ME_ expert 2.0 is available from the sourceforge server (*http://sourceforge.*

Published by Woodhead Publishing Limited, 2013

net/projects/me_expert) – one of the largest hosting services for open source software.

ME_expert 2.0 features:

- Simple GUI with options of input, output file, and starting computations,
- ANN interpreter included,
- ANN ensemble with average interpreter (EnA).

ME_expert is still under development (Figure 3.6). The current version 2.0 was launched to ensure basic functionality together with software portability to various OS. This was achieved by implementing only an ANN model and the simplest functionality of the input–output data system. Together with an EnA ensemble, this constitutes a full DSS able to aid ME formulation procedure. The choice of EnA versus EnV was decided by the major goal of the DSS use – it is dedicated to reduce laboratory experiments providing the most likely composition of ME in a particular experimental design. Thus, the system

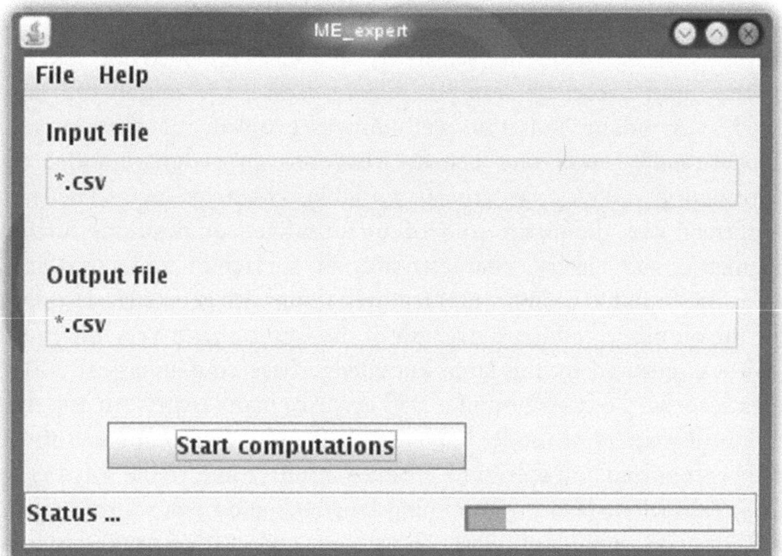

Figure 3.6 Simplistic GUI for version 2.0

characterized by higher non-ME prediction rate and, at the same time, lower false positive prediction rate is preferred in this task. Such a system is EnA.

ME_expert 3.0 (planned) features:

- GUI with graphical representation of Gibbs triangle,
- ANN and Weka interpreters,
- ANN and RF inference machines.

As it is planned, ME_expert 3.0 will use all the above described major models for ME formation. However, for the RF model there is an obstacle that would have to be overcome, namely the large size of the model configuration file, which is around 220 MB. Such a huge data size will cause trouble with application deployment through the Internet. This feature is in focus now and is a subject of current programming work.

3.4 Conclusions

It was demonstrated that both ANN and RF are suitable as DSS inference machines for ME formulation development. However, ANN were employed as predictive and data-mining tools, whereas RF were used only for prediction of ME phase boundaries. The ANN data-mining feature was based on the sensitivity analysis employed for reduction of the input vector. It was possible to reduce the initial 407 inputs to 17. Avoidance of the well-known problem of the 'curse of dimensionality' was one benefit from this procedure, another was information about the crucial variable characteristics. The latter confirmed the dominant role of quantitative composition; however, geometric and electric characteristics of surfactant and cosurfactant were also found to be important features along with geometric descriptors for the oil phase and ionic strength of the water phase. Versatility of the DSS was ensured by the large knowledge base containing ca. 300 000 data records. Construction of a DSS involves many issues. Among these, technical matters of model implementation into the computer software were recognized and solved to produce intuitive and stable software for DSS realization. Java programming language and open source software development paradigm were chosen in order to ensure maximum functionality and availability of the software. The latter is expressed in the independence from the OS as well as freedom of use for personal and commercial purposes as this is guaranteed by the GPL v3 license.

Published by Woodhead Publishing Limited, 2013

3.5 References

1. *A multiplatform and multilingual office suite, an open-source project*, OpenOffice 3.1, 2010 (*http://openoffice.org*).
2. Ahmat N, Ugail H, and Castro GG. Method of modelling the compaction behaviour of cylindrical pharmaceutical tablets. *Int J Pharm*, 2011, 405(1–2), 113–21.
3. Alanazi F, Fu ZF and Lu DR. Effective transfection of rabies DNA vaccine in cell culture using an artificial lipoprotein carrier system. *Pharm Res*, 2004, 21(4), 675–82.
4. Alany RG, Agatonovic-Kustrin S, Rades T and Tucker IG. Use of artificial neural networks to predict quaternery phase systems from limited experimental data. *J Pharm Biomed Anal*, 1999, 19, 443–52.
5. Alany RG, Rades T, Nicoll J, Tucker IG and Davies NM. W/O microemulsions for ocular delivery: Evaluation of ocular irritation and precorneal retention. *J Control Release*, 2006, 111, 145–52.
6. Ammar HO, Salama HA, Ghorab M and Mahmoud A.A. Nanoemulsion as a Potential Ophthalmic Delivery System for Dorzolamide Hydrochloride. *AAPS PharmSciTech*, 2009, 10(3), 808–19.
7. Attwood D and Florence TA. *Surfactant Systems, their Chemistry, Pharmacy and Biology*, Chapman & Hall, New York, 1983.
8. Balaban AT. Highly discriminating distance-based topological index. *Chem Phys Lett*, 1982, 89(5), 399–404.
9. Balogh J. Determining scaling in known phase diagrams of nonionic microemulsions to aid constructing unknown. *Adv Colloid Interface Sci*, 2010, 159(1), 22–31.
10. Barmpalexis P, Kanaze FI, Kachrimanis K and Georgarakis E. Artificial neural networks in the optimization of a nimodipine controlled release tablet formulation. *Eur J Pharm Biopharm*, 2010, 74(2), 316–23.
11. Barmpalexis P, Kanaze FI, Kachrimanis K and Georgarakis E. Solid dispersions in the development of a nimodipine floating tablet formulation and optimization by artificial neural networks and genetic programming. *Eur J Pharm Biopharm*, 2011, 77(1), 122–31.
12. Baroli B, López-Quintela MA, Delgado-Charro MB, Fadda AM and Blanco-Méndez J. Microemulsions for topical delivery of 8-methoxsalen. *J Control Release*, 2000, 69, 209–18.
13. Behzadi SS, Prakasvudhisarn Ch, Klocker J, Wolschann P and Viernstein, H. Comparison between two types of Artificial Neural Networks used for validation of pharmaceutical processes. *Powder Technology*, 2009, 195(2), 150–7.
14. Belic A, Skrjanc I, Bozic DZ, Karba R and Vrecer F. Minimisation of the capping tendency by tableting process optimisation with the application of artificial neural networks and fuzzy models. *Eur J Pharm Biopharm*, 2009, 73(1), 172–8.
15. Bewick V, Cheek L and Ball J. Statistics review 13: Receiver operating characteristic curves. *Crit Care*, 2004, 8(6), 508–12.
16. Bilski J. In: *The backpropagation learning with logarithmic transfer function*. Proceedings of the Fifth Conference Neural Networks and Soft

Computing. Zakopane, Poland, 6–10 June 2000. Conference Materials, pp. 71–7.
17. Bozi DZ, Vrecer F and Kozjek F. Optimization of diclofenac sodium dissolution from sustained release formulations using an artificial neural network. *Eur J Pharm Sci*, 1997, 5(3), 163–9.
18. Breiman L. Bagging predictors, *Mach Learn* 1996, 24(2), 123–40.
19. Breiman L. Random forests, *Mach Learn* 2001, 45 (1), 5–32.
20. Brevnov DA, Finklea HO and Ryswyk HV. Ac voltammetry studies of electron transfer kinetics for a redox couple attached via short alkanethiols to a gold electrode. *J Electroanal Chem*, 2000, 493, 100–7.
21. Calculator Plugins, Marvin 5.3.0, 2010, *ChemAxon – toolkits and desktop applications for cheminformatics* (*http://www.chemaxon.com*).
22. Chieng T-H, Gan L-M, Chew C-H, Ng S-C and Pey K-L. Microporous polymeric materials by polymerization of microemulsions containing different alkyl chain lengths of cationic surfactants. *Polymer*, 1996, 37(13), 2801–9.
23. Chieng T-H, Gan L-M, Teot W-K and Pey K-L. Porous polymeric membranes by bicontinuous microemulsion polymerization: effect of anionic and cationic surfactants. *Polymer*, 1996, 37(26), 5917–25.
24. Cho H-J, Balakrishnan P, Shim W-S, Chung S-J, Shim Ch-K and Kim D-D. Characterization and in vitro evaluation of freeze-dried microparticles composed of granisetron-cyclodextrin complex and carboxymethylcellulose for intranasal delivery. *Int J Pharm*, 2010, 400(1–2), 59–65.
25. Currie F, Holmberg K, and Westman G. Regioselective nitration of phenols and anisols in microemulsion. *Colloids Surf A Physicochem Eng Asp*, 2001, 182, 321–7.
26. Danielsson I and Lindman B. The definition of microemulsion. *Colloid Surf*, 1981, 3, 391–2.
27. Dehzangi A, Phon-Amnuaisuk S and Dehzangi O. Using random forest for protein fold prediction problem: An empirical study, *J Inf Sci Eng*, 2010, 26 (6), 1941–56.
28. Djekic L, Ibrica S and Primoraca M. The application of artificial neural networks in the prediction of microemulsion phase boundaries in PEG-8 caprylic/capric glycerides based systems. *Int J Pharm*, 2008, 361(1–2), 41–6.
29. Ee L.-S, Wang J, Ng S.-C and Gan L.-M. Low temperature synthesis of PZT powders via microemulsion processing. *Mater Res Bull*, 1998, 33(7), 1045–55.
30. Fang J, Stokes KL, Wiemann J and Zhou W. Nanocrystalline bismuth synthesized via an in situ polymerization–microemulsion process. *Mater Lett*, 2000, 42, 113–20.
31. Fanun M, Wachtel E, Antalek B, Aserin A and Garti N. A study of the microstructure of four-component sucrose ester microemulsions by SAXS and NMR. *Colloids Surf A Physicochem Eng Asp*, 2001, 180, 173–86.
32. Gan LM and Chew CH. Microporous polymer composites from microemulsion polymerization. *Colloids Surf A Physicochem Eng Asp*, 1997, 123–24, 681–93.

Published by Woodhead Publishing Limited, 2013

33. Gan L-M, Liu J, Poon L-P, Chew C-H and Gan L-H. Microporous polymeric composites from bicontinuous microemulsion polymerization using a polymerizable nonionic surfactant, *Polymer*, 1997, 38(21), 5339–45.
34. Gan LM, Zhang K and Chew CH. Preparation of silica nanoparticles from sodium orthosilicate in inverse microemulsions. *Colloids Surf A Physicochem Eng Asp*, 1996, 110, 199–206.
35. Gao F, Zhang Z, Bu H, Huang Y, Gao Z, et al. Nanoemulsion improves the oral absorption of candesartan cilexetil in rats: Performance and mechanism. *J Control Release*, 2011, 149(2), 168–74.
36. Garti N, Aserin A, Ezrahi S, Tiunova I and Berkovic, G. Water Behavior in Nonionic Surfactant Systems I: Subzero Temperature Behavior of Water in Nonionic Microemulsions Studied by DSC. *J Colloid Interface Sci*, 1996, 178, 60–8.
37. Garti N, Aserin A, Ezrahi S and Wachtel E. Water Solubilization and Chain Length Compatibility in Nonionic Microemulsions. *J Colloid Interface Sci*, 1995, 169, 428–36.
38. Garti N, Aserin A, Tiunova I and Fanun M. A DSC study of water behavior in water-in-oil microemulsions stabilized by sucrose esters and butanol. *Colloids Surf A Physicochem Eng Asp*, 2000, 170, 1–18.
39. Garti N, Aserin A, Wachtel E, Gans O and Shaul, Y. Water Solubilization in Nonionic Microemulsions Stabilized by Grafted Siliconic Emulsifiers, *J Colloid Interface Sci*, 2001, 233, 286–94.
40. Garti N, Yaghmur A, Aserin A, Spernath A, Elfakess R and Ezrahi, S. Solubilization of active molecules in microemulsions for improved environmental protection. *Colloids Surf A Physicochem Eng Asp*, 2004, 230, 183–90.
41. Guo R, Zhang Q, Qian J and Zou A. Hydrotrope and hydrotrope-solubilization action of penicillin-K in CTAB/n-C5H11OH/H2O system. *Colloids Surf A Physicochem Eng Asp*, 2002, 196, 223–34.
42. Gupta S and Moulik SP. Biocompatible microemulsions and their prospective uses in drug delivery. *J Pharm Sci*, 2008, 97, 22–45.
43. Haegel FH, Schlupen J, Schultze JW, Winkels S and Stromberg C. Anodic polymerization of thiophene derivatives from microemulsions and liquid crystals. *Electrochimica Acta*, 2001, 46, 3973–84.
44. Häger M, Holmberg K and Olsson U. Synthesis of an amphiphilic polymer performed in an oil-in-water microemulsion and in a lamellar liquid crystalline phase. *Colloids Surf A Physicochem Eng Asp*, 2001, 189, 9–19.
45. Hany SMA, Blagden N, York P, Amani A and Brook T. Artificial neural networks modelling the prednisolone nanoprecipitation in microfluidic reactors, *Eur J Pharm Sci*, 2009, 37(3–4), 514–22.
46. Hertz J, Krogh A and Palmer RG. *Introduction to Neural Calculations Theory, 2nd edition*, WNT, Warszawa, 1995.
47. Ho TK. The random subspace method for constructing decision forests. *IEEE Trans Pattern Anal Mach Intell*, 1998, 20(8), 832–44.
48. Hoar TP and Schulman JH. Transparent Water-in-Oil Dispersions: the Oleopathic Hydro-Micelle. *Nature*, 1943, 152, 102–3.
49. *GNU Operating System. http://www.gnu.org* Accessed 02.11.2011

50. Huuskonen J, Rantanen J and Livingstone D. Prediction of aqueous solubility for a diverse set of organic compounds based on atom-type electrotopological state indices, *Eur J Med Chem*, 2000, 35(12), 1081–8.
51. Kachrimanis K, Karamyan V and Malamataris S. Artificial neural networks (ANNs) and modeling of powder flow. *Int J Pharm*, 2003, 250(1), 13–23.
52. Kantaria S, Rees GD and Lawrence MJ. Formulation of electrically conducting microemulsion-based organogels, *Int J Pharm*, 2003, 250, 65–83.
53. Khiew PS, Huang NM, Radiman S and Ahmad S. Synthesis of NiS nanoparticles using a sugar-ester nonionic water-in-oil microemulsion, *Mater Lett*, 2004, 58, 762–7.
54. Kumar M, Misra A, Mishra AK, Mishra P and Pathak K. Mucoadhesive nanoemulsion-based intranasal drug delivery system of olanzapine for brain targeting. *J Drug Target*, 2008, 16(10), 806–14.
55. Kumar M, Pathak K and Misra A. Formulation and characterization of nanoemulsion-based drug delivery system of risperidone. *Drug Dev Ind Pharm*, 2009, 35(4), 387–95.
56. Kumar P and Mittal KL. *Handbook of Microemulsion Science and Technology*, CRC, 1999.
57. Lim GK, Wang J, Ng SC, Chew CH and Gan LM. Processing of hydroxyapatite via microemulsion and emulsion routes, *Biomaterials*, 1997, 18, 1433–9.
58. Liu X, Wang J, Gan L-M, Ng S-C and Ding J. An ultrafine barium ferrite powder of high connectivity from water-in-oil microemulsion, *J Magn Magn Mater*, 1998, 184, 344–54.
59. Malcolmson C and Lawrence MJ. Three-component non-ionic oil-in-water microemulsions using polyoxyethylene ether surfactants. *Colloids Surf B Biointerfaces*, 1995, 4, 97–109.
60. Martinez LA, Martínez CG, Klopotek BB, Lang J, Neuner A, et al. Nonradiative and radiative deactivation of singlet molecular oxygen in micellar media and microemulsions. *J Photochem Photobiol B Biol*, 2000, 58, 94–107.
61. Marvin 5.3.0, 2010, *ChemAxon – toolkits and desktop applications for cheminformatics* (*http://www.chemaxon.com*).
62. Mason TJ, Wilking JN, Meleson K, Chang CB and Graves SM. Nanoemulsions: formation, structure and physical properties. *J Phys Condens Matter*, 2006, 18, 635–66.
63. Mendyk A and Jachowicz R. ME_expert — a Neural Decision Support System as a Tool in the Formulation of Microemulsions, *Biocyber Biomed Eng* 2006, 26(4), 25–32.
64. Mendyk A and Jachowicz R. Neural network as a decision support system in the development of pharmaceutical formulation – focus on solid dispersions. *Expert Syst Appl* 2005, 28(2), 285–94.
65. Mendyk A and Jachowicz R. Unified methodology of neural analysis in decision support systems built for pharmaceutical technology. *Expert Syst Appl*, 2007, 32(4), 1124–31.
66. Mendyk A, Kleinebudde P, Thommes M, Yoo A, Szlęk J and Jachowicz R. Analysis of pellet properties with use of artificial neural networks. *Eur J Pharm Sci*, 2010, 41(3–4), 421–9.

Published by Woodhead Publishing Limited, 2013

67. Michie D, Spiegelhalter DJ and Taylor CC. (eds.) In: *Machine Learning, Neural and Statistical Classification.* Ellis Horwood Series Artificial Intelligence, 1994.
68. *Molecule File Converter, Marvin 5.3.0, 2010, ChemAxon – toolkits and desktop applications for cheminformatics (http://www.chemaxon.com).*
69. Monnoyer Ph, Fonseca A and Nagy JB. Preparation of colloidal AgBr particles from microemulsions. *Colloids Surf A Physicochem Eng Asp*, 1995, 100, 233–43.
70. Mou D, Chen H, Du D, Mao C, Wan J, et al. Hydrogel-thickened nanoemulsion system for topical delivery of lipophilic drugs. *Int J Pharm*, 2008, 353(1–2), 270–6.
71. Mukhopadhyay L, Mitra N, Bhattacharya PK and Moulik SP. Thermodynamics of Formation of Biological Microemulsion (with Cinnamic Alcohol, Aerosol OT, Tween 20, and Water) and Kinetics of Alkaline Fading of Crystal Violet in Them, *J Colloid Interface Sci*, 1997, 186, 1–8.
72. Murtoniemi E, Yliruusi J, Kinnunen P, Merkku P and Leiviska K, The advantages by the use of neural networks in modelling the fluidized bed granulation process, *Int J Pharm*, 1994, 108(2), 155–64.
73. Nałęcz M. (eds.), *Biocybernetyka i inżynieria biomedyczna, Tom 6 Sieci neuronowe.* Akademicka Oficyna Wydawnicza EXIT, Warszawa, 2000.
74. Neubert RH. Potentials of new nanocarriers for dermal and transdermal drug delivery. *Eur J Pharm Biopharm*, 2011, 77(1), 1–2.
75. Ohguchi Y, Kawano K, Hattori Y and Maitani Y. Selective delivery of folate-PEG-linked, nanoemulsion-loaded aclacinomycin A to KB nasopharyngeal cells and xenograft: effect of chain length and amount of folate-PEG linker. *J Drug Target*, 2008, 16(9), 660–7.
76. Palmer DS, O'Boyle NM, Glen RC and Mitchell JBO. Random forest models to predict aqueous solubility, *J Chem Inf Model*, 2007, 47 (1), 150–8.
77. Plewczynski D, Spieser S and Koch U. Performance of Machine Learning Methods for Ligand-Based Virtual Screening. *Comb Chem High Throughput Screen*, 2009, 12(4), 358–68.
78. Podlogar F, Gasperlin M, Tomsic M, Jamnik A and Rogac M.B. Structural characterisation of water-Tween 40/Imwitor 308-isopropyl myristate microemulsions using different experimental methods. *Int J Pharm*, 2004, 276, 115–28.
79. Polak S. *Optimization of the use of information for in vitro and in silico to predict in vivo Computational toxicology* – in silico drug safety assessment during the 3rd Annual Predictive Toxicology; 14–16 September 2011; Berlin, Germany.
80. Polak S, Glinka A, Wisniowska B and Mendyk A. *Influence on the physiological parameters on the ADP90 value simulated by human ventricular tissue model.* Eurotox 2011, Aug 28–31, Paris, France.
81. Polak S and Mendyk A. Artificial intelligence technology as a tool for initial GDM screening. *Expert Syst Appl* 2004, 26(4), 455–60.
82. Pons R, Carrera I, Caelles J, Rouch J and Panizza P. Formation and properties of miniemulsions formed by microemulsions dilution. *Adv Colloid Interface Sci*, 2003, 106, 129–46.

83. *Random Forest – classification description*, Random Forests Leo Breiman and Adele Cutler, *http://www.stat.berkeley.edu/~breiman/RandomForests/cc_home.htm.*
84. Richardson CJ, Mbanefo A, Aboofazeli R, Lawrence MJ and Barlow DJ. Prediction of Phase Behavior in Microemulsion Systems Using Artificial Neural Networks. *J Colloid Interface Sci*, 1997, 187(2), 296–303.
85. Rusanov AI. Equation of state and phase transitions in surface monolayer. *Colloids Surf A Physicochem Eng Asp*, 2004, 237, 105–11.
86. Sakiyama Y. The use of machine learning and nonlinear statistical tools for ADME prediction. *Expert Opin Drug Metab Toxicol*, 2009, 5 (2), 149–69.
87. Saltelli A, Ratto M, Tarantola S and Campolongo F. Sensitivity Analysis for Chemical Models. *Chem Rev*, 2005, 105(7), 811–28.
88. Sarker DK. Engineering of nanoemulsions for drug delivery. *Curr Drug Deliv*, 2005, 2(4), 297–310.
89. Savelli MP, Solans C, Pons R, Clausse M and Erra P. Keratin cystine reactivity in microemulsion media: influence of cosurfactant chain length. *Colloids Surf A Physicochem Eng Asp*, 1996, 119, 155–62.
90. Savelli MP, Solans C, Rodenas E, Pons R, Clausse M and Erra P. Kinetic study of keratin cystine reduction in W/O microemulsion media. *Colloids Surf A Physicochem Eng Asp*, 1998, 143, 103–10.
91. Schneider G. Neural networks are useful tools for drug design, *Neural Networks*, 2000, 13(1), 15–6.
92. Shah DO. (eds.) In: *Surface Phenomena in Enhanced Recovery*, Plenum Press, New York, 1981.
93. Shakeel F, Baboota S, Ahuja A, Ali J, Aqil M and Shafiq, S. Nanoemulsions as vehicles for transdermal delivery of aceclofenac. *AAPS PharmSciTech*, 2007, 14, 8(4), E104.
94. Shakeel F, Baboota S, Ahuja A, Ali J and Shafiq S. Enhanced anti-inflammatory effects of celecoxib from a transdermally applied nanoemulsion. *Pharmazie*, 2009, 64(4), 258–9.
95. Shakeel F, Baboota S, Ahuja A, Aqil M and Shafiq S. Celecoxib nanoemulsion: skin permeation mechanism and bioavailability assessment. *J Drug Target*, 2008, 16(10), 733–40.
96. Singh KK and Vingkar SK. Formulation, antimalarial activity and biodistribution of oral lipid nanoemulsion of primaquine. Int J Pharm, 2008, 22, 347(1–2), 136–43.
97. Sintov AC, Levy HV and Botner S. Systemic delivery of insulin via the nasal route using a new microemulsion system: In vitro and in vivo studies. *J Control Release*, 2010, 148(2), 168–76.
98. Sintov AC and Shapiro L. New microemulsion vehicle facilitates percutaneous penetration in vitro and cutaneous drug bioavailability in vivo. *J Control Release*, 2004, 95, 173–83.
99. Solans C, Esquena J, Forgiarini AM, Usón N, Morales D, et al. Nano-emulsions: formation, properties and applications. *Surfactant Science Series*, 2003, 109, 525–54.
100. Sonneville-Aubrun O, Simonnet JT and L'Alloret F. Nanoemulsions: a new vehicle for skincare products. *Adv Colloid Interface Sci*, 2004, 20, 108–9, 145–9.

Published by Woodhead Publishing Limited, 2013

101. Southworth H and O'Connell M. Data Mining and Statistically Guided Clinical Review of Adverse Event Data in Clinical Trials. *J Biopharm Stat*, 2009, 19(5), 803–17.
102. Stiglic G, Rodriguez JJ and Kokol P. In: *Rotation of Random Forests for Genomic and Proteomic Classification Problems, Software Tools and Algorithms for Biological Systems, Advances in Experimental Medicine and Biology*, Springer New York, 2011, 211–21.
103. Tadeusiewicz T. Elementary introduction to neural networks technique with exemplary programme. *PLJ Warszawa*, 1999, 1–51.
104. Tagne JB, Kakumanu S and Nicolosi RJ. Nanoemulsion preparations of the anticancer drug dacarbazine significantly increase its efficacy in a xenograft mouse melanoma model. *Mol Pharm*, 2008, 5(6), 1055–63.
105. Teixeira PC, Leite GM, Domingues RJ, Silva J, Gibbs PA and Ferreira JP. Antimicrobial effects of a microemulsion and a nanoemulsion on enteric and other pathogens and biofilms. *Int J Food Microbiol*, 2007, 118(1), 15–9.
106. Tenjarla S. Microemulsions: an overview and pharmaceutical applications. *Crit Rev Ther Drug Carrier Syst*, 1999, 16, 461–521.
107. Vyas TK, Shahiwala A and Amiji MM. Improved oral bioavailability and brain transport of Saquinavir upon administration in novel nanoemulsion formulations. *Int J Pharm*, 2008, 347(1–2), 93–101.
108. Wang C-C, Chen D-H and Huang T-C. Synthesis of palladium nanoparticles in water-in-oil microemulsions. *Colloids Surf A Physicochem Eng Asp*, 2001, 189, 145–54.
109. Wang L, Li X, Zhang G, Dong J and Eastoe J. Oil-in-water nanoemulsions for pesticide formulations. *J Colloid Interface Sci*, 2007, 314(1), 230–5.
110. Warisnoicharoen W, Lansley AB and Lawrence MJ. Nonionic oil-in-water microemulsions: the effect of oil type on phase behaviour. *Int J Pharm*, 2000, 198(1), 7–27.
111. *Weka Application Programming Interface (API) – http://weka.sourceforge.net/doc/.*
112. Winsor PA. Hydrotropy, solubilisation and related emulsification processes. *Trans Faraday Soc*, 1948, 44, 376–98.
113. Wisniowska B, Mendyk A, Polak M, Szlek J and Polak S. RandomForest based assessment of the hERG channel inhibition potential for the early drug cardiotoxicity testing. *Bio-Algorithms Med-Systems*, 2010, 6(12), 131–6.
114. Yu W, Zou A and Guo R. Hydrotrope and hydrotrope-solubilization action of Vitamin C. *Colloids Surf A Physicochem Eng Asp*, 2000, 167, 293–303.
115. Żurada JM, Malinowski A and Usui, S. Perturbation method for deleting redundant inputs of perceptron networks. *Neurocomputing*, 1997, 14, 177–93.

Expert system for the development and formulation of push–pull osmotic pump tablets containing poorly water-soluble drugs

Zhi-hong Zhang and Wei-san Pan, People's Republic of China

DOI: 10.1533/9781908818508.73

Abstract: The push–pull osmotic pump (PPOP) is a challenging technology in the drug delivery system (DDS) domain, and more and more institutes and companies are interested in this technology. A tool which could employ the technology and the experience of experts to design the formulations of PPOP would be helpful and convenient to reduce the cost and shorten the time of PPOP development. As yet, there is no expert system available for the formulation of controlled release dosage forms. This chapter describes such a tool, designed to employ the knowledge of human experts to help those who have no or little knowledge about PPOP and want to develop such products. Generally, an expert system contains three major components: a man–machine interface, a knowledge base, and an inference engine. Here, the knowledge base including database and rule base was built based on available experiences of professionals and experimental data. The prediction model of release behaviors was built using a back-propagation (BP) neural network. The formulation design model was established based on the prediction model of release behaviors, which was the nucleus of the inference engine. Finally, the expert system program was constructed by VB.NET associating with SQL Server.

Key words: push–pull osmotic pump (PPOP), expert system, artificial neural network, formulation design, poorly water-soluble drugs.

4.1 Introduction

Oral extended release dosages have a number of well-known advantages over other dosage forms, such as reduction of drug administration times, stabilization of the blood drug level/reduction lower side effects, enhancement of the frictional conformability of patients, etc. Oral osmotic pump tablets (OPT) are considered a perfect dosage form in the oral extended release domain, as OPT can control drug release at constant rates, which means that the blood drug level is stable and side effects are minimized. In recent years, there has been a sharply increasing interest in the development of OPT. About 20 OPT have been developed for commercial use globally.

OPT have existed for over 40 years, and various types of oral osmotic pumps have been developed and studied to deliver drugs possessing different aqueous solubility. The first type, the elementary osmotic pump tablet (EOP), was invented in the 1970s (Theeuwes and Higuchi, 1972; Theeuwes, 1975). Drugs with moderate water solubility could easily be made into EOP. Another kind of osmotic pump tablet suitable for the delivery of water-soluble drugs is the porosity osmotic pump tablet (Verma et al., 2000). Such osmotic pump tablets contain leachable water-soluble components in their membranes, thus delivery orifices are formed when the water-soluble components dissolve.

More and more drugs have been developed with better curative effect that are poorly water-soluble. As they cannot be dissolved in water, they cannot produce osmotic pressure by themselves. Increasing drug solubility was considered to be a good choice for improvement of drug release, such as converting the active pharmaceutical ingredients (API) into ionic substances by reacting with or adding alkali/acid (Lu et al., 2002; Ouyang et al., 2005), using (SBE) 7m-β-CD as a solubilizer (Okimoto et al., 1999, 2004). This is ideal for such poorly water-soluble drugs to be released in the form of suspension. The monolithic osmotic tablet system (MOTS, Liu et al., 2000) is a good example, in which polymers are used as suspending agents. However, drug sedimentation and incomplete drug release might occur if the viscosity, osmotic capacity, or swell capacity inside the system are incorrect. The push–pull osmotic pump tablets (PPOP) presented by Theeuwes in the 1970s (Theeuwes, 1978) are still the most practical way to deliver poorly water-soluble drugs from osmotic pump systems. Most commercially available osmotic pump products containing poorly water-soluble drugs are of this kind, such as nifedipine push–pull osmotic pump tablets (Procardia XL®, Pfizer and Adalat®, Bayer) and glipizide push–pull osmotic pump tablets (Glucotrol®, Pfizer).

Compared with development of new drug substances, development of drug delivery systems (DDS) has distinct advantages, such as a shorter R&D period and lower cost. Thus, more companies now regard DDS as important. PPOP is one of the hottest technologies. However, not all companies can master the PPOP technology. Most companies who want to develop PPOP still have to spend a lot of money over a long time, even though they could ask professional people for help. Therefore, a tool employing the regularities of PPOP technology and the experience of experts in designing PPOP formulations would be helpful and convenient to reduce the cost and shorten the time of PPOP development. Hence, our 'expert system' was planned and designed.

An expert system, which is one of the most popular subjects in the artificial intelligence domain, is a knowledge-based system that draws on the knowledge of human experts captured in a knowledge base and then emulates experts' thoughts to solve problems in the selected domains (Cai and Xu, 2004; Rowe and Roberts, 1998). Generally, an expert system contains three major components: a man–machine interface, a knowledge base, and an inference engine. The man–machine interface is the communication window for the people and the system, which means that the tool can receive the input information and display the results. The knowledge base is the place where all knowledge accumulated pertaining to the selected domain is stored. The inference engine, which is also called inference machine or reasoning machine, can use the stored knowledge to manipulate relevant problems. Expert systems can be developed using conventional computer languages, special purpose languages, or developed shells/toolkits. It is easier and more convenient to build up an expert system using special purpose languages and developed shells/toolkits than conventional computer languages. However, conventional languages such as PASCAL, Basic and C have the advantages of wide applicability and full flexibility to create the control and inference strategies.

The first report referencing the use of expert systems in pharmaceutical product formulations was published on 27 April 1989 in the London *Financial Times* (see Rowe and Roberts, 1998). Since then, several companies and academic institutes have reported their experiences in this area. Table 4.1 displays the published expert systems in pharmaceutical product formulations (Aguilar et al., 2009; Aleksander and Renata, 2007; Batrman et al., 1996; Cai and Xu, 2004; Lai et al., 1996; Perez et al., 2006; Rowe, 1993; Rowe and Roberts, 1998; Rowe et al., 1995; Yannis, 1998; Zhi-hong Zhang et al., 2011).

Table 4.1 Published applications of pharmaceutical product-formulation expert systems

Company/institution (System name)	Domain	Developed/first reported year
University of Heidelberg (Galenical Development System)	Aerosols, capsules, tablets, IV injections	1990
Boots Company	Topicals	1990
Cadila Laboratories	Tablets	1992
Zeneca Pharmaceuticals	Tablets/parenterals/film coatings	1993/1995/1998
University of London/ Capsugel	Capsules	1996
Sanofi Research	Capsules (HGC)	1996
University of London	Liposomes	1998
University of Barcelona (SeDeM Diagram)	Tablets	2006
Shenyang Pharmaceutical University	Push–pull osmotic pump tablets	2011

Our team has studied PPOP over 10 years, and gained much experience. An expert system which could apply such experience to help those who have no or little knowledge about PPOP and want to develop such products would be advantageous. As well as the reductions and savings it can provide, this expert system is the beginning of the application of man-made artificial intelligence on DDS. It is expected to initiate more and more experts to share their knowledge on DDS using artificial intelligence tools.

4.2 Description of the tool

The tool is similar to most computer programs. First, the users have to start the program and login to the system. The first interface is shown in Figure 4.1.

The system will record and manage the 'USER's and 'CODE's. And the system will record and manage the projects when users build them up (Figure 4.2).

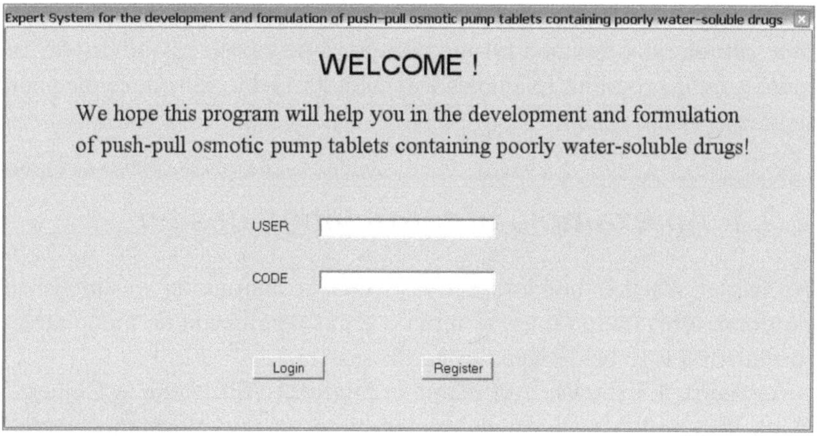

Figure 4.1 Welcome interface of the tool

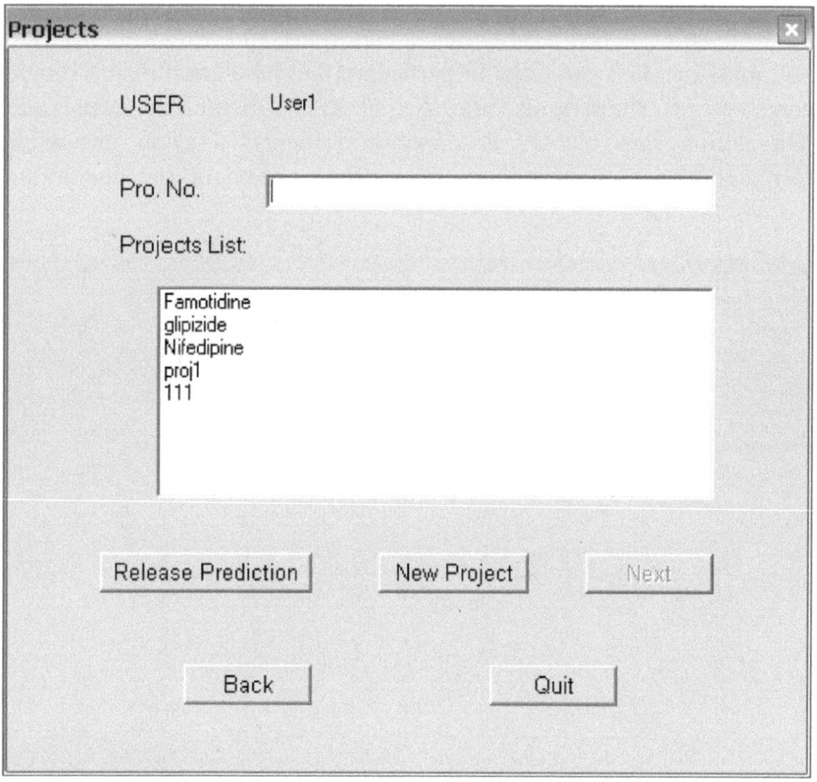

Figure 4.2 Interface of projects management

From Figure 4.2, it can be seen that the system can predict the release of a formulation, design a formulation for a new project, and display or finish a built program. Examples will be described to introduce the main functions of the system.

4.2.1 An example of formulation design

No matter whether building a new project or continuing an unfinished program, information must be input if a push–pull osmotic pump tablet formulation is to be designed using the system.

As Figure 4.3 shows, 'API Name in English,' 'API Name in Chinese,' 'Mol. Wt.' and 'Mol. Formula' are required for the information record and management in the database. Information must be input into the spaces with '*'; if any are left blank, the system cannot deal with the data correctly. Other information about API is used for the inference procedure of formulation design.

The dissolution test information is important, and blanks in the group box must be filled correctly. In particular, the dissolution media should correspond to the data of 'Solubility of API in dissolution media' and 'Dissolution rate of API in dissolution media*', or an unsuitable formulation could result. The collocation method of the dissolution

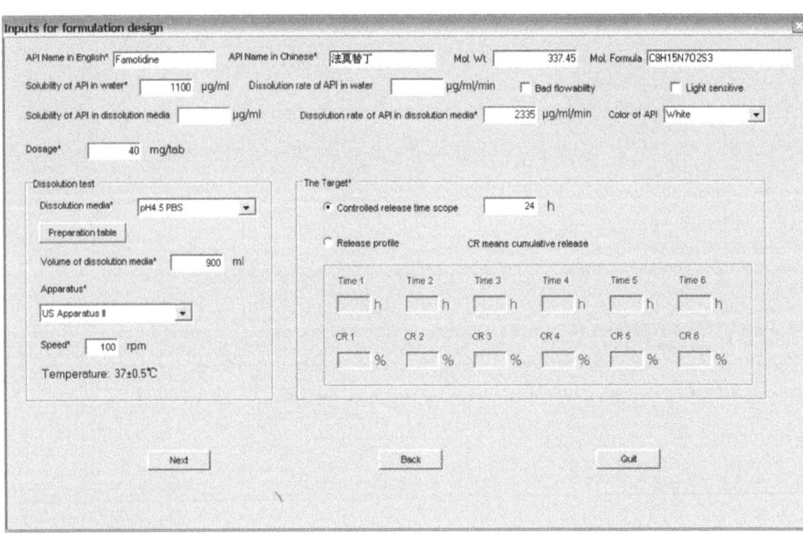

Figure 4.3 Information input interface for formulation design

Published by Woodhead Publishing Limited, 2013

media will be displayed when the 'Preparation table' button is clicked. There is a selection of new dissolution media at the end of the combo box of dissolution media, which could add a new dissolution medium and the collocation method into the system. Only apparatus I and apparatus II in USP are included in this version, because these two apparatuses are the most extensively used. More apparatuses will be added to this tool when they are applied well and extensively to the dissolution test.

In this tool, two ways are accepted to describe the target as displayed in Figure 4.3. One way is controlled release time scope, which describes the expected controlled release time of the user. If the user employs this way, he/she just needs to check the radio button of controlled release time scope and enter one number in the corresponding textbox. The other way is release profile, which describes the expected cumulative release of the user at each time point. If the user employs this way, he/she needs to check the radio button of release profile and enter times and expected cumulative release in the corresponding textboxes. When one way is chosen, the other way is unavailable.

In this example, famotidine, the blood concentration half-life of which is about 3 hours (Chen et al., 2007), is chosen as a candidate. Famotidine is a third-generation H_2 receptor blocking agent, used to treat peptic ulcers of the stomach and duodenum. It is good to deliver famotidine from controlled release dosage forms, especially from osmotic pump tablets. The data needed were input, as shown in Figure 4.3.

After inputting the required information, the user can choose excipients, as shown in Figure 4.4.

From Figure 4.4, it can be seen that the user can choose excipients for each component. Each component has several selections in the corresponding combo box. In this example, PEO Coagulant was selected as swelling agent. Auto was chosen for other components of tablet core, which meant that the system would select the excipients for the formulation. Moreover, the tooling for the compression of tablet core could be decided at this interface. Dimple was selected for the tooling style, and auto was selected for the tooling diameter in this example. Cellulose acetate is the default material of coating in the system, which was chosen as the coating material in this example. It can be seen also from Figure 4.4 that the orifice size was selected by the system.

When the button marked 'Next' was clicked, the system gave out the formulations and a general procedure in the next step (Figure 4.5).

The formulation of tablet core containing drug layer and push layer was displayed on the left side. Also, the tablet size, core hardness, orifice diameter, and the coating weight gain were shown in this area. Meanwhile,

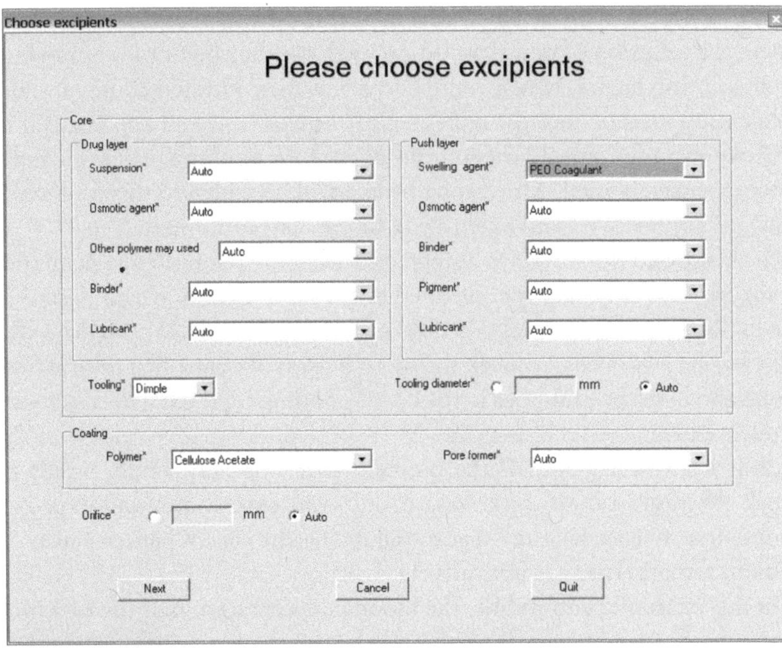

Figure 4.4 Interface for choosing excipients

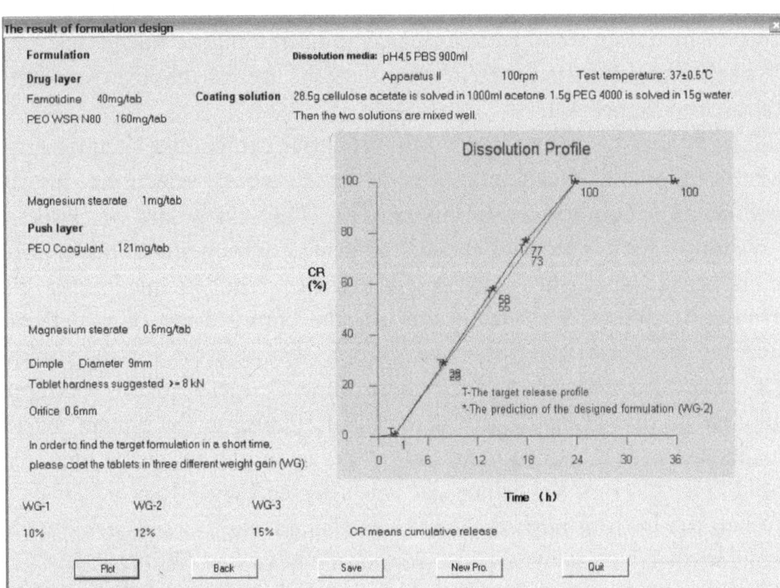

Figure 4.5 Interface for displaying the formulation design result

Published by Woodhead Publishing Limited, 2013

the example of the collocation method of coating solution appeared at the top-right, accompanied by the dissolution condition. The dissolution profiles were plotted when the button 'plot' was clicked. As Figure 4.5 shows, the profile marked with 'T' was the target release profile which was the one the user expected. And the profile marked with '*' was the predicted release profile of the designed formulation with WG-2, which was 12% in this example. In this step, the user can decide to save the project and quit the system and do the experiment, or start a new project. In this example, the project was saved and the experimental study was done. The dissolution test was carried out under the conditions displayed in Figure 4.5, and the sampling time was on the basis of the profile in Figure 4.5 and the time points in the next step in continuing the unfinished project (Figure 4.6).

When continuing the unfinished project of this example, the built project of famotidine was chosen and the button 'next' was clicked. Then the interface for the input of experimental result was shown (Figure 4.6). This interface displayed the formulation and dissolution condition for checking. The important part of this interface is the experimental data input. The user should type the coating weight gain in

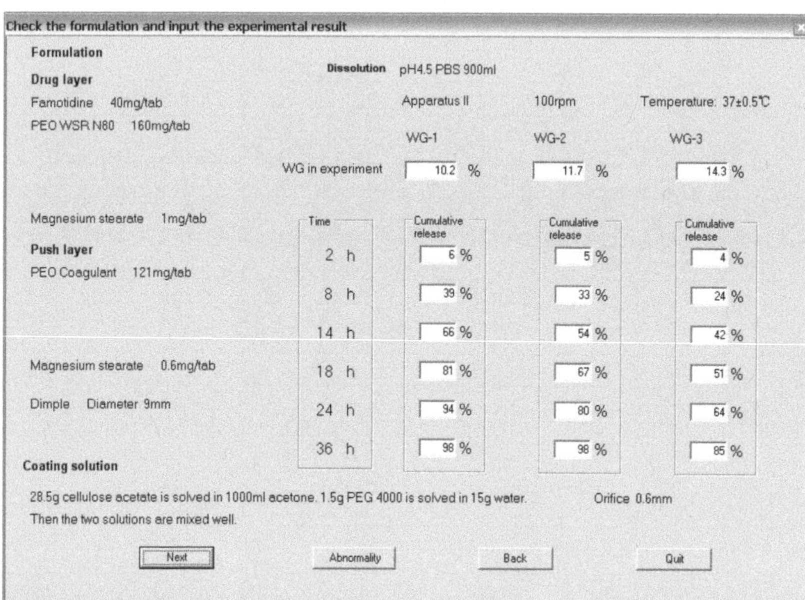

Figure 4.6 Interface for the input of experimental results

the experiment and the corresponding cumulative release in dissolution test in the homologous textbox. After inputting the data from our experiment, the next step is as shown in Figure 4.7.

In this interface, the dissolution profile of the experimental formulation of three different coating weight gains and the target profile were plotted in the identical scheme after clicking the button plot. Moreover, the similarity factors (f_2) between the experimental cumulative release profile and the target profile were displayed following the symbols of the experimental profile. The f_2 factor can be calculated as follows (Shah et al., 1998):

$$f_2 = 50\log\left\{\left[1+\left(\frac{1}{5}\right)\sum_{t=1}^{5}(E_t - T_t)^2\right]^{-\frac{1}{2}}\times 100\right\}$$

Here E_t and T_t stand for the dissolution value at time t of the experimental profile and the target profile, respectively. The former five

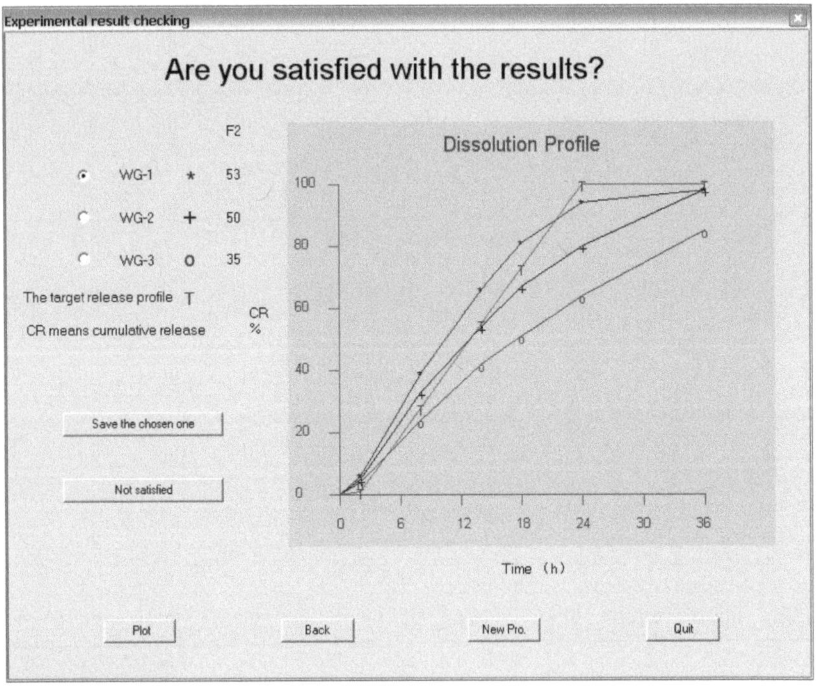

Figure 4.7 Interface for the experimental result checking

Published by Woodhead Publishing Limited, 2013

points were taken in the equation for calculation. If the similar factor (f_2) is not less than 50, the two drug release profiles are considered similar. It can be seen from Figure 4.7 that WG-1 and WG-2 were considered similar to the target. WG-1 was selected according to the visualized profiles. Then the project was finished. When the user next logs in to the system, he/she can see the formulation and experimental dissolution result by selecting this program and clicking the button 'next' (Figure 4.8).

4.2.2 An example of release prediction

Here gliclazide was taken as an instance. Gliclazide is a second-generation sulfonylurea oral blood glucose-lowering drug. Gliclazide can improve blood clotting and postpone the complications of diabetes, and is commonly used in the diabetic II treatment (Li Wei et al., 2008). It has been found that one extended release matrix tablet of 30 mg gliclazide per day can achieve a satisfactory therapeutic effect (Zhi-hong

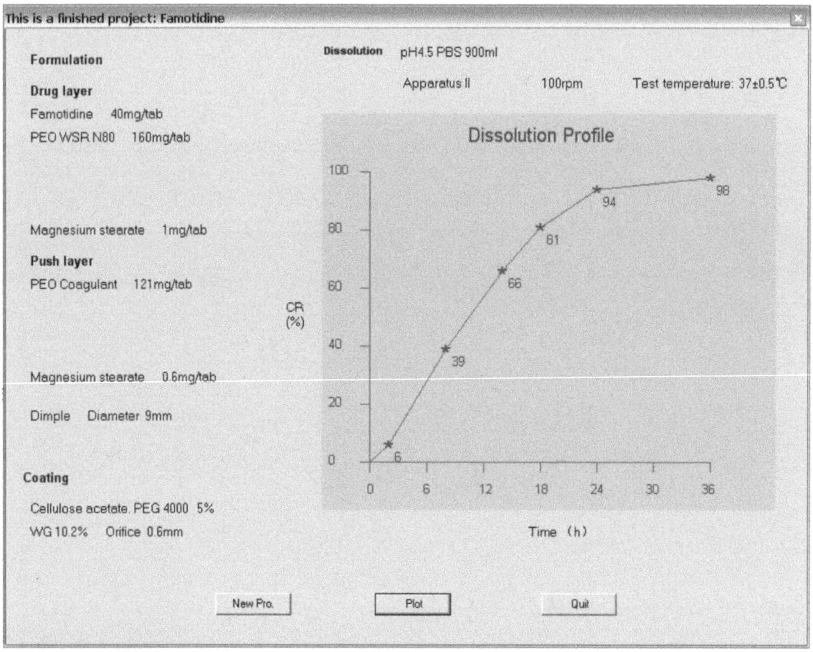

Figure 4.8 Interface for displaying the finished program

Zhang et al., 2009). In order to execute the release prediction action, click the button 'Release Prediction' in the projects management interface (see Figure 4.2), then the interface displayed in Figure 4.9 is open.

The textboxes at the top of the interface are for the data collection of the API which are the same as those at the top of the information input interface for formulation design (Figure 4.3). At the bottom left is a group box for information collection of the tablet core formulation, outline form, and hardness. Moreover, a group box for information collection of coating construction and a group box for the input of dissolution test condition are on the right-hand side. The API information, formulation, and dissolution test condition were entered as in Figure 4.9. In the next step, the system gave out the potential release profile (Figure 4.10).

4.2.3 An example of troubleshooting

Sometimes an abnormality might occur. In this example, acyclovir was employed as a candidate. Acyclovir is a nucleoside antiviral drug, which is able to inhibit the generation of several DNA virals.

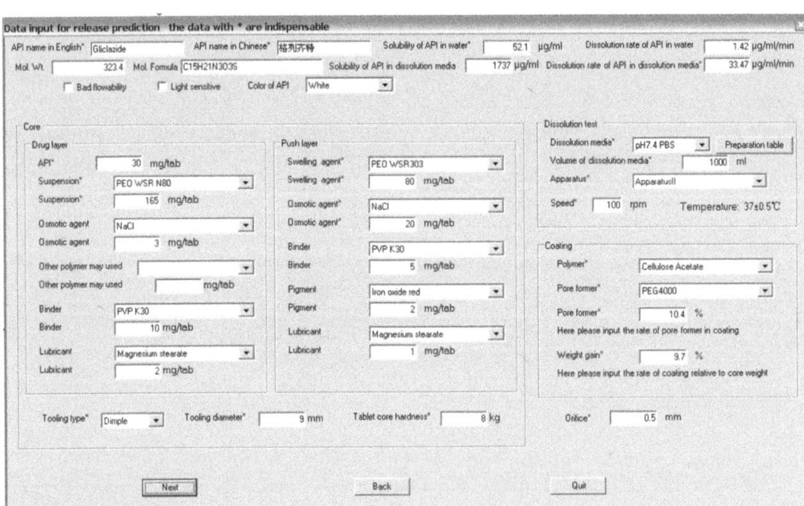

Figure 4.9 Interface for the release prediction information input

Published by Woodhead Publishing Limited, 2013

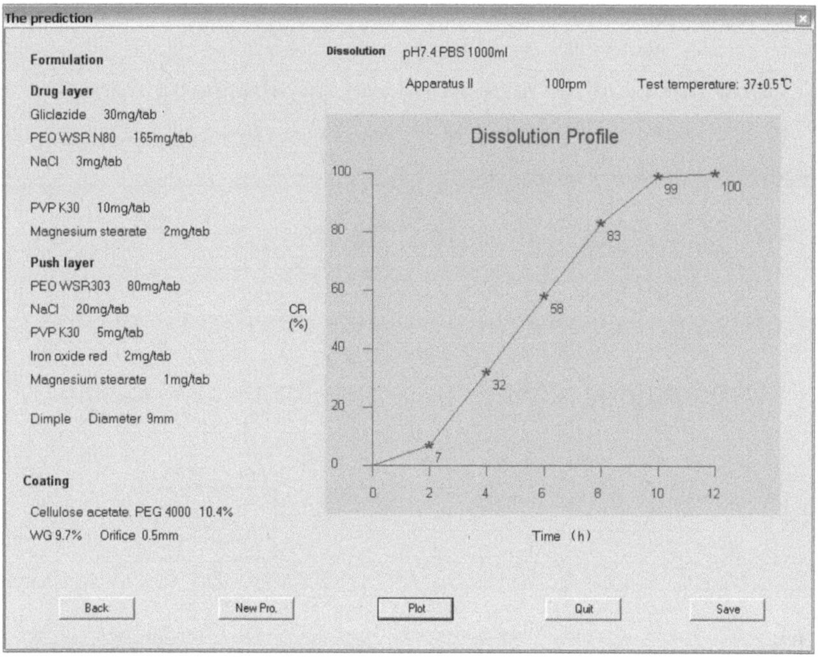

Figure 4.10 Interface of the release prediction results

The drug concentration in blood can reach 1.4–4.0 μmol·l^{-1} in 1–2 hours after oral administration. Acyclovir is suitable for extended release dosage forms. Our expert system was applied to design the push–pull osmotic pump tablet formulation. However, in the experimental study, the coating was broken during the dissolution test. Therefore the troubleshooting model was activated by clicking the button 'Abnormality' in the interface for the input of experimental results (refer to Figure 4.6).

As shown in Figure 4.11, after receiving the answers to a series of questions, the system raised a suggestion (or suggestions) which indicated that there might be something wrong with the tooling we had used to compress the tablets. It was found that significant circles of protection were rounding the edge of each side of the tablets when the PPOP tablets were checked, which meant that a crack occurred between the punch and the die. A new batch of the same formulation was prepared using a new tooling. No protection or claw was observed at any edge of the tablets, and the coating was no longer broken during the dissolution test.

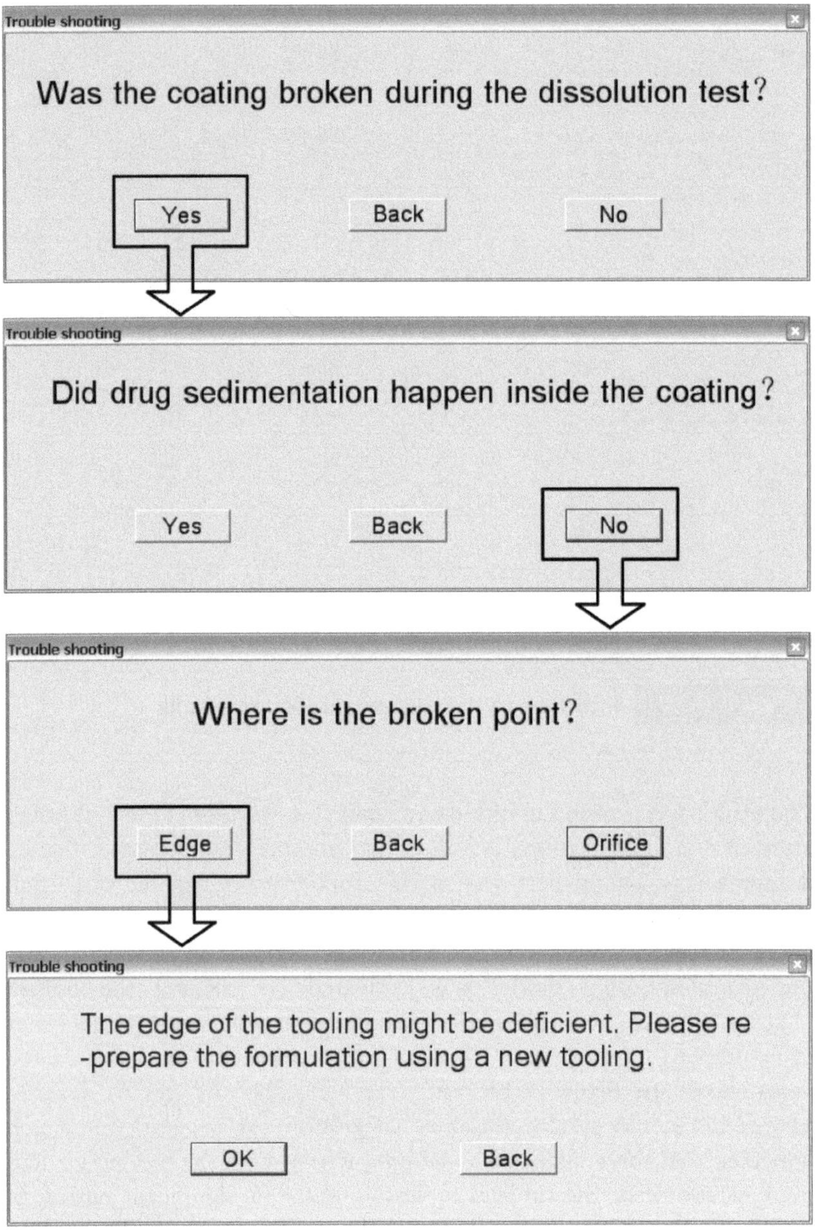

Figure 4.11 An example of troubleshooting

Published by Woodhead Publishing Limited, 2013

4.3 Methodology of the tool

4.3.1 The structure of the tool

Like most of the tools which are called expert systems, this tool consists of a man–machine interface which is also called an explanatory interface, a knowledge base which usually contains rules and data, and an inference engine which does the reasoning work. The general structure of this tool is displayed in Figure 4.12.

4.3.2 The workflow of the tool

Figure 4.13 shows the steps in the workflow of the tool. The steps until 'Project No.' were used for the management of the users and projects. The user login interface is shown in Figure 4.1. The user should register if it is the first time he/she has used the tool or the username is not recorded in the database. The interface of projects management shows after successful registration. The interface is different from that shown in Figure 4.2 as no project is in the list. It can be seen from Figure 4.13 that the tool has three main functions: release prediction, formulation design, and troubleshooting, which were described in the examples. These functions will be discussed in more detail, but, first, we turn to the database and the rule base as they are the base of the functions.

4.3.3 The database

The database is one of the important parts of the knowledge base. The database consists of six parts which are built and managed using SQL

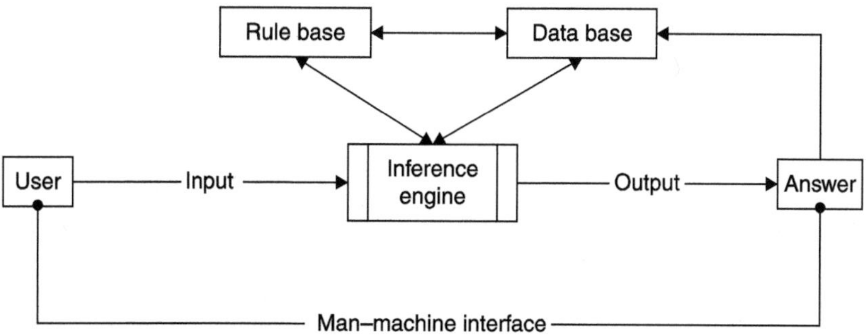

Figure 4.12 Structure of the tool

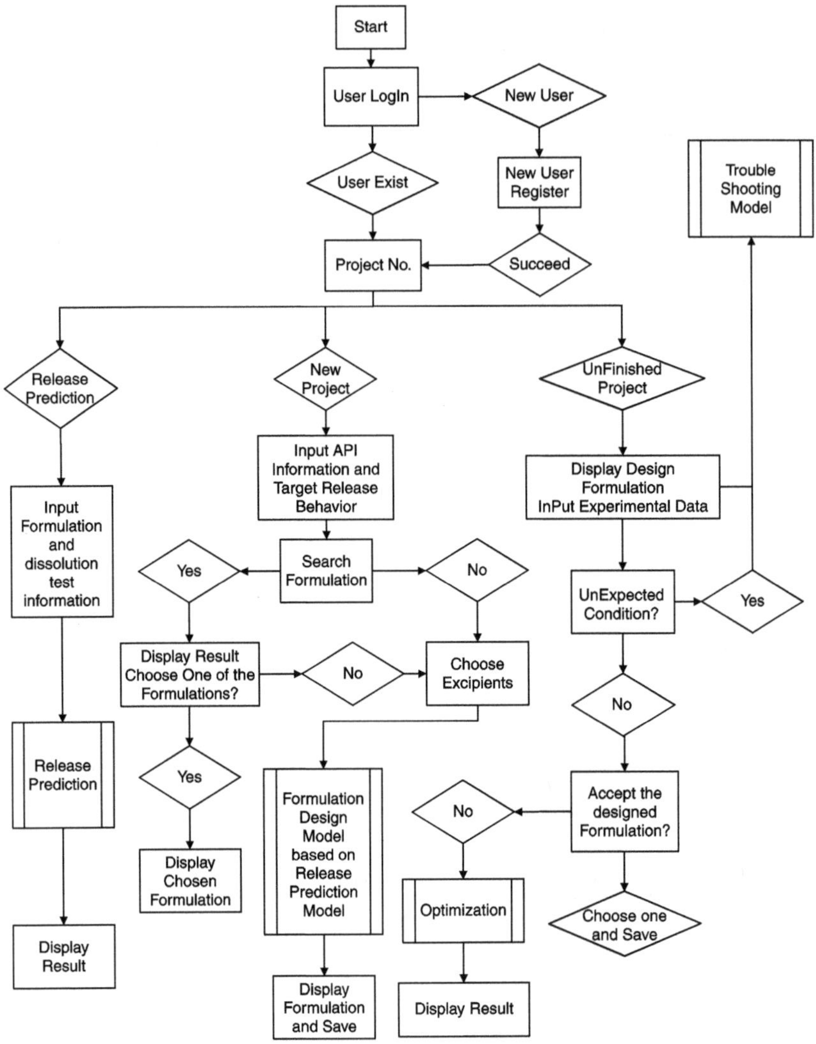

Figure 4.13 **Workflow of the tool**

Server. The table of UserEs is used to record and manage the users and codes, and is related to the table of FProjES by the key of UserName. The table of FProjES is used to record and manage the projects of the users, which means that this table can record the formulations and results of the projects which have been built by the users. Here, the results stored are the experimental data when the projects are finished, or the predicted results when the projects are unfinished. Experimental formulations, dissolution conditions, and drug release profiles are stored in the table of

Published by Woodhead Publishing Limited, 2013

Formulation. The difference between the table of FProjES and the table of Formulation is that the data in FProjES are related to projects and may be invalidated, whereas the data in Formulation are validated and could be applied to reason out.

Properties of API, such as solubility, dissolution rate, and color, are recorded in the table of API. The properties of excipients such as solubility and expansion are recorded in the table of Excipients. These two tables are related to the tables of FProjES and Formulation by the keys of EEnglishiName (the English name of the excipients) and APINameE (the English name of the API), respectively. The dissolution media and the collocation methods are stored in the table of DMPM. Synchronization between different tables was set, and the relations between different tables are shown in Figure 4.14. A large quantity of formulations, excipients, dissolution results, etc., were imported into the database by the designers when the tool was built. As the tool is used, the database will expanded, i.e. it could be considered that the system learns as it is used.

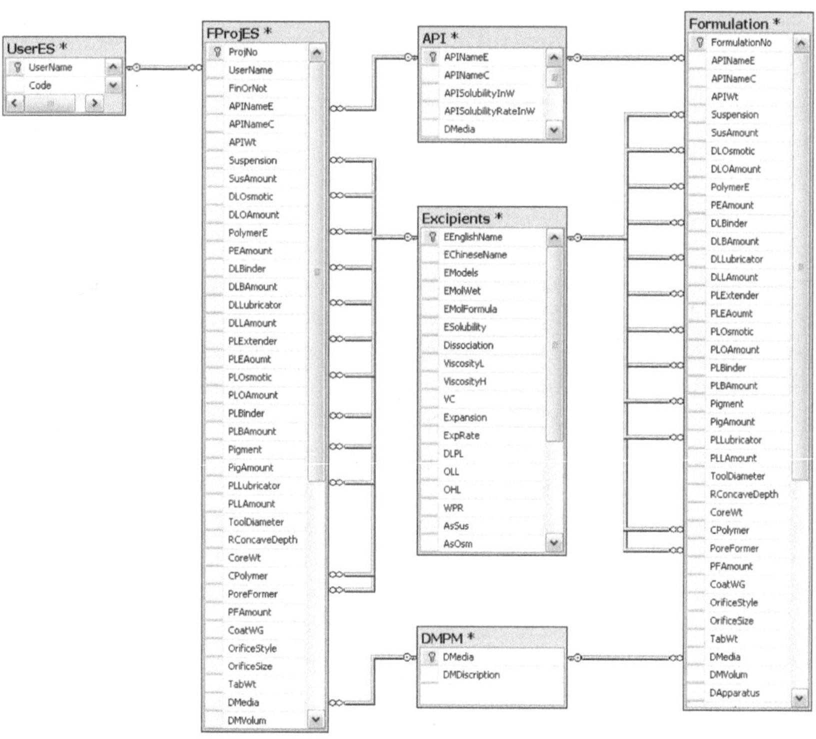

Figure 4.14 Relations of tables in the database

4.3.4 The rule base

The rule base is another important part of the knowledge base. Unlike the database, the rule base is not an entity in this tool. It is the description of the whole rules which were employed in the tool. The rules obtained from the experimental research and the experience of the professionals exist in two ways in this tool. Some of the rules which are numerical and serial are stored in the database. For instance, it is found that the amount of suspension used in the drug layer is limited according to different excipients, which means that drug sedimentation and incomplete drug release would occur if the polymer used as suspension is insufficient, as discussed in the introduction of this chapter. Different polymers have different properties such as solubility in water, the viscosity of the aqueous solution, etc., which result in different suspending capacities of the polymers.

The other rules which cannot be stored in the database are planted in the main structure of the program. For example, it used to be considered important that the orifice should be formed only on the drug side of PPOP. After a paper was published detailing how to overcome side identification in PPOP by making orifices on both layers (Zhi-hong Zhang et al., 2009), this was no longer considered necessary. So in our tool it is no longer set that the orifice should be formed only on the drug side.

Another example concerns the API. Many aspects of the API, including the molecular structure, crystal form, particle size, etc., affect the drug release from an oral solid dosage form, especially when the API is poorly water-soluble. Some of the relations are irregular. For example, the relations between drug release and crystal forms and between drug release and molecular structures cannot be described numerically using computer language. For some APIs, crystal form I is better than form II in dissolution, whereas for others crystal form I is worse than form II. Moreover, many APIs have no crystal form I or II, but have crystal form a. Some of the relations between the property of API and the drug release are regular. For instance, it is known that dissolution might be improved when the particle size of the poorly water-soluble drug becomes smaller. However, the relation between particle size and drug release cannot be evaluated in the same numerical standard. Different poorly water-soluble drugs have different dissolution even though they have the same particle size. Furthermore, the particle size cannot influence the drug release independent of other properties of the API-like crystal form. Fortunately, the relationship between the drug release and the solubility and dissolution rate of the API is regular and can be evaluated in the same numerical standard. The solubility and dissolution rate of the API influence the drug release independent of other properties of the API, which shows that the dissolution releases are influenced by other properties of the API. In this tool, the solubility and dissolution rate of the API is designed in the input interface and employed in the reasoning.

In the following, the inference engine will be introduced. In this tool, the inference engine is not a corporeally independent structure, which is consistent with several reasoning models. Human beings are able to generate long chains of reasoning which produce inferences, including metaphysical reasoning. If thinking can be seen as a psychological function, reasoning is a set of cognitive functions. The categorization of different kinds of reasoning is to focus on reasoning which produces prediction versus reasoning which explains observations. Classification of the different kinds of reasoning has produced a large number of definitions, such as algebraic, analogical, automated, bounded, case-based, causal, circular, clinical, commonsense, critical, deductive, default, demonstrative, diagnostic, formal, forward, and fuzzy, which frequently contrast with each other.

4.3.5 The release prediction model

This model is the kernel of the release prediction action. And it is the important foundation of the formulation design model. The release prediction model was constructed based on the artificial neural network (ANN), which is good at dealing with non-linear problems. It was found in the preceding experimental studies that the relationship between the cumulative release and the formulation composition was highly non-linear.

ANN are essentially mathematical models defining a function $f: X \rightarrow Y$ or a distribution over X or both X and Y. Sometimes ANN are also intimately associated with a particular learning algorithm or learning rule. ANN have many different classifications:

1. Defined by actions: successive type or discrete type, stochastic pattern or systematic pattern, static or dynamic state, etc.
2. Defined by teaching modes: feed forward (prorsad in other words) or back-propagation (BP) ANN.
3. Defined by approximation properties: overall approximation or partly approximation.
4. Defined by learning algorithm: supervised learning, unsupervised learning or reinforcement learning ANN.

BP, which was developed by Werbos and popularized by Rumelhart and McClelland and (Jatinder and Randall, 1999), is a common method of teaching ANN how to perform a given task. It is a supervised learning method which is a generalization of the delta rule. BP requires that the activation function used by the artificial neurons be differentiable. In this tool, a BP ANN which has three layers was employed.

Structure of the ANN of the release prediction model

The first layer is an input layer including input neurons, which send data via synapses to the second layer of neurons. The input neurons are of formulation aspects including the API properties (like solubilities and dissolution rates), dosages, properties of excipients (like solubilities, viscosities, and osmosis), the amount of excipients in the formulation, the coating weight gain, tablet core hardness, orifice, etc. According to the experiences and preceding experimental studies, those aspects which were considered to significantly influence the drug release were designed in the input neurons.

The second layer is also called the hidden layer. The number of neurons in this layer will influence the error and learning time of the ANN. The more neurons in this layer, the less error, but the greater time of learning. Following trial and error, 10 neurons were designed in the second layer as an optimization.

The data are sent via more synapses to the third layer of output neurons. Data which could describe the drug release profile were designed in the output neurons in this tool.

More complex ANN have more layers or more neurons in each layer. The synapse store parameters are called 'weights', which manipulate the data in the calculations.

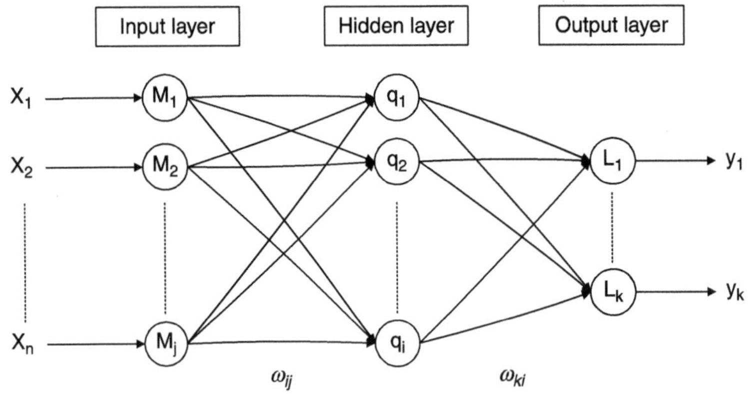

Figure 4.15 **Structure of BP neural networks in this tool**

Published by Woodhead Publishing Limited, 2013

Learning of the ANN

Learning means using a set of observations to find $f^* \in F$, which solves the task. In this tool, F is the mathematical model definition of a function: $X \rightarrow Y$, where X is the formulation aspects and Y is the description of the release profile. In other words, learning means finding the interconnection pattern (weights) between different layers of neurons.

The formulations, procedures, and dissolution profiles pre-stored in the database, which were obtained from experimental study, were used as the observations for network training.

Accomplishment of the release prediction

Two steps are in progress when the release prediction function is applied. First, the system searches the database to find out whether the formulation and the procedure and dissolution test information have been recorded. Before the searching is started, the system checks the input data to make sure that the data are acceptable by the system according to the rules. If some of the data are out of the acceptable range of the system, it would break off the processing and cancel the steps. If there is a matching record in the database, the stored dissolution profile will be displayed as the prediction result. If there is no requisite record in the database, the release prediction ANN model described above will be activated and then the dissolution profile of prediction is displayed.

4.3.6 Formulation design

This workflow is activated when a new project is established and the API information and target release behavior are input, which means it is activated by clicking the button 'next' in the information input interface for formulation design (refer to Figure 4.3). Formulation design includes some steps as shown in Figure 4.13.

Search formulation in the database

Searching formulation in the database could be considered as the first step. However, before this, the system checks the input data to make sure that the data are acceptable by the system according to the rules. If some of the data are out of the acceptable range of the system, it will break off the processing and cancel the steps.

When the input data are all acceptable, the system starts searching according to the target release behavior. If no formulation is found with a release profile similar to the target release profile, the system will display the interface for choosing excipients (Figure 4.4). After the excipients are chosen, the formulation design model will be activated.

The formulation number and the dissolution profile are displayed if a formulation is found with release profile similar to the target release profile. Sometimes more than one formulation including procedure and dissolution test are displayed. At this moment, the user decides the direction in which the system will go. If the user is satisfied by one of the displayed results and chooses one, the detail of the chosen result will be displayed including formulation, procedure, and dissolution test. Then the experimental study can be carried out. However, if no displayed result satisfies the user, the system has to move into the phase of choosing excipients (Figure 4.4).

Choosing excipients

This step is activated in two ways. When no requested formulation is found in the database, the system will go to the step of choosing excipients automatically. When requested formulations are found but none are chosen, the system will move to the step of choosing excipients by the user. In this step, the system receives the properties of the excipients and the information on the tooling and orifice. That information would be used in the inference in the formulation design model.

Formulation design model

Initialization of the formulation

The first action of the formulation design model is getting an initial formulation based on the information of API, excipients, and the rules. When this action is over, the categories of the excipients are decided. In the following actions, only the amount of the excipients in the formulation will be changed.

Regulation of the weight of tablet core

The tablets of the initial formulation might be too large to be swallowed. Or the tablets might be so small that the tablet weight variation would be hard to control in manufacturing. So the weight of the tablet core should be adjusted to an acceptable range. There are two ways in which this tool regulates the weight of the tablet core, employed based on selection by the user in the step of choosing excipients.

Published by Woodhead Publishing Limited, 2013

Auto regulation

When the user chooses 'auto' of the tooling diameter in the interface for choosing excipients, regulation of the weight of the tablet core will be carried out automatically, which means that the system will optimize the tablet weight within a wide range according only to the rules. This will be executed as follows.

(i) The tablet core weight of the initial formulation is calculated. Then go to (ii).

(ii) The suspension in the drug layer is increased by 10% if the weight of the tablet core is less than 300 mg. All other excipients in the tablet core are altered by the same rate. Then go to (iii).

 - If the weight of the tablet core is between 300 mg and 400 mg, it moves to the next step, which is going to modify the formulation in order to find the one which could release the drug as expected.
 - If the weight of the tablet core is over 400 mg, the push layer is reduced to 40% of the drug layer, which means that the push layer is reduced to 40%/60% of its initial usage amount, including the swelling agent, osmotic agent, binder, pigment, and lubricant in the push layer. The initial usage amount of the push layer is 60% of the drug layer according to the rules. Then go to (iv).

(iii) The tablet core weight of the modified formulation is calculated. Then go to (ii).

(iv) The tablet core weight of the modified formulation is calculated. If the core weight is no more than 800 mg, then it moves to the next step which is going to modify the formulation in order to find the one which could release the drug as expected.

 - If the core weight is larger than 800 mg, the push layer is reduced to 25% of the drug layer, which means that the push layer is reduced to 25%/60% of its initial usage amount. And then the tablet core weight of the modified formulation is calculated. If the core weight is still larger than 800 mg this time, the system will finish the process and display a message to inform the user that the system is unable to find the target formulation. Or it moves to the next step, which is going to modify the formulation in order to find the one which could release the drug as expected.

The workflow is displayed in Figure 4.16.

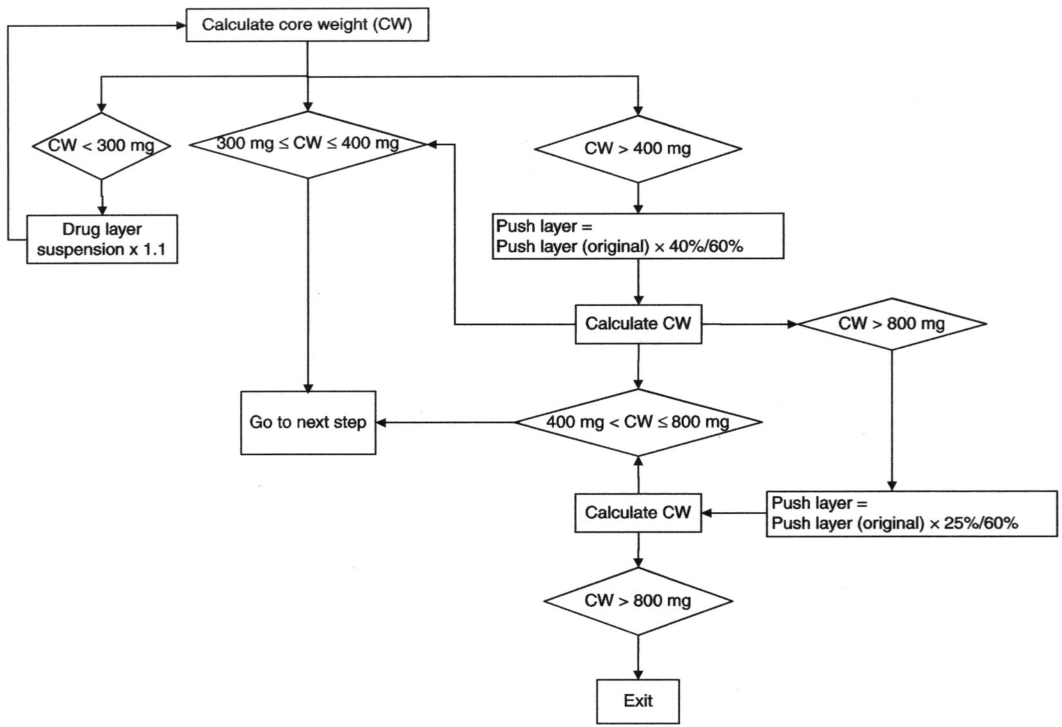

Figure 4.16 Workflow of core weight modification (auto core weight limit). Exit: the system cannot get an acceptable result, then exits the processes and informs the user. Go to next step: the system gets an acceptable result, and then moves to the next step

What happens when the tooling diameter is selected

When the user chooses one of the tooling diameters in the interface for choosing excipients other than auto, regulation of the weight of tablet core will be carried out in this way, which means that the system will optimize the tablet weight in the selected range. This is executed as follows.

(i) The minimum and the maximum tablet weights are decided according to the rules and the user selection of the tooling diameter. The tablet core weight of the initial formulation is calculated. Then go to (ii).

(ii) The suspension in the drug layer is increased by 10% if the weight of the tablet core is less than the minimum. All other excipients in the tablet core are altered by the same rate. Then go to (iii).

- If the weight of the tablet core is between the minimum and the maximum, it moves to the next step, which is going to modify the formulation in order to find the one which could release the drug as expected.
- If the weight of the tablet core is over the maximum, the push layer is reduced to 40% of the drug layer, which means that the push layer is reduced to 40%/60% of its initial usage amount, including the swelling agent, osmotic agent, binder, pigment, and lubricant in the push layer. The initial usage amount of the push layer is 60% of the drug layer according to the rules. Then go to (iv).

(iii) The tablet core weight of the modified formulation is calculated. Then go to (ii).

(iv) The tablet core weight of the modified formulation is calculated. If the core weight is no more than the maximum, then it moves to the next step, which is going to modify the formulation in order to find the one which could release the drug as expected.

- If the core weight is larger than the maximum, the push layer is reduced to 25% of the drug layer, which means that the push layer is reduced to 25%/60% of its initial usage amount. And then the tablet core weight of the modified formulation is calculated. If the core weight is still larger than the maximum this time, the system will finish the process and display a message to inform the user that the system is unable to find the target

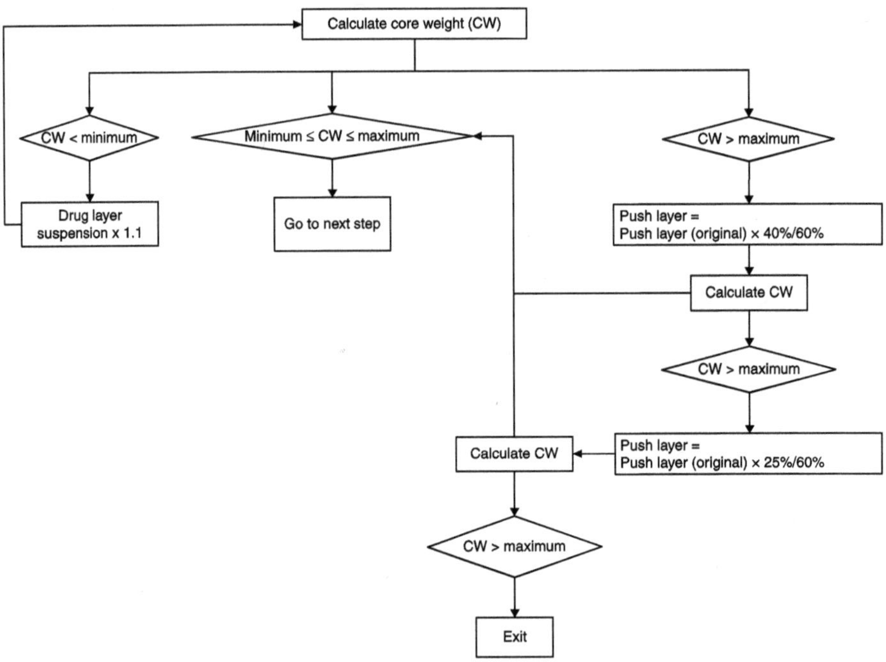

Figure 4.17 Workflow of core weight modification (tooling diameter is selected other than auto). Exit: the system cannot get an acceptable result, then exits the processes and informs the user. Go to next step: the system gets an acceptable result, and then moves to the next step

formulation. Or it moves to the next step, which is going to modify the formulation in order to find the one which could release the drug as expected.

The workflow is displayed in Figure 4.17.

Modify the formulation to look for the one which could release the drug as expected based on the release prediction model

This action is started when a formulation is found with acceptable tablet core weight. It is a long process, and works as introduced below. The workflow is displayed in Figure 4.18.

First, the dissolution profile of the formulation obtained in the regulation of the weight of tablet core is simulated using the release prediction model. Then the similar factor (f_2) between the predicted

Published by Woodhead Publishing Limited, 2013

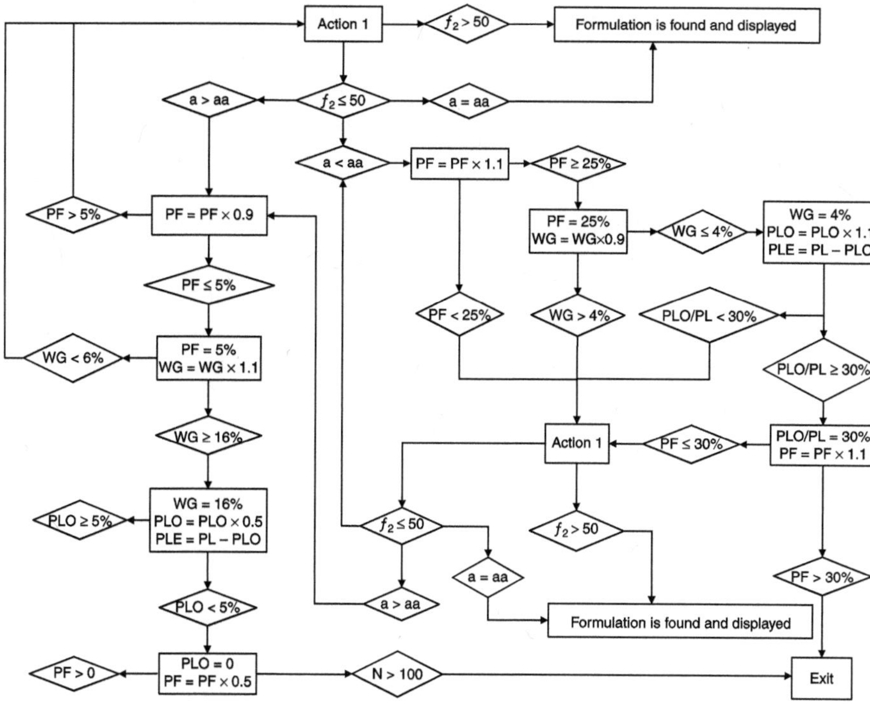

Figure 4.18 **Workflow of formulation modification. Action I: predict drug release using prediction model and calculate the f_2 between the dissolution profile of designed formulation and the target dissolution profile; PLO: the quality of osmotic agent used in push layer; PLE: the quality of extender used in push layer; PL: the quality of push layer; WG: coating weight gain; PF: the percentage of pore former used in the coating; a: release rate of designed formulation; aa: target release rate; N: the times of formulation modified; Exit: the system cannot get an acceptable result, then exits the processes and informs the user**

profile and the target dissolution profile is calculated. If f_2 is larger than 50, the system considers the predicted profile similar to the target, which means that the target formulation is found, and the formulations, dissolution condition, predicted profile, etc., are displayed in a new window. Here, the deviation of the prediction model is considered, so the standard is raised a little. According to the literature (Shah et al., 1998), the two drug release profiles are considered similar when the similar factor (f_2) is not less than 50.

If f_2 is not larger than 50, the system considers that the predicted profile is different from the target. In this situation, there are three subconditions: the first is that the predicted release rate of designed formulation is larger than the release rate of the target profile; the second is that the predicted release rate of designed formulation is smaller than the release rate of the target profile; the third is that the predicted release rate of designed formulation is the same as the target profile.

When the predicted release rate of designed formulation is the same as the target profile, it will be considered that the target formulation has been found, and the formulations, dissolution condition, predicted profile, etc., are displayed in a new window.

In the first subcondition that the predicted release rate of designed formulation is larger than the release rate of the target profile, the system will adopt a series of measures to reduce the release rate until it is no longer in this condition. The first aspect of the modified formulation is the usage amount of the pore former. The pore former in the coating is reduced by 10% when the pore former is more than 5% of the coating. When the pore former is reduced to no more than 5% of the coating, it is fixed on 5% of the coating and then the coating weight gain will be increased by 10% until the coating weight gain is no less than 16% of the tablet core. Then the pore former is fixed on 5% of the coating and the coating weight gain is fixed on 16% of the tablet core, and the osmotic agent in the push layer is reduced by 50% while the reduced amount is replaced by the PEO in the push layer, which means that the tablet core weight is not changed. When the osmotic agent in the push layer is reduced to less than 5% of push layer, the osmotic agent in the push layer is cancelled and the pore former is reduced by 50% again. The drug release profile is changed little when the pore former is near to zero. In order to avoid the endless loop, when the formulation is modified over 100 times before the target formulation is found, the system will finish the process and inform the user that the formulation could not be found.

In the second subcondition that the predicted release rate of designed formulation is smaller than the release rate of the target profile, the system will adopt a series of measures to increase the release rate until it is no longer in this condition. Here, the first aspect modified is also the usage amount of the pore former. In this condition, the pore former in the coating is increased by 10% when the pore former is less than 25% of the coating. When the pore former is increased to 25% and more of the coating, the content of pore former in the coating stays at 25% and

Published by Woodhead Publishing Limited, 2013

then the coating weight gain is reduced to 90% until it is no more than 4% of the tablet core. After that, the content of pore former in coating and coating weight gain of the tablet core stay at 25% and 4%, respectively, the osmotic agent in the push layer is stepped up to 110% while the PEO in the push layer is reduced to balance the push layer weight, which means that the tablet core weight is not changed. When the osmotic agent in the push layer is increased to no less than 30% of push layer, the osmotic agent in the push layer stays at 30% and the pore former is increased by 10% again. If the pore former gets to over 30% of the coating before the target formulation is found, the system will finish the process and inform the user that the formulation could not be found.

The formulation optimization model

The experimental results of the designed formulation might differ from the target release profile. This model is designed for formulation optimization based on the experimental data. If the user is not satisfied by any of the experimental results (refer to Figure 4.7), this model is activated. This model mainly adjusts the coating to modify the dissolution. As is designed in this tool, the three samples which are used to do the dissolution test are all the same except for the coating weight gain. When the optimization model is activated, the coating weight gains of the three samples are taken as independent variables; and f_2 between the dissolution profiles of the three samples and the target profile are calculated and treated as the dependent variables. Then a quadric equation is established. It is found that f_2 would be large when the two profiles get close, and f_2 would be lower down either when the experimental profile is faster than the target or when the experimental profile is slower than the target. So the quadric equation is employed here. In the next step, the maximum of the quadric equation is calculated by the system and the homologous coating weight gain is discovered, which is the result of the optimization. Finally, the formulation of the optimized coating weight gain is displayed in a new window.

The troubleshooting model

This model will be activated either when the button 'Abnormality' is clicked (see Figure 4.6) or when the system recognizes that the experimental result is too far from the expected results. This model is a search tree. The problems which have been observed and the solutions

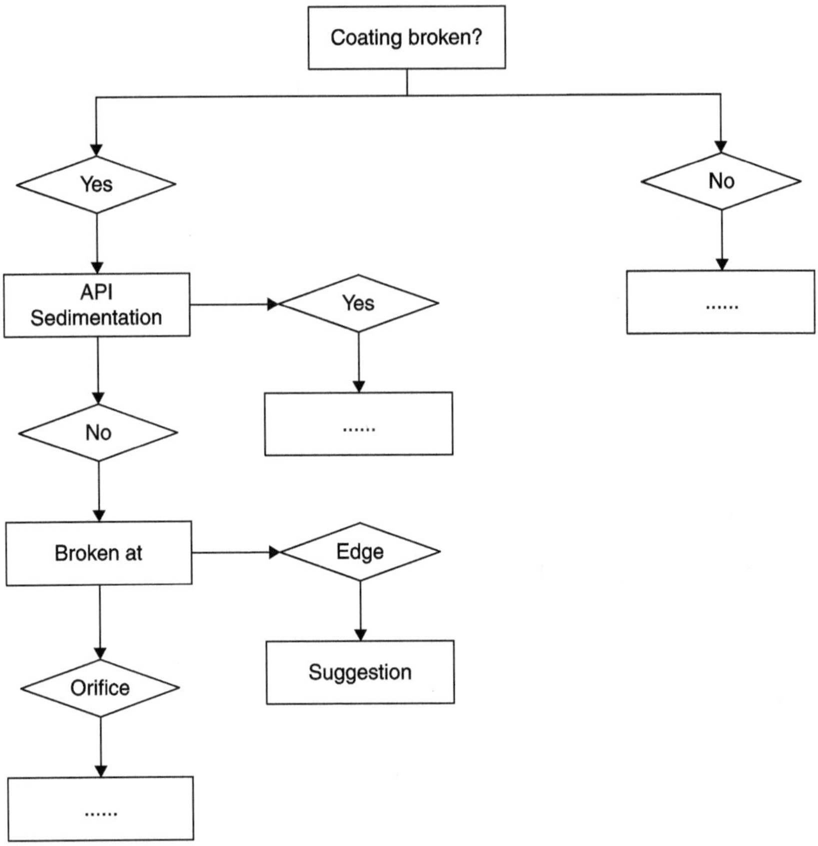

Figure 4.19 Part of the search tree

are designed in this tree. The forward direction deduction rule is employed to reason out the results.

Figure 4.19 shows the workflow of the example in 4.2.3. This figure is a part of the search tree. When the unexpected condition of broken coating is raised, two ways are provided which are the two branches connected to this node in the tree. When one way is selected, the system catches the next node of the tree which has two branches also. In the example, the system moved along the nodes and branches according to selections by the user, and reached a leaf which was one of the ends of the tree. The suggestion (Figure 4.19) obtained was 'The edge of the tooling might be deficient. Please re-prepare the formulation using a new tooling.'

Published by Woodhead Publishing Limited, 2013

4.4 Conclusions

Hundreds of PPOP formulations of poorly water-soluble drugs with extremely different dosages were studied and regularities of formulation components and manufacture procedures were extracted. The database, rules, prediction model of release behavior, formulation design model, optimization model, troubleshooting model, and man–machine interface were built. Then the expert system for the development and formulation of push–pull osmotic pump tablets containing poorly water-soluble drugs was established, which is the tool as introduced here.

Some conclusions can be reached from the above discussion. First, the tool is applicable and could help people to find target PPOP formulations in a very short period of time. This means that the tool could shorten the PPOP development cycle, which could indicate a resultant reduction in development cost. This is a goal pursued by all formulation R&D scientists and manufacturers. The tool furnishes three useable implements. The prediction action could help people to predict the dissolution profile of the formulations, which was applied and considered convenient in use. The optimization model could optimize the formulation based on the experimental data, which means that the system could improve the formulation according to its experimental performance. The troubleshooting model could help people to deal with any unexpected conditions, and is on trial and considered to be helpful. It is also indicated that this tool has the ability to learn, which means that it will improve as it is applied.

4.5 Discussions and future work

The designed expert system is not only expected to shorten the developing cycle, but also to inspect the current viewpoints of the PPOP. Problems will be discovered either in the tool or the viewpoints of the PPOP. This expert system is not perfect, and many improvements could be made in future.

4.5.1 Lower down the deviation between the predictions of the tool and the experimental results

First of all, this tool is still declinational, especially in the prediction model. It could be found in the example of formulation design (refer to

4.2.1) that the experimental result of the designed formulation is different from the predicted dissolution profile. The prediction of the designed formulation (Figure 4.5), which is almost the same as the target release profile, is the predicted dissolution profile of the formulation (WG-2) which is the expected one as designed by the system. The experimental dissolution profiles indicated that the dissolution profile of formulation (WG-2) is apparently different from the target release, although the f_2 between the formulation (WG-2) and the target is 50. Although the dissolution profile of formulation (WG-1) is clearly similar to the target release profile, the f_2 between the formulation (WG-1) and the target is 53.

The first thing which could be done in future to reduce the declination of the system is to expand the capacity of the database. Although many data have been recorded in the tool, which contains hundreds of formulations containing several poorly water-soluble drugs, the formulations are not abundant according to the discussion above. This tool is designed to be able to remember the formulations and the experimental dissolution profiles which are brought about during applications by users. However, the increase in formulations and experimental dissolution profiles will not be fast enough. Furthermore, the formulations which are produced during the applications are not systematized or regularized enough for training of the ANN. In future, more poorly water-soluble drugs should be selected and systematized formulations should be inspected and added to the database besides those produced during the applications. Expedition of the database will have two advantages. There will be more candidates in the searches when the prediction or the formulation design is carried out; the results will be accurate if it is found in the database. And the deviations of the weights will be low when more systematical and regular data are employed in the ANN training, which means that the prediction would be closer to the experimental results.

The second thing that could be done is to ameliorate the training of the ANN. The ANN was trained using all the data in the database, which could be considered as general training. When more formulations are saved in the system, especially when formulations containing more API are saved, this modification could be carried out. The formulations containing API with properties close to the API in the new project using the tool should be chosen in the ANN training, so that the deviation will be smaller. Amelioration of the ANN will also reduce the training time.

4.5.2 Add or improve the rules

Previously called rule base, in this tool, some of the rules are saved in the database whereas some of the rules are designed in the program sentence. The rule base is not a visible structure, so it is not used to describe the rules. When more APIs and formulations are studied, new rules might be observed. New rules should be fused into the system. In addition, the existing rules might be modified as more and more API and formulations are studied. For example, the tool could design the formulations for API with dosages no larger than 200 mg per tablet. When some API have dosages over 200 mg and the formulations are studied and loaded into the system, the rule of the dosage range could be expanded. For another example, new excipients, especially the coating material, will be studied, and then the new excipients will be added to the system. The properties of the new excipients might be different from those already in the system, so the rules of the excipients might be modified.

4.5.3 About the manufacturing process

In this tool, the commonly used manufacture procedure is acquiescent. First the blends of drug layer and push layer are prepared; then the blends of the two layers are made into double layer tablets by direct compression; after that the tablets are coated by a semi-permeable membrane; and, finally, an orifice is formed in the membrane of the drug layer. However, a procedure other than direct compression might be applied because of the manufacturing facilities. So more procedures and the parameters should be studied and added into the system in future. Moreover, the coating of semi-permeable membrane might be translucent or opaque when improper parameters are used. So the coating procedure should be studied.

4.5.4 Enlarge the capacity of troubleshooting model

This tool has the capacity to deal with unexpected phenomena. However, new clauses still might be added into the troubleshooting model. When more API, excipients, formulations, and procedures are studied, more unexpected phenomena will show up, which indicates that the troubleshooting model should be able to deal with more unexpected problems. So the new unexpected phenomena and the resolutions could be added into the model.

4.5.5 Independence of the optimization model

At present, the optimization model can be used only after the formulation design is finished and the experimental dissolution data are input. It is realized that users might already have the formulations and only need to do the optimization. So it would be convenient if this model could be activated standalone.

Another problem will be raised when the optimization model is independent. The user might request that the system perform optimization by inputting a series of formulations which are different other than coating weight gain. What if the formulations are all the same except for the content of pore former? So in the future, more optimization policies should be studied. For instance, an optimization model with two variables such as content of pore former and coating weight gain could exist in the improved system.

4.5.6 Ameliorate the interfaces and networking

This tool is still a uniprocessor version. It cannot easily be separated and applied. The wider application would be very good for this tool, because more problems and shortcomings would be found in the applications which are the foundations for the improvement of the system. Networking will do much to help. If the tool could be used over the Internet, many more users could use it at the terminals all over the world.

Three things should be considered. First, the interfaces should be modified to adapt to networking. Decoration of the interfaces will be carried out. Then non-disclosure of the projects should be reconstructed, which is very important for the companies. The third thing is how to discriminate the information input by the users. Users might input fake information, especially information on API, in order to keep their current programs secret. If fake information is input to the system, this could result in complications when searching is carried out and when the ANN is training.

Published by Woodhead Publishing Limited, 2013

4.5.7 Reflection of current thinking

If thinking and reasoning of human beings can be observed in a computer program, current thinking could be tested. In particular, the rules and regularities could be inspected during application of this tool. It is expected to reflect the current thinking and the current formulation design policies of PPOP. It is also expected to throw out a minnow to catch a whale, in the hope that more advanced technologies will be introduced to pharmaceutics.

4.6 References

Aguilar JE, Garcia E, Perez P, Suñé-Negre JM, Miñarro M and Ticó JR. (2009) The use of the SeDeM Diagram expert system to determine the suitability of diluents-disintegrants for direct compression and their use in formulation of ODT. *Eur J Pharm Biopharm*, 73, 414–23, ISSN: 0939-6411.

Aleksander M and Renata J. (2007) Unified methodology of neural analysis in decision support systems built for pharmaceutical technology. *Expert Syst Appl*, 32, 1124–31, ISSN: 0957-4174.

Batrman SD, Jerome V and Mark R. (1996) The Development and Validation of a Capsule Formulation Knowledge-Based System. *Pharm Technol*, 20, 174–84, ISSN: 1543-2521.

Cai ZX and Xu GY. (2004) *Artificial Intelligence: Principles and Applications*. Tsinghua University Press, Beijing.

Chen CX, Li SM, Li HJ and Sun YH. (2007) Preparation of monolithic osmotic pump tablets of famotidine. *Chin New Drug J*, 16, 1035–8, ISSN: 1003–3734.

Jatinder ND Gupta and Randall S. Sexton (1999) Comparing backpropagation with a genetic algorithm for neural network training. *Omega*, 27, 679–84, ISSN: 0305–0483.

Lai S, Podczeck F, Newton JM and Daumesnil R. (1996) An expert system to aid the development of capsule formulation. *Pharm Technol Eur*, 10, 60–8, ISSN: 0164–6826.

Li Wei, Zhang Zhi-hong, Du Ga-ni, Nie Shu-fang, Yang Xing-gang and Pan Wei-san. (2008) Preparation of gliclazide push-pull osmotic pump system. *Chin New Drugs J*, 17, 233–6, ISSN: 1003–3734.

Liu L, Khang G, Rhee JM and Lee HB. (2000). Monolithic osmotic tablet system for nifedipine delivery. *J Control Release*, 67, 309–22, ISSN: 0168–3659.

Lu EX, Jiang ZQ, Zhang QZ and Jiang XG. (2002) Preparation of controlled release coated tablets of naproxen sodium. *Chin Pharm J*, 37, 841–4, ISSN: 1001–2494.

Okimoto K, Rajewski RA and Stella VJ. (1999) Release of testosterone from an osmotic pump tablet utilizing (SBE) 7m-β-CD as both a solubilizing and an osmotic pump agent. *J Control Release*, 58, 29–38, ISSN: 0168–3659.

Okimoto K, Tokunaga Y, Ibuki R, Irie T, Uekama K, et al. (2004). Applicability of (SBE) 7m-β-CD in controlled-porosity osmotic pump tablets (OPTs). *Int J Pharm*, 286, 81–8, ISSN: 0378–5173.

Ouyang DF, Nie S, Li W, Guo H, Liu H and Pan WS. (2005) In vitro and in vivo evaluation of two extended release preparations of combination metformin and glipizide. *Drug Dev Ind Pharm*, 31, 677–85, ISSN: 0363–9045.

Perez P, Suñé-Negre JM, Miñarro M, Roig M, Fuster R, et al. (2006) A new expert systems (SeDeM Diagram) for control batch powder formulation and preformulation drug products. *Eur J Pharm Biopharm*, 64, 351–9, ISSN: 0939–6411.

Rowe RC. (1993) Expert systems in solid dosage development. *Pharm Ind*, 55, 1040.

Rowe RC, Wakerly MG, Roberts RJ and Grundy RU. (1995) Expert Systems for Parenteral Development. *PDAJ, Pharm Sci Technol*, 49, 257–61.

Rowe RC and Roberts RJ. (1998) Artificial intelligence in pharmaceutical product formulations: knowledge-based and expert systems. *Pharm Sci Technol Today*, 1, 153–9.

Shah VP, Tsong Y, Sathe P and Liu J. (1998) In Vitro Dissolution Profile Comparison-Statistics and Analysis of the Similarity Factor, f2. *Pharma Res*, 15, 889–96, ISSN: 1735–0328.

Theeuwes F and Higuchi T. (1972) *Osmotic dispensing device for releasing beneficial agent*. US Patent 3,845,770.

Theeuwes F. (1975). Elementary osmotic pump. *J Pharm Sci*, 64, 1987–91, ISSN: 1520–6017.

Theeuwes F. (1978) *Osmotic system for delivering selected beneficial agents having varying degrees of solubility*. US Patent 4 111 201, 5 Sep.

Verma R, Mishra B and Garg S. (2000) Osmotically Controlled Oral Drug Delivery. *Drug Dev Ind Pharm*, 26, 695–708, ISSN: 0363–9045.

Yannis LL. (1998) A computer-based expert system designs and analyzes a 2(k-p) fractional factorial design for the formulation optimization of novel multicomponent liposomes. *J Pharm Bio Aral*, 17, 133–40, ISSN: 0731–7085.

Zhi-hong Zhang, Hong-ye Dong, Bo Peng, Hong-fei Liu, Chun-lei Li, et al. (2011) Design of an expert system for the development and formulation of push-pull osmotic pump tablets containing poorly water-soluble drugs. *Int J Pharm*, 410, 41–7, ISSN: 0378–5173.

Zhi-hong Zhang, Wei Li, Shu-fang Nie, Xin Tang, Bo Peng, et al. (2009) Overcome side identification in PPOP by making orifices on both layers. *Int J Pharm*, 371, 1–7, ISSN: 0378–5173.

Published by Woodhead Publishing Limited, 2013

5

SeDeM Diagram: an expert system for preformulation, characterization and optimization of tablets obtained by direct compression

Josep M. Suñé Negre, Manuel Roig Carreras, Roser Fuster García, Encarna García Montoya, Pilar Pérez Lozano, Johnny E. Aguilar, Montserrat Miñarro Carmona and Josep R. Ticó Grau, University of Barcelona, Spain

DOI: 10.1533/9781908818508.109

Abstract: SeDeM expert system is an innovative tool which allows characterization of a powdered substance. This information is used to identify strengths and weaknesses for development of tablets by direct compression. The tool allows successful design of tablets, avoiding unnecessary studies and trials, and reducing the lead time of development. In addition, SeDeM expert system provides a mathematical formula to obtain the final formulation of tablets by direct compression in an easy way containing the minimum excipient (one) with a minimum test. The information provided is categorised as dimension, compressibility, flowability/powder flow, lubricity/stability, and lubricity/dosage—this can be provided in graphical form, the SeDeM Diagram. The methodology information can be used in further studies using Quality by Design. In this chapter, the methodology is described along with some examples. It has been widely demonstrated in pharmaceutical labs that this is a robust tool. This tool was developed at the University of Barcelona.

Key words: direct compression, expert system, preformulation tool, prediction of tablets, analysis of powder.

5.1 Introduction

The pharmaceutical industry aims to manufacture medicines at the optimum cost, adapting processes to requirements such as GMP (good manufacturing practice), HSE (Health, Safety and Environment), etc. To reach this optimum cost, methodology is selected which yields robust and optimized products in terms of productivity. Direct compression technology is an attractive way in which to develop tablets, as the lead times for manufacturing are low, and requirements for equipment, solvents, and residues are reduced.

In the development of a formulation using direct compression technology, it is important to have a tool that allows identification of potential formulas and rejection of those that require a transformation of the granules prior to the compression phase. SeDeM expert system was designed and developed with this in mind at the Pharmaceutical Technology Department of the University of Barcelona. SeDeM expert system is an innovative and useful tool, which provides information about the suitability of obtaining tablets by direct compression (Figure 5.1). In addition, this methodology can be used in already commercialized formulas to identify any variability in the required final properties of the compression phase when one ingredient is changed, for example in the selection of a new supplier of an excipient.

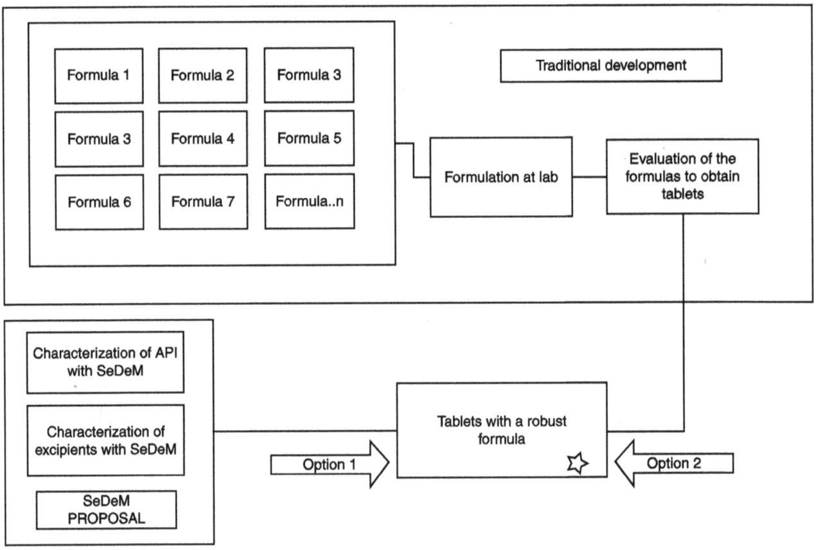

Figure 5.1 Strategy for development

Published by Woodhead Publishing Limited, 2013

SeDeM expert system is applied in preformulation and formulation studies of medicines, but it can also be used to evaluate the properties of commercialized products in solid dosage forms. This methodology can be applied to elucidate the physical profile of powdered substances (active pharmaceutical ingredients (API) and excipients or final mixture) used to formulate drugs by direct compression technology (Suñé et al., 2005; Suñé et al., 2008a,b; Suñé et al., 2011a,b; García et al., 2010; Pérez et al., 2006; Aguilar et al., 2009). SeDeM expert system allows construction of an Index of Good Compressibility, within which profiles can be created listing advantages and deficiencies in powdered substances to be used in direct compression, hence the system contributes to deciding whether or not the direct compression method is appropriate for a particular substance (Suñé et al., 2011).

Characterization of powdered substances by SeDeM facilitates identification of any characteristics that require amendment in order to obtain tablets by direct compression. This system thus provides information that will ensure the robust design of the formulation in the final product.

This new method is based on selection and application of several parameters that the formulation must fulfill to ensure a successful tablet elaborated by direct compression. The following criteria are applied:

1. The formulation must be representative and appropriate for the requirements of compression technology.
2. The execution of the experimental methodology and calculus must be readily applicable.

After determining the profile of the drug substance and the proposed excipients, this methodology proposes a mathematical formula for easy determination of the proportion of the ingredients required for the final formulation.

5.2 Parameters examined by SeDeM expert system

SeDeM uses 12 tests (Suñé et al., 2005; Suñé et al., 2008, Suñé et al., 2011a,b; García et al., 2010; Pérez et al., 2006; Aguilar et al., 2009) to decide whether a powder is suitable for direct compression.

- Bulk density (Da),
- Tapped density (Dc),

- Inter-particle porosity (Ie),
- Carr index (IC),
- Cohesion index (Icd),
- Hausner ratio (IH),
- Angle of repose (α),
- Flowability (t″),
- Loss on drying (%HR),
- Hygroscopicity (%H),
- Particle size (%Pf),
- Homogeneity index (Iθ).

These tests are grouped into five factors on the basis of the physical characteristics of the powder and the functionality of the drug:

- Dimensional Parameter. Bulk density (Da) and Tapped density (Dc). These affect the size of the tablet and its capacity to pile up. In addition, these tests are used in the calculation of other mathematical indexes for determination of the compressibility parameter.
- Compressibility Parameter. Inter-particle porosity (Ie), Carr index (IC) and Cohesion index (Icd). These affect the compressibility of the powder.
- Flowability/Powder Flow Parameter. Hausner ratio (IH), Angle of repose (α) and Flowability (t″). These influence the flowability of the powdered substance when compressed.
- Lubricity/Stability Parameter. Loss on drying (%HR) and Hygroscopicity (%H). These affect the lubricity and future stability of the tablets.
- Lubricity/Dosage Parameter. %Particles <50 mcm and Homogeneity index. These influence the lubricity and dosage of the tablets.

Table 5.1 shows the five parameters, with the abbreviations, units, formulas and incidence on compression.

5.2.1 Methodology required by SeDeM to study a powdered substance

Pharmacopoeia methodologies are used to calculate these parameters. However, when this is not possible, a common strategy used in

Published by Woodhead Publishing Limited, 2013

Table 5.1 **Parameters and tests used by SeDeM**

Incidence factor	Parameter	Symbol	Unit	Equation
Dimension	Bulk density	Da	g/ml	Da = P/Va
	Tapped density	Dc	g/ml	Dc = P/Vc
Compressibility	Inter-particle porosity	Ie	–	Ie = Dc – Da/Dc × Da
	Carr index	IC	%	IC = (Dc – Da/Dc) 100
	Cohesion index	Icd	N	(Experimental)
Flowability/ powder flow	Hausner ratio	IH	–	IH = Dc/Da
	Angle of repose	(α)	°	tg α=h/r
	Powder flow	t″	s	Experimental
Lubricity/stability	Loss on drying	%HR	%	Experimental
	Hygroscopicity	%H	%	Experimental
Lubricity/dosage	Particles < 50 µm	%Pf	%	Experimental
	Homogeneity index	(Iθ)	–	* Iθ= Fm / 100 + Δ Fmn

pharmaceutical technology development is applied. The methods used for each test are described below (Pérez et al., 2006):

- Bulk density (Da): The method is described in Section 2.9.34 of the *European Pharmacopeia* (*European Pharmacopeia*, 2011).
- Tapped density (Dc): The volume taken is the value obtained after 2500 strokes using a settling apparatus with a graduated cylinder (voluminometer).
- Inter-particle porosity (Ie) of the powder mixture (Font, 1962) is calculated from the following equation: Ie = Dc – Da/Dc × Da.
- Carr index (IC%) (Córdoba et al., 1996; Rubinstein, 1993; Torres and Camacho, 1991; Wong and Pilpel, 1990). This is calculated from Da and Dc as: IC = (Dc – Da/Dc)100.
- Cohesion index (Icd): This index is determined by compressing the powder, preferably in an eccentric press. First of all the mean hardness (N) of the tablets is calculated, the raw powder is tested, but if it cannot be compressed, 3.5% of the following mixture is added to the mix: talc 2.36%, Aerosil® 200 0.14% and magnesium stearate 1.00%.

- Hausner ratio (IH) (*European Pharmacopeia*, 2011; Rubinstein, 1993). The method is described in Section 2.9.34 of the *European Pharmacopeia* (*European Pharmacopeia*, 2011). This is calculated from Da and Dc as: IH = Dc/Da.
- Angle of repose (α) (Rubinstein, 1993; Muñoz, 1993). The method is described in Section 2.9.36 of the *European Pharmacopeia* (*European Pharmacopeia*, 2011). This is the angle of the cone formed when the product is passed through a funnel with the following dimensions: height 9.5 cm, upper diameter of spout 7.2 cm, internal diameter at the bottom, narrow end of spout 1.8 cm. The funnel is placed on a support 20 cm above the table surface, centered over a millimeter-grid sheet on which two intersecting lines are drawn, crossing at the centre. The spout is plugged and the funnel is filled with the product until it is flush with the top end of the spout when smoothed with a spatula. Remove the plug and allow the powder to fall onto the millimeter sheet. Measure the four radii of the cone base with a slide caliper and calculate the mean value (r). Measure the cone height (h). Deduce α from $\tan(\alpha) = h/r$.
- Flowability (t″): The method is described in Section 2.9.16 of the *European Pharmacopeia* (*European Pharmacopeia*, 2011). It is expressed in seconds and tenths of a second per 100 grams of sample, with a mean value of three measurements.
- Loss on drying (%HR): This is measured by the method described in Section 2.2.32 in the *European Pharmacopeia* (*European Pharmacopeia*, 2011). The sample is dried in an oven at 105°C ± 2°C, until a constant weight is obtained.
- Hygroscopicity (%H): Determination of the percentage increase in sample weight after being kept in a humidifier at a relative humidity of 76% (± 2%) and a temperature of 22°C ± 2°C for 24 h.
- Percentage of particles measuring < 50 μm (%Pf): Particle size is determined by means of the sieve test following the General method 2.9.12 of the *European Pharmacopeia* (*European Pharmacopeia*, 2011). The value returned is the % of particles that pass through a 0.05-mm sieve when vibrated for 10 min at speed 10 (CISA® vibrator).
- Homogeneity index (Iθ): This is calculated according to the General method 2.9.12 of the *European Pharmacopeia* (*European Pharmacopeia*, 2011).

To determine particle size by means of the sieve test, the grain size of a 100 g sample is measured by subjecting a sieve stack to vibration for

10 min at speed 10 (CISA® vibrator). The sieve sizes used are 0.355 mm, 0.212 mm, 0.100 mm and 0.05 mm. The percentage of product retained in each sieve is calculated and the amount that passes through the 0.05 mm sieve is measured. The percentage of fine particles (<50 µm) (%Pf) was calculated as described above. Note that if this percentage is higher than that calculated in the complete sieve test, it is because some of the particles adhere to the product retained in the sieves during the grain-size test, and the percentage of <50 µm particles found may be lower than the true figure. The following equation is then applied to the data obtained.

$$*I\theta = \frac{Fm}{100 + (dm - dm\text{-}1)Fm\text{-}1 + (dm+1 - dm)Fm+1 + (dm - dm\text{-}2)Fm\text{-}2 + (dm+2 - dm)Fm+2 + \ldots + (dm - dm\text{-}n)Fm\text{-}n + (dm+n - dm)Fm+n} \quad [5.1]$$

where:

$I\theta$, Relative homogeneity index. Particle-size homogeneity in the range of the fractions studied;

Fm, percentage of particles in the majority range;

Fm-1, percentage of particles in the range immediately below the majority range;

Fm+1, percentage of particles in the range immediately above the majority range;

n, order number of the fraction studied under a series, with respect to the major fraction;

dm, mean diameter of the particles in the major fraction;

dm-1, mean diameter of the particles in the fraction of the range immediately below the majority range;

dm+1, mean diameter of the particles in the fraction of the range immediately above the majority range.

5.2.2 Scientific rationale for acceptable limit values for each parameter applied to SeDeM

Having obtained the values as described above, certain limits are set (Table 5.2) on the basis of the parameters chosen and the values described in the *Handbook of Pharmaceutical Excipients* (Rowe et al., 2006), or alternatively on the basis of experimental tests.

Table 5.2 **Limit values accepted for the SeDeM Diagram parameters**

Incidence	Parameter	Acceptable range
Dimension	Bulk density	0–1 g/ml
	Tapped density	0–1 g/ml
Compressibility	Inter-particle porosity	0–1.2
	Carr index	0–50 (%)
	Cohesion index	0–200 (N)
Flowability/powder flow	Hausner ratio	3–1
	Angle of repose	50–0 (°)
	Powder flow	20–0 (s)
Lubricity/stability	Loss on drying	0–10 (%)
	Hygroscopicity	20–0 (%)
Lubricity/dosage	Particles < 50 μ	50–0 (%)
	Homogeneity index	0–2 × 10–2

The rationale to establish the limits for each parameter is:

- Da, Dc, Ie and IC are calculated from the extreme values (excluding the most extreme values) described in the *Handbook of Pharmaceutical Excipients* (Rowe et al., 2006). For the Carr Index, limits are based on references in *Tecnologia Farmaceutica* by S. Casadio (Casadio, 1972) and on monograph 2.9.36 of *European Pharmacopeia* (*European Pharmacopeia*, 2011).
- Icd. The limit is determined empirically from compression tests on many powdered substances, based on the maximum hardness obtained without producing capped or broken tablets. This hardness is then established as the maximum limit. The minimum value is '0'. This value implies that no tablets are obtained when the powders are compressed.
- IH, Powder flow, repose angle. The limits are set on the basis of the monographs described in the *Handbook of Pharmaceutical Excipients* (Rowe, 2006), and monograph 2.9.36 of *European Pharmacopeia* (*European Pharmacopeia*, 2011) or other references in *Tecnologia Farmaceutica* by S. Casadio (Casadio, 1972).
- %HR. The limits are established on the basis of the references cited elsewhere, such as *Farmacotecnia teórica y práctica* by José Helman (Helman, 1981). The optimum humidity is between 1% and 3%.

Hygroscopicity is based on the *Handbook of Pharmaceutical Excipients* (Rowe et al., 2006): based on manitol (not hygroscopic) and sorbitol (highly hygroscopic).

- Particle size. The limits are based on the literature. These sources (Rowe et al., 2006) report that rheological and compression problems occur when the percentage of fine particles in the formulation exceeds 25%. The limits for the Homogeneity index ($I\theta$) are based on the distribution of the particles of the powder (see Table 5.3, indicating the size of the sieve (in mm), average particle size in each fraction and the difference in average particle size in the fraction between 0.100 and 0.212 and the others). A value of 5 on a scale from 0 to 10 was defined as the minimum acceptable value (MAV), as follows:
  - The major fraction (Fm) corresponds to the interval from 0.100 to 0.212 mm, because it falls in the middle of the other fractions of the table. This interval is calculated as the proportion in which the powder particles are found in each fraction considered in the table (as described above). Those particles located in the major fraction (Fm) in a proportion of 60% are considered to represent the MAV of 5. The distributions of the other particles are considered to be Gaussian. The limits for the Homogeneity index are set between 0 and 0.02.

5.2.3 Conversion of the limits considered in each parameter of SeDeM into the radius (r) of the SeDeM Diagram

The numerical values of the parameters of the powder, which are obtained experimentally (v) as described above, are placed on a scale from 0 to 10,

Table 5.3 Distribution of particles in the determination of $I\theta$

Sieve (mm)	Corresponding fraction	Average of the diameter of the fraction	Corresponding diameter (dm ... dm ± n)	Dif dm with the major component
0.355–0.500	Fm + 2	427	dm + 2	271
0.212–0.355	Fm + 1	283	dm + 1	127
0.100–0.212	Fm	156	dm	0
0.050–0.100	Fm–1	75	dm–1	81
<0.050	Fm–2	25	dm–2	131

considering 5 as the MAV. The correspondence of the value of the parameters with this scale takes into account the limit values (see 5.2.2), using the factors indicated in Table 5.4. When all radius values are 10, the SeDeM Diagram takes the form of a circumscribed regular polygon, drawn by connecting all the radius values of the parameters with linear segments. Table 5.4 shows the factors used for calculating the numerical value of each parameter required for the SeDeM method. The exceptional values that appear below 1 are considered values corresponding to non-sliding products.

Initially, relative humidity was calculated based on the establishment of three intervals because the percentage relation obtained from the measurement of the humidity of the substance does not follow a linear relation with respect to the correct behavior of the dust. Humidity below 1% makes the powder too dry, and electrostatic charge is induced, which affects the rheology. Furthermore, low humidity percentages do not allow compression of the substance (moisture is necessary for compacting powders). Moreover, more than 3% moisture causes caking, in addition to favoring adhesion to punches and dyes. Consequently, it was considered that this parameter should present

Table 5.4 **Conversion of limits for each parameter into radius values (r)**

Incidence	Parameter	Limit value	Radius (r)	Factor applied to v
Dimensions	Bulk density	0–1	0–10	10v
	Tapped density	0–1	0–10	10v
Compressibility	Inter-particle porosity	0–1.2	0–10	10v/1.2
	Carr index	0–50	0–10	v/5
	Cohesion index	0–200	0–10	v/20
Flowability/ powder flow	Hausner ratio	3–1	0–10	(30 − 10v)/2
	Angle of repose	50–0	0–10	10 − (v/5)
	Powder flow	20–0	0–10	10 − (v/2)
Lubricity/ stability	Loss on drying	10–0	0–10	10-v
	Hygroscopicity	20–0	0–10	10 − (v/2)
Lubricity/ dosage	Particles < 50 μ	50–0	0–10	10 − (v/5)
	Homogeneity index	0–2 × 10–2	0–10	500v

optimal experimental values from 1% to 3% (Braidotti and Bulgarelli, 1974). Nevertheless, experience using the SeDeM Diagram has demonstrated no significant variations in the results, so the previous three intervals of relative humidity can be simplified to the calculation of the parameter, thus finally the linear criterion of treatment of results is adopted (Suñé et al., 2011).

5.2.4 Graphical representation of the SeDeM Diagram

When all radius values are 10, the SeDeM Diagram takes the form of a circumscribed regular polygon, drawn by connecting the radius values with linear segments. The results obtained from the earlier parameter calculations and conversions are represented by the radius. The figure formed indicates the characteristics of the product and of each parameter that determines whether the product is suitable for direct compression. In this case, the SeDeM Diagram is made up of 12 parameters, thus forming an irregular 12-sided polygon (Figure 5.2).

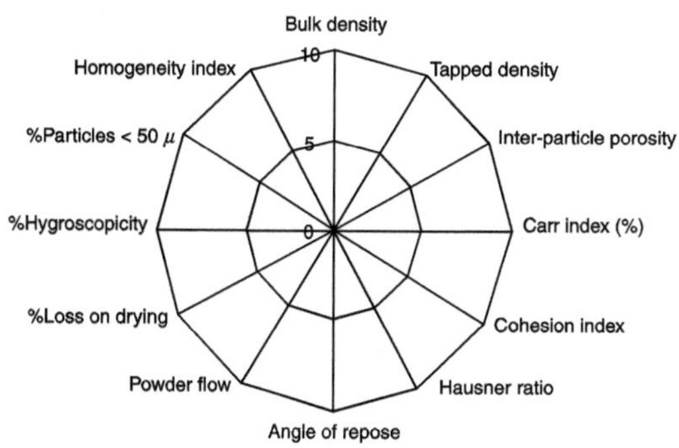

Figure 5.2 **The SeDeM Diagram with 12 parameters**

5.2.5 Acceptable limits for indexes

To determine whether the product is suitable for direct compression using a numerical method, the following indexes are calculated based on the SeDeM Diagram:

- Parameter index $IP = \dfrac{n^\circ P \geq 5}{n^\circ Pt}$ [5.2]

  where:

  n° P ≥ 5: Indicates the number of parameters whose value is equal to or higher than 5,

  n° Pt: Indicates the total number of parameters studied.

The acceptability limit would correspond to:

- Parameter profile index IPP = Average of (r) all parameters [5.3]
- Parameter profile index IPP = Average of (r) all parameters [5.4]

  Average (r) = mean value of the parameters calculated.

The acceptability limit would correspond to: IPP = media (r) = 5

- Good compressibility index $IGC = IPP \times f$ [5.5]

  $f = \text{Reliability factor} = \dfrac{\text{Polygon area}}{\text{Circle area}}$ [5.6]

The acceptability limit would correspond to: $ICG = IPP \times f = 5$. The reliability factor indicates that the inclusion of more parameters increases the reliability of the method (Figure 5.3).

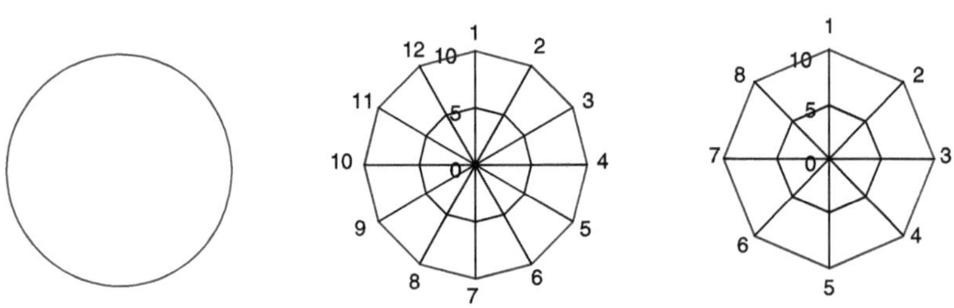

Figure 5.3 On the left, graph with ∞ parameters (maximum reliability), f = 1. In the centre, graph with 12 parameters (no. of parameters in this study), f = 0.952. On the right, graph with eight parameters (minimum reliability), f = 0.900

Published by Woodhead Publishing Limited, 2013

5.3 Practical applications of SeDeM expert system

5.3.1 Determination of suitability of an API for direct compression technology

A characterization of an active product ingredient in powder form (API CPSMD0001) is carried out using SeDeM expert system to determinate whether it is suitable for direct compression.

Twelve parameters are proposed by the SeDeM method. Thus we obtained the numerical values as given in Table 5.5 corresponding to the radius of the diagram and the values of the mean incidence. All the values in Table 5.5 are the average of two determinations. The radius values are represented in the diagram shown in Figure 5.4.

To obtain the indices of acceptance or qualification for formulation by direct compression, the formulas corresponding to the parametric

Table 5.5 **Application of the SeDeM method to API CPSMD0001 in powdered form and calculation of radius**

Incidence factor	Parameter	Symbol	Unit	Value (v)	(r)	Mean incidence
Dimension	Bulk density	Da	g/ml	0.450	4.50	5.06
	Tapped density	Dc	g/ml	0.562	5.62	
Compressibility	Inter-particle porosity	Ie	–	0.443	3.69	5.89
	Carr index	IC	%	19.929	3.99	
	Cohesion index	Icd	N	263.0	10.0	
Flowability/ powder flow	Hausner ratio	IH	–	1.249	5.84	6.53
	Angle of repose	(α)	°	17.550	6.49	
	Powder flow	t	S	5.500	7.25	
Lubricity/ stability	Loss on drying	%HR	%	1.140	5.70	6.21
	Hygroscopicity	%H	%	6.570	6.72	
Lubricity/ dosage	Particles <50 μm	%Pf	%	19.000	6.20	4.93
	Homogeneity index	$(I\theta)$		0.0073	3.65	

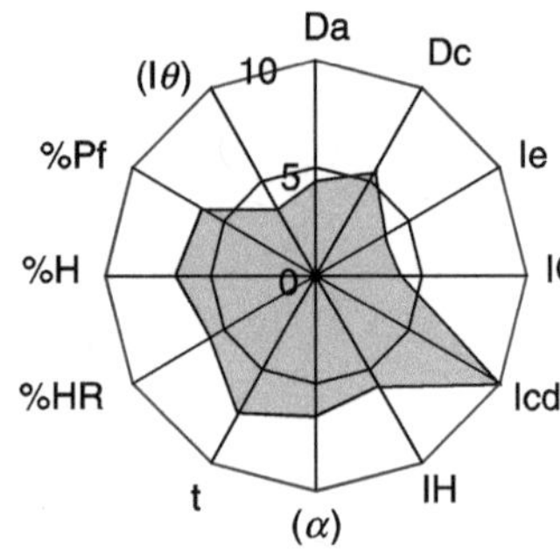

Figure 5.4 SeDeM Diagram for API CPSMD0001

index were applied from the numerical results of the radius as shown in Table 5.5. The results of the acceptance indices are shown in Table 5.6.

On the basis of the results of the radius corresponding to the SeDeM Diagram, the parametric profile was > 5. This value implies that the API CPSMD0001 is suitable for direct compression. However, in order to discern the appropriateness of this substance for this formulation technology, we analyzed the five groups of individual factors classified by the type of incidence in this compression.

In the case study above, only the parameters involved in the general factor of denominated incidence lubricity/dosage presented values below 5 (median = 4.93). This finding implies deficient rheological qualities focused on particle form and distribution, but as in this specific case the value is near to 5, then it is not a big negative impact during experimentation at the lab. The homogeneity index and distribution of the particles is expected to be improved when mixed with an appropriate excipient which would make up for this lower value. These deficiencies are reflected graphically in the SeDeM Diagram, which shows that a large shaded area (activity area) (the greater the shaded area, the more suitable the

Table 5.6 SeDeM acceptance index for API CPSMD0001

Parameter index	0.67
Parametric profile index (mean r of all parameters)	5.80
Good compression index (IGC)	5.52

Published by Woodhead Publishing Limited, 2013

characteristics for direct compression) is present for most of the parameters. Thus, it indicates that the powder is suitable for direct compression.

In this regard, the SeDeM method (Table 5.5) yielded the following information for API CPSMD0001: it is a dusty substance with correct dimensional characteristics (Da and Dc); it shows moderately acceptable compressibility (IE, IC, Icd), which can be improved with the addition of excipients of direct compression; it shows very good fluidity/flowability (IH, α, t″) and, as the values are very close to 5, it could be said that this is the correct lubrication/dosage (%Pf, Iθ). Given these characteristics, API CPSMD0001 is suitable for compression with the addition of standardized formula of lubricant.

The results given in this example demonstrate that the SeDeM method is reliable in establishing whether powdered substances have suitable profiles to be subjected to direct compression. Consequently, SeDeM is a tool that will contribute to preformulation studies of medicines and help to define the manufacturing technology required. Indeed, the application of the SeDeM Diagram allows determination of the direct compression behavior of a powdered substance from the index of parametric profile (IPP) and the index of good compression (IGC), in such a way that an IPP and an IGC equal to or over 5 indicate that the powder displays characteristics that make it suitable for direct compression, adding only a small amount of lubricant (3.5% of the magnesium stearate, talc and Aerosil® 200). Also, with IPP and IGC values between 3 and 5, the substance will require a direct compression diluent excipient suitable for direct compression. In addition, it is deduced that techniques other than direct compression (wet granulation or dry granulation) will be required for API with IPP and IGC values below 3.

Use of the SeDeM expert system is not restricted to active products as it can also be used with new or known excipients or mixtures of final blends to assess their suitability for application as adjuvants in direct compression (it is very important to do this when a change is made in supplier of an excipient). Thus, knowledge of excipient profiles, with their corresponding parameters, will allow identification of the most suitable excipient to correct the characteristics of API registering values under 5.

Of note, the greater the number of parameters selected, the greater the reliability of the method, in such a way that to obtain a reliability of 100%, the number of parameters applied would have to be infinite (reliability factor = 1). The number of parameters could be extended using additional complementary ones, such as the true density, the index of porosity, the electrostatic charge, the specific surface, the adsorption power, % of lubrication, % friability, and the index of elasticity. However, although improving the reliability of the method, the inclusion of further parameters would be to the detriment of its simplicity and rapidity, as complementary parameters are difficult to apply.

5.3.2 Application of SeDeM to determine the amount of excipient required for compression of an API that is not suited to direct compression

Experimental determination of the parameters of the SeDeM method for a range of API and excipients allows definition of their corresponding compressibility profiles and their subsequent mathematical treatment and graphical expression (SeDeM Diagram). Various excipient diluents can be analyzed to determine whether a substance is appropriate for direct compression, and the optimal proportion of excipient required for designing a suitable formulation for direct compression based on the SeDeM characteristics of the API (Suñé et al., 2008a). Thus, the SeDeM method is a valid tool with which to design the formulation of tablets by direct compression.

As previously explained, the SeDeM expert system provides information about whether a powdered substance is appropriate for use to obtain tablets by direct compression. When this is not possible, as the IGC is below 5, this innovative expert system provides a mathematical formula allowing determination of the composition of the final formulation and the percentage required of each component, meaning that this expert system provides qualitative and quantitative design for future successful formulations. The mathematical equation can be applied to five parameters (dimension, compressibility, flowability/powder flow, lubricity/stability, lubricity/dosage) considered deficient by the SeDeM system. The mathematical equation is applied to correct a deficient parameter of the API. The equation proposed (Eq. 5.7) allows calculation of the amount of excipient required to compress the API on the basis of the SeDeM radius considered minimum (5) for each parameter of incidence that allows correct compression.

$$CP = 100 - \left(\frac{RE - R}{RE - RP} \times 100 \right) \qquad [5.7]$$

Published by Woodhead Publishing Limited, 2013

where:

CP = % of the corrective excipient,

RE = mean-incidence radius value (compressibility) of the corrective excipient,

R = mean-incidence radius value to be obtained in the blend,

RP = mean-incidence radius value (compressibility) of the API to be corrected.

The unknown values are replaced by those calculated required for each substance in order to obtain R = 5 (5 is the minimum value considered necessary to achieve satisfactory compression). For example, if a deficient compressibility parameter for an API requires correction, Eq. 5.7 is applied by replacing the terms RE and RP with the values calculated for each substance with the purpose of obtaining R = 5, thus obtaining the optimal excipient to design a first drug formulation and the maximum amount required for a comprehensive understanding of the proposed formula. From this first formulation, research can get under way for the final optimization of the formulation, taking into consideration the biopharmaceutical characteristics required in the final tablet (disintegration, dissolution, etc). We thus present a method to establish details of the formulation of a given drug by direct compression. This strategy is summarized in Figure 5.5.

Practical application of the mathematical equation to calculate the amount of excipient required for a deficient API to be subjected to direct compression technology

According to Figure 5.5, when an API requires an appropriate formula for direct compression, it must be characterized following the SeDeM Diagram. Furthermore, a series of excipients used for direct compression are also characterized using the diagram. If the API has deficient dimension parameters (< 5), it is mixed with an excipient with a satisfactory dimension parameter (> 5), thereby correcting the deficiency when they are mixed in the final blend. The excipient required in the smallest amount to correct this parameter should be used, as this results in tablets of an appropriate weight. The amount of excipient is determined by the mathematical equation provided by the SeDeM system (Eq. 5.1).

Here we describe an example using an API IBUSDM0001 and four diluents and one co-processed excipient used for direct compression. The

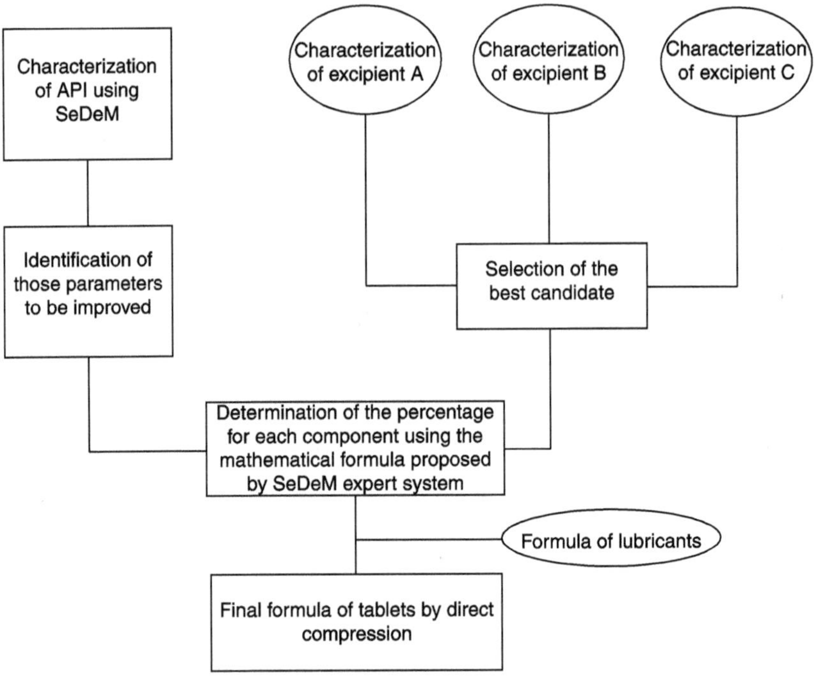

Figure 5.5 Determination using the SeDeM expert system of the percentage of each component required in the final formulation of a tablet by direct compression

corresponding parameters and the radius mean values obtained with samples of this substance are shown in Table 5.7, and the parameters and the radius mean values of six excipient diluents used in direct compression are shown in Table 5.8 (Suñé et al., 2008a).

The SeDeM Diagram for API IBUSDM0001 (Figure 5.6, Table 5.7) indicates that this substance has deficient dimension ($r = 3.39$), compressibility ($r = 4.46$) and flowability/powder flow ($r = 1.90$) parameters. Consequently, to apply direct compression to API IBUSDM0001, formulation with an excipient is required to enhance the compressibility factor. This excipient is identified by the SeDeM system.

In order to select the excipient and the concentration used to correct the deficiencies and, in particular, the compressibility, we applied the mathematical equation of SeDeM expert system (Eq. 5.7): replacing the unknowns (RE and RP) with the values calculated for each substance (RE for excipients and RP for API) with the aim of obtaining $R = 5$. Results are shown in Table 5.9.

Published by Woodhead Publishing Limited, 2013

Table 5.7 **Parameters, mean incidence and parametric index for IBUSDM0001**

Incidence factor	Parameter	Symbol	Unit	Value (v)	(r)	Mean incidence
Dimension	Bulk density	Da	g/ml	0.296	2.96	3.39
	Tapped density	Dc	g/ml	0.381	3.81	
Compressibility	Inter-particle porosity	Ie	–	0.754	6.28	4.46
	Carr index	IC	%	22.310	4.46	
	Cohesion index	Icd	N	52.600	2.63	
Flowability/ powder flow	Hausner ratio	IH	–	1.287	5.71	1.90
	Angle of repose	(α)	°	–	0.00	
	Powder flow	t	s	–	0.00	
Lubricity/ stability	Loss on drying	%HR	%	0.960	4.80	7.40
	Hygroscopicity	%H	%	0.00	10.0	
Lubricity/ dosage	Particles <50 µm	%Pf	%	16.500	6.70	7.93
	Homogeneity index	$(I\theta)$		0.0183	9.15	
Parameter index				0.42		
Parametric profile index (mean r of all parameters)				4.71		
Good compression index (IGC)				4.48		

Avicel® PH102 or Avicel® 200 were the most suitable excipients to correct the deficit (dimension) of API IBUSDM0001 with the lowest concentration (39.00% in both cases, Table 5.9).

To better understand the SeDeM system, the graphical representations of the profiles of the API and the excipient can be superposed. Figure 5.7 shows how the deficiencies of an API would be compensated when formulated. The dashed line corresponds to the excipient that theoretically provides the final mixture with the characteristics to be compressed. In this way, the information provided by the SeDeM system allows the formulator to start working with excipients that have a high probability of providing a suitable formulation, thus reducing the lead time of the formulation.

Table 5.8 Radius parameters, mean incidence and parametric index for excipients direct compression

	Parameters (radius)												Factor					INDEX
Excipient	Da	Dc	Ie	IC	Icd	IH	A	t"	%HR	%H	%pf	(Iθ)	Dimension	Compressibility	Flowability/powder flow	Lubricity/stability	Lubricity/dosage	IGC
Avicel® PH102 Lot 7201C	3.73	5.05	5.83	5.22	10.00	5.49	3.90	0.00	2.76	8.48	4.48	3.75	4.39	7.02	3.13	5.62	4.12	**4.66**
Avicel® 200 Lot M343C	3.88	4.91	4.49	4.18	10.00	5.79	6.30	6.61	4.75	7.47	8.31	2.10	4.39	6.22	6.23	6.11	5.20	**5.46**
Vivapur® 12 Lot 6601260202	3.62	5.38	7.53	6.54	10.00	5.05	4.47	7.00	3.89	6.19	5.30	2.70	4.50	8.02	5.51	5.04	4.00	**5.37**
Microcel® MC 250 Lot 1960/4	4.06	5.62	5.70	5.55	10.00	5.39	4.87	8.50	2.97	8.48	6.80	1.75	4.84	7.08	6.25	5.73	4.28	**5.53**
Pharmaburst® C1 Lot 04K111	4.50	5.62	3.69	3.99	10.00	5.84	6.49	7.25	5.70	6.72	6.20	3.65	5.06	5.89	6.53	6.21	4.93	**5.53**

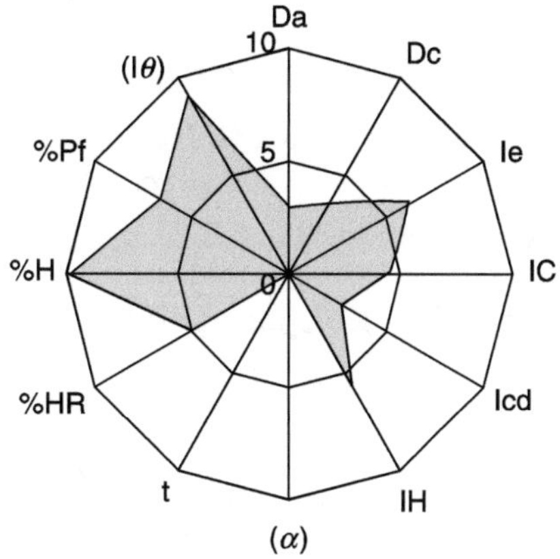

Figure 5.6 SeDeM Diagram for API IBUSDM0001

Table 5.9 Amount of excipient required to be mixed with the API to obtain a dimension factor equal to 5

Excipient	Avicel® PH102	Avicel® 200	Vivapur® 12	Microcel® MC 250	Pharmaburst® C1
RE	4.395	4.39	4.50	4.84	5.06
RP (API)	3.39	3.39	3.39	3.39	3.39
R	5.00	5.00	5.00	5.00	5.00
% excipient	39.00	39.00	54.95	88.97	96.41

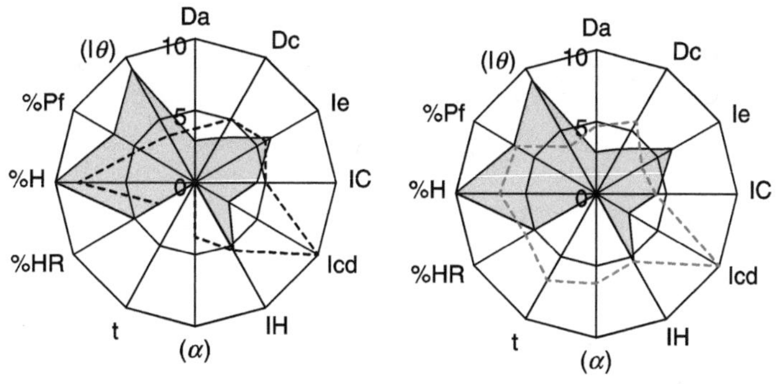

Figure 5.7 Dashed line indicates the excipient that provides suitable dimension to the final mixture with the API (in shadow). Two excipients are shown, both covering the deficiencies of the API

5.3.3 Application of the SeDeM system to quality control of batches of a single API or excipient used for direct compression

The SeDeM system is also appropriate for verification of the reproducibility of manufacturing standards between batches of the same powdered raw material (API or excipient). Indeed, superposing the SeDeM Diagrams of each batch, the degree of similarity or difference between the same API on the basis of the established parameters can determine its appropriateness for compression.

The SeDeM method is also a useful tool for the study of the reproducibility of a manufacturing method used for a powdered substance and, thus of the validation of systematic variation during elaboration. A manufacturing process gives rise to variations in the final product and these variations must fall within limits or established specifications. By applying the SeDeM method to study reproducibility between batches of the same API or excipient, specifications in the different parameters can be established to ensure the same quality of the product regardless of the batch analyzed. In addition, these specifications must be used for the establishment of particular limits for quality control applications. To achieve this goal it is necessary to study the parameters of the SeDeM Diagram, applying the same statistic analyses required to establish the pharmacotechnical equivalence between batches. Correct reproducibility between batches will ensure the reproducibility and the quality of the tablets formulated with this API or excipient, regardless of the batch used.

Figure 5.8 shows the SeDeM Diagrams of two batches from the same API of ibuprofen. In this case the mark and the indices were very similar. This control has the advantage that the method has the capacity to detect variations in particle size between batches of the product. This capacity thus contributes to the formulation of the pharmaceutical forms and their correct dissolution. In addition, this differentiation allows easy analysis when a change of supplier is proposed.

5.3.4 Application of the SeDeM method to differentiate the excipient in the same chemical family

The SeDeM system also allows differentiation between excipients of the same chemical family that differ in physical characteristics (see Figure 5.9). These characteristics will determine their use in a formulation for direct

Published by Woodhead Publishing Limited, 2013

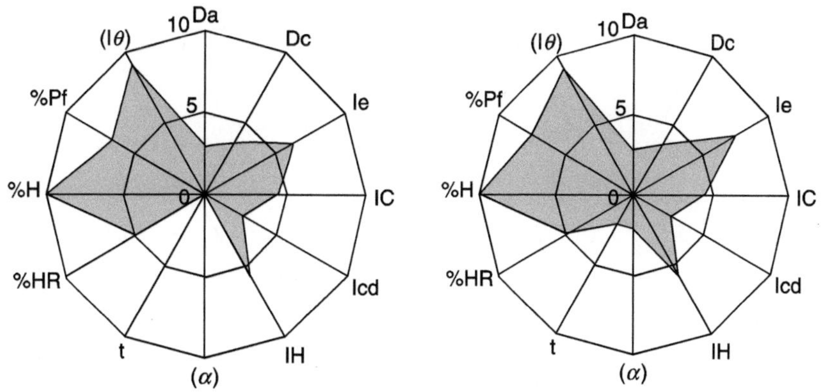

Figure 5.8 SeDeM Diagram of two batches of ibuprofen

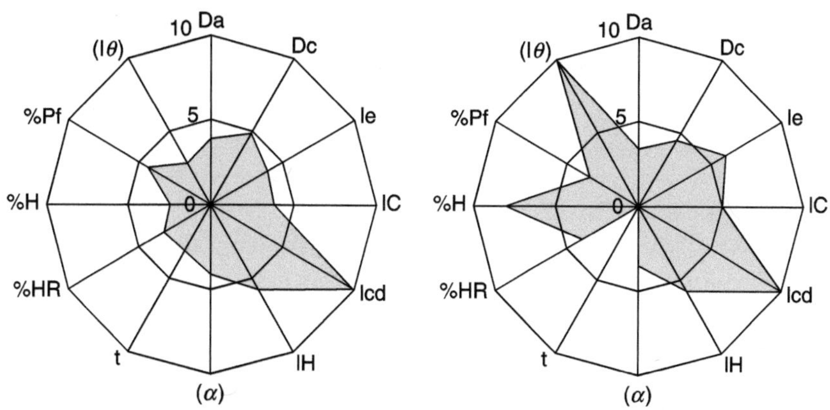

Figure 5.9 SeDeM Diagram for two kinds of Avicel. Left: Avicel PH102 IGC = 4.19. Right: Avicel PH101 IGC = 5.01

compression of a given API. The SeDeM expert system can help to differentiate raw material from different suppliers, which permits evaluation of different suppliers assuring successful implementation in the commercial scale batches and successful validation.

5.3.5 Application of the SeDeM Diagram to differentiate excipients of the same functional type

The SeDeM expert system also allows differentiation between excipients of the same functional type, for example disintegrant sodium

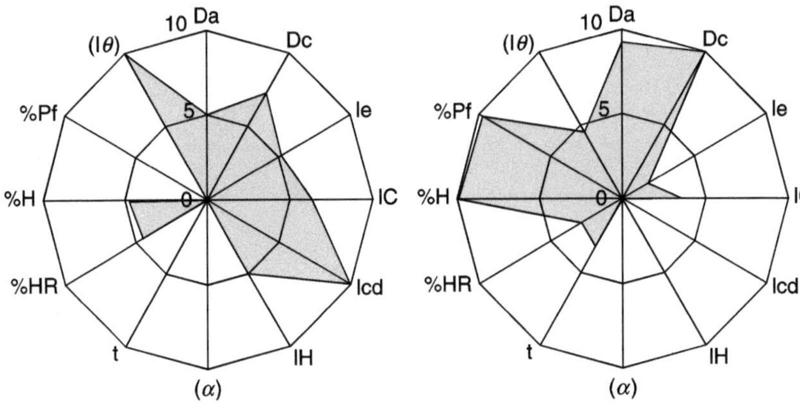

Figure 5.10 **SeDeM diagram for disintegrant excipients. Left: Sodium crosscarmellose (Nymcel ZSD16 IGC = 4.60). Right: Sodium starch glicolate (Brenncel-DIS. IGC = 4.90)**

crosscarmellose and sodium starch glicolate (Figure 5.10). The SeDeM characterization provides the information required to predict the difficulties encountered for compression.

By quantifying the 12 tests provided by the system, deficient values for compression can be defined; on the basis of these values, an adequate (applying the same SeDeM Diagram) substance can be selected to improve the compressibility in the final mixture of the disintegrants and the API. Figure 5.10 shows the characterization of two disintegrants using the SeDeM technique, where the differences between them in relation to their major or minor compression capacity are shown, although all are used because of their disintegrant function (Aguilar et al., 2009).

5.4 Conclusions

Herein, we describe an original methodology for preformulation and powder substance characterization. This method facilitates studies on design and development of formulations for the production of tablets by direct compression.

The SeDeM expert system is a useful tool because, in addition to considering the type of components, it also provides recommendations on intrinsic properties, such as the characteristics and morphology of particles. We propose that given the accuracy of the information provided

Published by Woodhead Publishing Limited, 2013

by this system, formulations will have a higher probability of being successfully compressed.

This method characterizes the individual components of a formulation and applies a mathematical analysis to determine the exact amount of each in the final formulation.

The formulation provided will be valid for direct compression. This manufacturing procedure offers many advantages from a production perspective. In addition to being faster than other techniques, it is straightforward as it reduces the number of steps during the manufacturing process.

In addition, SeDeM has the advantage of providing formulation with the lowest amount of excipients as it combines the API with only one excipient and the standard formula of lubricants, thus avoiding use of unnecessary excipients, such as diluents, binders and agglutinants.

The information given by the SeDeM system contributes to Quality by Design development. Consequently, this innovative tool is consistent with the current requirements of regulatory health authorities such as the FDA and ICH.

SedeM expert system is a tool which can be used for the design of solid formulations avoiding unnecessary trials, but also can be used for selection of new excipients or new suppliers in existing and commercial formulations.

SeDeM expert system permits identification of differences in excipients of the same chemical families but from different suppliers.

SeDeM expert system permits evaluation of commercial formulations and provides information for optimization, also for transfer of product in finished products from different manufacturing sizes.

5.5 References

Aguilar-Díaz JE, García-Montoya E, Pérez-Lozano P, Suñé-Negre JM, Miñarro M and Ticó JR. (2009) The use of the SeDeM Diagram expert system to determine the suitability of diluents-disintegrants for direct compression and their use in formulation of ODT. *Eur J Pharm Biopharm*, 73, 414–23, ISSN: 0939-6411.

Braidotti L and Bulgarelli D. (1974) *Tecnica Farmaceutica.* (1ª ed), Lleditrice Scientifica LG Guadagni, Milan.

Brittain, H.G. (1997). On the Physical Characterization of Pharmaceutical Solids. *Pharm Techn*, 1, 100–6, ISSN: 1543-2521.

Casadio S. (1972) *Tecnologia Farmaceutica.* (2ª ed), Cisalpino-Goliardica Ed., Milan Córdoba Borrego, M.; Moreno Cerezo, J.M.; Córdoba Díaz, M.

Córdoba Díaz, D. (1996). Preformulación y desarrollo galénico de nuevas formulaciones por compresión directa con agentes hidrotrópicos. *Inf Farm*, 4, 65–70, ISSN: 0213-5574.

European Pharmacopeia. (2011) (7th ed), Council of Europe, ISBN: 978-92-871-6053-9, Strasbourg.

Font Quer P. (1962) *Medicamenta: guía teórico práctica para farmacéuticos y médicos*. (6th ed), Labor Ed., Barcelona (1), 340–1.

García-Montoya E, Suñé-Negre JM, Pérez-Lozano P, Miñarro Carmona M and Ticó Grau JR. (2010) Metodología de preformulación galénica para la caracterización de sustancias en relación a su viabilidad para la compresión: Diagrama SeDeM. *Farmespaña Industrial*, enero/febrero, 58–62, ISSN: 1699-4205.

Helman J. (1981) *Farmacotecnia teórica y práctica*. Compañía Internacional Continental. ISBN: 950-06-5081-9, Méjico 6: 1721.

Muñoz Ruíz A, Muñoz Muñoz N, Monedero Perales MC, Velasco Antequera MV and Jiménez Castellanos Ballesteros MR. (1993) Determinación de la fluidez de sólidos a granel. Métodos (I). *Ind Farm*, 1, 49–55, ISSN: 0213-5574.

Pérez Lozano P, Suñé Negre JM, Miñarro M, Roig M, Fuster R, et al. (2006) A new expert system (SeDeM Diagram) for control batch powder formulation and preformulation drug products. *Eur J Pharm Biopharm*, 64, 351–9, ISSN: 0939-6411.

Rowe RC, Sheskey PJ and Owen SC. (2006) *Handbook of Pharmaceutical Excipients* (5th ed), American Pharmaceutical Association. Pharmaceutical Press, ISBN: 0-85369-381-1, London.

Rubinstein MH. (1993) *Pharmaceutical Technology (Tabletting Technology)*. (1st Ed), SA de Ediciones, ISBN:978-0136629580, Madrid.

Suñé Negre JM, Pérez Lozano P, Miñarro M, Roig M, Fuster R, et al. (2005) Nueva metodología de preformulación galénica para la caracterización de sustancias en relación a su viabilidad para la compresión: Método SeDeM. *Cienc Tecnol Pharm*, 15, 3, 125–36, ISSN:1575-3409.

Suñé Negre JM, Pérez Lozano P, Miñarro M, Roig M, Fuster R, et al. (2008a) Characterization of powders to preformulation studies with a new expert system (SeDeM diagram). *Proceedings of 6th World Meeting on Pharmaceutics, Biopharmaceutics and Pharmaceutical Technology*, Barcelona, April 2008.

Suñé Negre JM, Pérez Lozano P, Miñarro M, Roig M, Fuster R, et al. (2008b) Application of the SeDeM Diagram and a new mathematical equation in the design of direct compression tablet formulation. *Eur J Pharm Biopharm*, 69, 1029–39, ISSN: 0939-6411.

Suñé Negre JM, Roig-Carreras M, Fuster-Garcia R, Hernández-Pérez C, Ruhí-Rovira R, et al. (2011a). Optimization of parameters of the SeDeM Diagram Expert System: Hausner ratio (HI) and relative humidity (%HR). *Eur J Pharm Biopharm*, 79, 464–72. ISSN: 0939-6411.

Suñé Negre JM, Roig-Carreras M, Fuster-Garcia R, Hernández-Pérez C, Ruhí-Rovira R, et al. (2011b) SeDeM diagram: A new expert system for the formula. In: Petrica Vizureanu (Ed.), *Expert Systems for human, materials and automation*. Rijeka (Croacia): Intech Open Access Publisher. ISBN 978-953-307-334-7, 17–34.

Published by Woodhead Publishing Limited, 2013

Torres Suárez AI and Camacho Sánchez MA. (1991) Planteamiento de un programa de preformulación y formulación de comprimidos. *Ind Farm*, 2, 85–92, ISSN: 0213-5574.

Wong LW and Pilpel N. (1990) The effect of particle shape on the mechanical properties of powders. *Int J Pharm*, 59, 145–54, ISSN: 0378-5173.

6

New SeDeM-ODT expert system: an expert system for formulation of orodispersible tablets obtained by direct compression

Johnny Edward Aguilar, Encarna García Montoya, Pilar Pérez Lozano, Josep M. Suñe Negre, Montserrat Miñarro Carmona and José Ramón Ticó Grau, University of Barcelona, Spain

DOI: 10.1533/9781908818508.137

Abstract: SeDeM-ODT expert system is an innovative tool for predicting whether or not an excipient or mixture of powders containing API and excipients is suitable to obtain a buccal dispersible tablet by direct compression. This preformulation tool identifies the index of good compressibility and orodispersibility (IGCB index), unique to each powder or mixture of powders and based on the SeDeM expert system. The IGCB index indicates if a mixture of powder can be compressed by direct compression and, at the same time, indicates if the resulting tablets would be suitable for use as orodispersible tablets. SeDeM ODT and SeDeM expert systems are excellent tools to optimize tablet fabrication. These tools allow a reduction in the number of unnecessary experiments in the laboratory because they provide information on rheology, compactibility properties, etc. In addition, these tools also provide information that can be used for a better understanding of the formulation design.

Key words: IGCB, disintegrant, SeDeM-ODT, preformulation, bucodispersible tablets, direct compression, ODT.

6.1 Introduction

Orally disintegrating tablets are solid dosage forms which are formulated with the aim of improving the disintegrating and dissolution rates of a pharmaceutical product. In order to achieve rapid disintegration rates, the tablet formulation must provide high porosity, low density and a low hardness (Berthoumieu et al., 2010; Bandari et al., 2008). This dosage form is chosen when the patient has difficulty in swallowing (Lindgren et al., 1993), and is also suitable for use in geriatric and pediatric patients, or for those who suffer from conditions such as dysphagia (Sastry et al., 2000). Sometimes there are formulations which were initially formulated in another type of dosage form but were then changed into oral disintegrating tablets because of the benefits offered by such formulations. Orally disintegrating tablets are also called orodispersible tablets, quick disintegrating tablets, mouth dissolving tablets, fast disintegrating tablets, fast dissolving tablets, rapid dissolving tablets, porous tablets, and rapimelts (Fu et al., 2004; Fernandes et al., 2009). However, of all the above terms, the *United States Pharmacopoeia* (USP) approved these dosage forms as orally disintegrating tablets or ODTs (*Guidance for Industry: Orally Disintegrating Tablets*, 2008). Recently, the *European Pharmacopoeia* 7th ed has used the term orodispersible tablet for tablets that disperse inside the mouth readily and within 3 min before swallowing (*European Pharmacopoeia*, 2011a). The United States Food and Drug Administration (FDA) defined ODT as 'a solid dosage form containing a medicinal substance or active ingredient which disintegrates rapidly usually within a matter of seconds when placed upon the tongue' (*Guidance for Industry: Orally Disintegrating Tablets*, 2008).

Orally disintegrating tablets offer all the advantages of solid and liquid dosage forms together with special advantages, which include (Seager, 1998; Habib et al., 2000; Dobetti, 2003; Brown, 2003):

- As ODT are unit solid dosage forms, they provide good stability, accurate dosing, easy manufacturing, small packaging size, and they are easily handled by patients (Seager, 1998; Habib et al., 2000; Dobetti, 2003; Brown, 2003).
- ODT present no risk of obstruction of the gastrointestinal tract, which is beneficial for patients who do not have access to water such as patients who are traveling.
- Easy administration for pediatric, geriatric, and inpatients (especially for mentally retarded and psychiatric patients).

Published by Woodhead Publishing Limited, 2013

- The rapid disintegration of the resulting tablets results in a quick dissolution of the drug and fast absorption that provide a rapid onset of action (Behnke et al., 2003).
- The bioavailability of drugs that are absorbed in the mouth, pharynx, and esophagus is increased (Jaccard and Leyder, 1985; Dollo et al., 1999; Gafitanu et al., 1991).
- Pregastric absorption of drugs avoids hepatic metabolism, which reduces the dose and increase the bioavailability of the drug (Clarke et al., 2003).

Various processes are employed to obtain ODT tablets such as lyophilization, molding, cotton candy process, spray drying, mass extrusion, compaction, and other patented technologies (Bandari et al., 2008). These technologies require specific equipments and expensive processes compared with the standard manufacturing process; also some additional special packaging is required. When possible, the most interesting way for the pharmaceutical industry to obtain orodispersible tablets is by direct compression because the process is shorter and the technology is cheaper, as no high technology machines are required because the process consists of blending raw materials.

For these reasons, the work described in this chapter focused on developing an expert system to obtain useful information for development of orodispersible tablets by direct compression. The SeDeM-ODT expert system predicts the aptitude of a mixture of powder to produce conventional tablets by direct compression (Aguilar et al., 2012). In addition, this tool also provides information about the strengths and weaknesses of the powder or mixture of powders. This information can be used to optimize the initial formulation or ultimately reveal that it is not necessary to invest additional time in development and optimization of the formulation (Suñé et al., 2005; Pérez et al., 2006; Suñé et al., 2008; Aguilar et al., 2009; García et al., 2010; Suñé et al., 2011).

This expert system is an improvement on traditional development (see Figure 6.1), as it is more accurate and avoids unnecessary trials, because it provides an ODT formulation based on both primary laboratory tests and mathematical calculations. SeDeM-ODT not only takes into account the type of components, but also provides a recommendation based on their intrinsic properties such as the inherent characteristics and morphology of the particles, therefore the proposed formulation will have a high probability of being successfully compressed and having fast disintegration. Additionally, SeDeM-ODT can provide useful information for use in direct compression, reducing the number of required steps during the development process (e.g. avoiding granulation) (Aguilar et al., 2012).

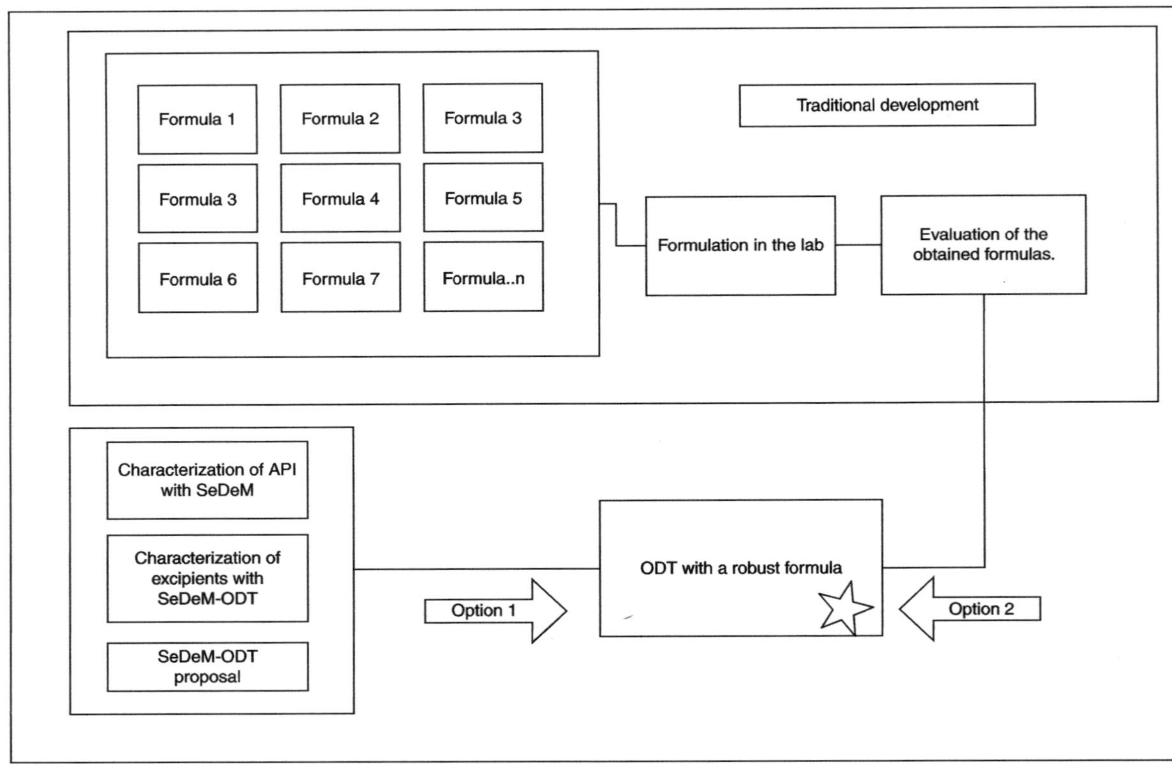

Figure 6.1 Traditional development of ODT against SeDeM-ODT expert system

In addition, the expert system has the advantage of optimizing the number of excipients in the formulations. It can provide formulations with only one excipient to be combined with the API and the standard formulation of lubricants, avoiding other unnecessary excipients, for example diluents (Aguilar et al., 2012).

The resulting information about the formulation can be used in the final analysis for better process understanding when Quality by Design development is being carried out, therefore this innovative tool is aligned with the actual requirement of the regulatory health authorities such as FDA and ICH (Aguilar et al., 2012).

6.2 Characterization of powders using the SeDeM-ODT method

The new expert system SeDeM-ODT helps to calculate the index of good compressibility and bucodispersibility (IGCB) for powdered substances. A value of ≥5 indicates that a powder could be compressed by direct compression and that the resulting tablet would have good bucodispersible properties (see Figure 6.2).

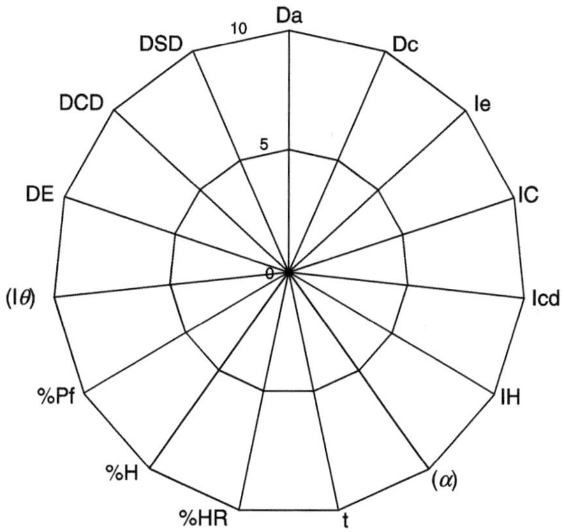

Figure 6.2 Diagram of SeDeM-ODT

The SeDeM-ODT methodology is composed of six factors, which come from 15 main parameters. Five of these factors are identical to those in the SeDeM expert system proposed by Suñe et al. (Aguilar et al., 2012; Suñé et al., 2005; Pérez et al., 2006; Suñé et al., 2008; Aguilar et al., 2009; García et al., 2010; Suñé et al., 2011). The additional parameter is the disgregability factor (see Tables 6.1, 6.2 and 6.3 and Figure 6.2).

Calculation of the five factors (dimensions, compressibility, flowability/powder flow, lubricity/stability, lubricity/dosage) from the previous

Table 6.1 Parameter and equations used for SeDeM-ODT expert system

Factor/incidence	Parameter	Symbol	Unit	Equation
Dimension	Bulk	Da	g/ml	$Da = P/V_a$
	Tapped density	Dc	g/ml	$Dc = P/V_c$
Compressibility	Inter-particle porosity	Ie	–	Ie = Dc – Da/Dc x Da
	Carr index	IC	%	IC = Dc – Da x 100/Dc
	Cohesion index*	Icd	N	Experimental
Flowability/ powder flow	Hausner ratio	IH	–	IH = Dc/Da
	Angle of repose	(α)	°	tg α = h/r
	Powder flow	t"	s	Experimental
Lubricity/stability	Loss on drying	%HR	%	Experimental
	Hygroscopicity	%H	%	Experimental
Lubricity/dosage	Particles <50	%Pf	%	Experimental
	Homogeneity index†	($I\theta$)	–	*$I\theta$ = Fm + Δ Fmn/100
Disgregability	Effervescence	DE	min	Experimental‡
	Disintegration with disc	DCD	min	Experimental‡
	Disintegration without disc	DSD	min	Experimental‡

*Hardness (N) of the tablets obtained with the product in question, alone or blended with lubricants if highly abrasive.

† Determine particle size. In accordance with the percentages of the different particle size fractions.

‡ See Tables 6.2 and 6.3.

Published by Woodhead Publishing Limited, 2013

Table 6.2 **Conversion of limits required for disgregability factor into radio values (v)**

Factor	Parameter	Limit value v (min)	Radius	Factor applied to v
Disgregability	Effervescence	0–5	10–0	See Table 6.3
	Disintegration time with disc (DCD)	0–3	10–0	
	Disintegration time without disc (DSD)	0–3	10–0	

Table 6.3 **Calculations to obtain radio value**

Description	Effervescence	DCD	DSD
Experimental range expressed in min	0–5	0–3	0–3
Range of the radio	10–0	10–0	10–0
r=formula to obtain radio (X=experimental value)	(5-X)*2	(3-X)*3.333	(3-X)*3.333

DCD, disintegration time with disc; DSD, disintegration time without disc.

SeDeM tool is based on experimental study and quantitative determination of the characterization parameters of substances in powder form that provide the necessary information about the suitability of these substances for obtaining tablets by direct compression technology. The parameters are as follows: bulk density (Da), tapped density (Dc), inter-particle porosity (Ie), Carr index (IC), cohesion index (Icd), Hausner ratio (IH), angle of repose (α), powder flow (t"), loss on drying (%HR), hygroscopicity (%H), particle size (%Pf) and homogeneity index ($I\theta$). These parameters are determined by means of the SeDeM Diagram method, based on known equations duly validated and reproducible experimental tests (Aguilar et al., 2012; Suñé et al., 2005; Pérez et al., 2006; Suñé et al., 2008; Aguilar et al., 2009; García et al., 2010; Suñé et al., 2011).

SeDeM-ODT includes a new factor: disgregability. The scientific rationale for the disgregability parameter is based on three parameters that combine to give an idea of the disintegration per se of the excipient.

Following the previous methodology, we chose three pharmacopoeia tests: effervescence (disintegration for effervescent tablets), disintegration with disc and disintegration without disc.

6.2.1 Effervescence test

According to Monograph 701 *USP32–NF27* (USP 32, 2009b) and *European Pharmacopeia* <0478> 7th ed (*European Pharmacopeia*, 2011a), one tablet is placed in a vessel containing 200 ml of purified water at 15–25°C and it is observed whether the tablet is dissolved or dispersed in the water so that no agglomerates of particles remain within 5 min. It is clear that this test is not specific for bucodispersible tablets, but it is a good indicator of the behavior of a tablet when it is bucodispersible; if a tablet disaggregates in less than 5 min, there is a high probability this is a bucodispersible tablet. Additionally, this test is interesting because the medium is water which has a pH similar to saliva. According to Tables 6.2 and 6.3, the experimental values obtained will be converted into a radius which has a maximum value when the disintegration is faster than 1 min, and the model will assign a value of 0 when the tablet does not disintegrate in a time less than or equal to 5 min.

6.2.2 Disintegration time with disc

According to Monograph 701 *USP32–NF27* (USP 32, 2009a) and *European Pharmacopeia* 7th ed (*European Pharmacopeia*, 2011b), the specification is ≤3 min. The specific technique is disintegration time without disc, but this test is also included as it simulates a mechanical action inside of the mouth which improves the disintegration of the tablets. According to Tables 6.2 and 6.3, the experimental values obtained in this test are converted into a radius which follows a linear model which is higher when the tablet disintegrates fast. In the case of tablets which do not disintegrate in time below or equal to 3 min, a 0 value is assigned.

6.2.3 Disintegration time without disc

According to Monograph 701 *USP32–NF27* (USP 32, 2009b) and *European Pharmacopeia* 7th ed (*European Pharmacopeia*, 2011b), the specification is ≤3 min. This is a specific technique for evaluation of bucodispersible tablets. According to Tables 6.2 and 6.3, the experimental values obtained in this test are converted into radiuses that follow a linear model which is higher when disintegration is faster. For tablets that do not disintegrate in a period of time below or equal to 3 min, a 0 value is given.

6.3 Determination of the IGCB

The index was developed based on the fact that if all radius values are 10, the IGCB Diagram makes a shape of a circumscribed regular polygon, drawn by connecting the radius values with linear segments. The figure formed indicates the characteristics of the product and each parameter that determine whether or not the product is suitable for use as bucodispersable tablets, because of its good properties for compression and good disintegration characteristics. In this special case the IGCB diagram is made up of 15 factors, which would form an irregular 15-sided polygon (Figure 6.1). The method also gives a numerical index to express whether the powdered substance could be used to form bucodispersable tablets. Three indexes must be calculated in a numerical form: the parameter index (IP) (Eq. 6.1), the parameter profile index (IPP) (Eq. 6.2) and the index of good compressibility and bucodispersability (IGCB) (Eq. 6.3).

$$\text{Parameter index (IP)} = \frac{\text{N°P} \geq 5}{\text{N°Pt}} \qquad [6.1]$$

N° P ≥ 5 = Number of parameters with value ≥ 5.

N° Pt = Total number of studied parameters.

The acceptability limit would correspond to: IP ≥ 0.5

$$\text{Parameter profile index (IPP)} = \text{mean r of all studied parameters} \qquad [6.2]$$

The acceptance limit is: IPP = mean r ≥ 5.

The index of good compressibility and bucodispersibility (IGCB) is calculated as follows:

$$\text{IGCB} = \text{IPP} \times f \qquad [6.3]$$

where f is a reliability factor and is calculated as follows:

$$f = \text{polygon area/circle area} \qquad [6.4]$$

In this case (15 sides), so $f = 0.971$. The acceptability limit will be IGCB ≥ 5.

Differences between IGC and IGCB will be noted when a powder has good aptitude for compression but bad disgregability; in this case, the powder will have an IGC greater than 5, but when the IGCB is calculated it will be lower than 5. On the other hand, if a powder has good aptitude for compression and good disgregability properties, the IGCB will increase with respect to the IGC. Thus, the new tool (SeDeM-ODT) will select more accurately than the old SeDeM method the excipients that could be used to make orodispersible tablets by direct compression.

6.4 Design of ODT formulations using SeDeM-ODT expert system

As summarized in Figure 6.3, to design a suitable ODT formulation, the SeDeM-ODT expert system proposes the following sequence:

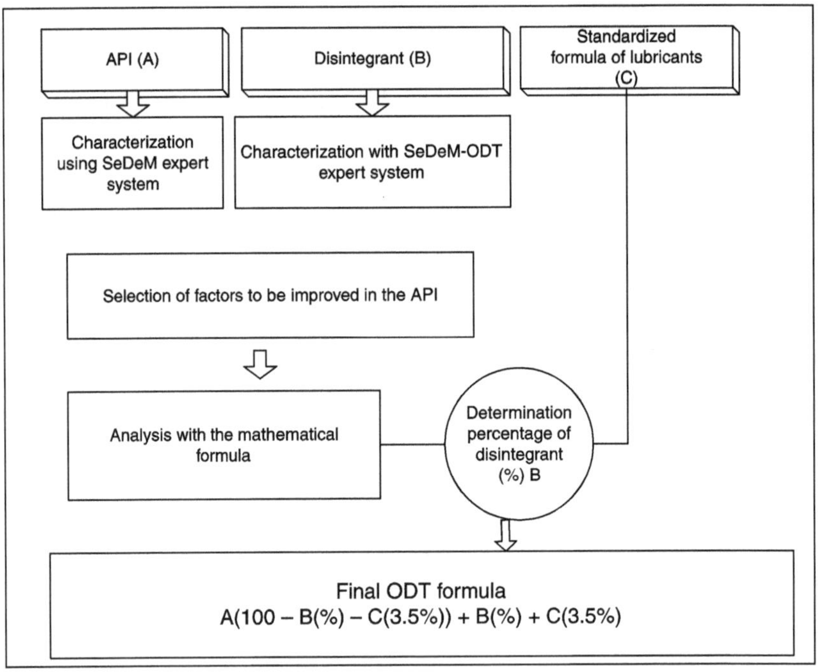

Figure 6.3 Development of oral disintegrating tablets using SeDeM-ODT expert system

Published by Woodhead Publishing Limited, 2013

1. Perform characterization of the API using SeDeM expert system. The scientific rationale of not using SeDeM-ODT expert system for analysis of the API is that it is not expected that the API will have disgregability properties, but its compressibility properties must be evaluated, as bucodispersibility properties are provided by the disintegrant. The bucodispersible properties will be produced for the combination of API and excipient.
2. The disintegrants must be characterized by SeDeM-ODT expert system and those with IGCB near to, equal to or higher than 5 identified.
3. The less than optimal factors obtained must be improved after performing characterization of the API. A mathematical evaluation will be performed for each factor to be improved according to Eq. 6.5, which is used for selection of the excipient as well as the concentration required in order to correct the poor characteristics observed in the API. Eq. 6.5 was originally specifically designed for this purpose by Suñe et al. (Aguilar et al., 2012; Suñé et al., 2005; Pérez et al., 2006; Suñé et al., 2008; Aguilar et al., 2009; García et al., 2010), and is intended for use in calculating the amount of excipient required to compress the API, based on the SeDeM-ODT radius obtained for the API and the excipients.

   $$CP = 100 - ((RE - R)/(RE - RP) \times 100) \qquad [6.5]$$

   where:

   CP = % of the corrective excipient,

   RE = mean-incidence radius value (compressibility) of the corrective excipient,

   R = mean-incidence radius value to be obtained in the blend. It is recommended that R = 5 (5 is the minimum value regarded as necessary in order to achieve good compression),

   RP = mean-incidence radius value (compressibility) of the API to be corrected.

   Once the unknown values in Eq. 6.5 have been replaced with the calculated values required for each substance in order to obtain R = 5, the CP or percentage of excipient recommended by the expert system can be calculated for an ODT tablet.
4. Eq. 6.5 will provide the percentage of excipient which must be added to the standardized formula of lubricants proposed by Suñe et al. (Suñé et al., 2005; Pérez et al., 2006; Suñé et al., 2008; Aguilar et al.,

2009; García et al., 2010; Suñé et al., 2011) composed as detailed in Table 6.4.

5. Finally, the remaining percentage will correspond to the API taking into account the strength required.

Table 6.4 Standardized formula of lubricants

Talc	2.36%
Aerosil 200	0.14%
Magnesium stearate	1.00%

6.4.1 Methodology

The following is the methodology for formulation of a suitable orodispersible tablet.

Select an API and carry out its characterization using SeDeM expert system. When the characterization of the API is finished, several disintegrants which might be suitable candidates must also be characterized using the SeDeM expert system; the disintegrants are selected based on previous published studies taking into account the characteristics of the API (Aguilar et al., 2009).

Characterization of API is performed using SeDeM expert system, but the characterization of the selected disintegrants must be performed using the SeDeM-ODT expert system in order to determine if these excipients have orodispersible properties.

After determining the IGCB of the disintegrants, excipients that have values ≥ 5 will be considered. SeDeM-ODT recommends excipients with IGCB ≥ 5 for use as unique disintegrants, which could be used in combination with the API and the standardized formula of lubricant without adding any diluents to obtain ODT tablets.

6.4.2 Design of the ODT formulations

After performing characterization of the API and excipients using the SeDeM expert system, the factors which need to be improved in the API must be determined, and analyzed in detail. This could determine whether the flowability/powder flow is improved as its lubrication is expected to

Published by Woodhead Publishing Limited, 2013

be improved with the standardized formula of lubricants (Suñé et al., 2005; Pérez et al., 2006; Suñé et al., 2008; Aguilar et al., 2009; García et al., 2010; Suñé et al., 2011).

The selected disintegrant candidates must be characterized using SeDeM-ODT expert system and a mathematical analysis according to Eq. 6.5 between the worst factors of the API against the same factors in each of the selected disintegrant candidates. The mathematical formula will provide the percentage of excipient (disintegrant candidate) required to obtain ODT tablets (CP value).

6.4.3 Formulation of bucodispersible tablets

To prepare bucodispersible tablets of the selected API and disintegrant candidates, the design and development of the formulation should be based on the following condition: strength required is, e.g. 500 mg, and only one excipient and no diluents will be added. The percentage of disintegrant to be added will be determined by mathematical analysis (Eq. 6.5) and should be as low as possible. The fixed formula of lubricants recommended by the expert system is added.

The selected formulas will be prepared as follows:

- weigh all the raw compounds except lubricants,
- weigh the lubricants and put this mixture aside,
- sieve the mixture of API + disintegrant without excipients through a 600 μm sieve,
- mix the API + disintegrant mixture without excipients using a Turbula® mixer for 10 min,
- add the lubricants and mix again for 2 min.

The resulting formulation will be compressed in a continuous eccentric press, mounted with a 19 × 10 mm punch set.

6.4.4 Method of characterization of the modeled bucodispersible tablets

Disintegration

The test of disintegration is carried out according to a USP method with disc and without disc. The acceptance criterion is that tablets must be disintegrated in $T \leq 3$ min (USP 32, 2009b; *European Pharmacopeia*, 2011b).

Dissolution profile

According to the USP method, samples must be taken at the following times: 1, 2, 3, 4, 5, 15, 30 and 60 min (the endpoint will be determined by the pharmacopoeia method). This test must be performed using USP-II equipment in the required conditions for the formulation: representative samples must be taken at each time point, the samples must be filtered and read using suitable equipment such as HPLC, spectrophotometer, etc.

Preparation of standard

Preparation of the standard solution must be performed according to the corresponding monograph defined for the API.

Acceptance criteria

The following are recommended for evaluating whether or not a formulation can be considered suitable for used as an ODT: $Q \geq 80\%$ in 3 min and $Q \geq 100\%$ in 5 min, where Q = percentage of dissolution.

Hardness

This is performed according to USP <1217> (USP 32, 2009d) and *European Pharmacopeia* (*European Pharmacopeia*, 2011c), using Erweka® TBH30 equipment.

Friability

This is performed according to USP <1216> (USP 32, 2009e) and *European Pharmacopeia* (*European Pharmacopeia*, 2011d) using Erweka® TA10 equipment. The friability was evaluated if weight variation was $\leq 1\%$.

6.5 Results and discussion

The SeDeM-ODT model predicts formulations which can produce tablets by direct compression and which can disperse in a few minutes. SeDeM-ODT could conclude that a higher percentage of disintegrant is required than that recommended by the majority of published studies.

Published by Woodhead Publishing Limited, 2013

This recommendation is useful as this approach cannot be applied to all disintegrants. There could be cases where a high percentage of disintegrant is used; however, the disgregability property would be reduced with respect to the same disintegrant used in smaller quantities.

6.5.1 Characterization of disintegrants using new expert system SeDeM-ODT

Factors requiring improvement will be identified, but it could be decided that it is not necessary to improve the factor flowability/powder flow, as it is expected that this factor will increase when the standardized formula of lubricant is added to the formulations.

When a disintegrant candidate has an IGCB near to 5, it must be analyzed in detail. If it is noted that the disgregability factor is higher than 5 and the compressibility factor is also higher than 5, the candidate must not be discarded as it could be used to obtain ODT by direct compression although its IGCB is lower than 5.

6.5.2 Design of ODT formulations

The percentage of the excipients takes into account the strength (therapeutic dose of the drug substance) and the final weight of the tablet, which must be ≤30% (CP value). This recommended percentage aims to avoid production of large tablets.

Sometimes, percentages of excipients with negative CP values are obtained. These must be discarded because they cannot be introduced in the SeDeM expert system formula. When a negative value is obtained, it means that the excipient has a lower radius parameter value than the API, and therefore the excipient makes the formulation less suitable for direct compression. Thus, it is impossible to formulate with only this excipient in the formulation.

The SeDeM-ODT expert system can identify and predict cases where excipients belong to the same chemical families, but contain different particle sizes. In cases where the excipient has smaller particle size (below 50 μm), the tablet captures water by swelling, and the tablet divides but the disintegration is not total. This could be as a result of the kind of disintegrants; where the swelling is produced, it could make further entrance of water difficult. For these specific situations an additional study is recommended considering a lower percentage of this specific excipient or combination with excipients of the same chemical family having a higher particle size.

In addition, SeDeM-ODT expert system can identify differences in excipients from different suppliers; therefore this expert system could help to ensure a successful validation as it can be used in initial studies of new suppliers for existing formulations.

6.5.3 Discussion of results

It can be concluded that the SeDeM-ODT expert system is helpful in reducing the lead-time of ODT development, as the tool informs about those formulations which will not form ODT. SeDeM-ODT expert system is a preformulation and formulation tool for ODT, which has been demonstrated by the authors to be a useful, effective, trustworthy, and reproducible tool to develop ODT in an easier and faster way. The obtained ODT tablets are effective as the SeDeM-ODT expert system evaluates the specific properties of these kinds of tablets.

SeDeM-ODT expert system provides information about the capacity of a disintegrant to be used in direct compression, which results in tablets with bucodispersibility characteristics. SeDeM-ODT expert system helps to obtain ODT by direct compression using only one excipient (one disintegrant) in the formulation together with the standardized mixture of lubricants and the API.

It was proved that disintegrants with a disgregability factor greater than 5 impact the IGCB in a positive way against IGC and vice versa, as the SeDeM-ODT expert system evaluates the specific properties of ODT tablets. So, the strategy for designing ODT shown in Figure 6.3 is effective.

When they are used at high percentages, some disintegrants could produce tablets with characteristics opposite to those expected. Therefore, the SeDeM-ODT expert system only recommends disintegrants which will produce an increase of disgregability and informs to avoid those producing the opposite effect. Hence, unnecessary trial formulations are avoided when SeDeM-ODT expert system is used, reducing the lead-time of ODT development.

6.6 References

Aguilar-Díaz JE, García-Montoya E, Pérez-Lozano P, Suñé-Negre JM, Miñarro M and Ticó JR. (2009) The use of the SeDeM Diagram Expert System to

Published by Woodhead Publishing Limited, 2013

determine the suitability of diluents-disintegrants for direct compression and their use in formulation of ODT. *Eur J Pharm Biopharm* 73, 414–23.

Aguilar-Díaz JE, García-Montoya E, Suñé-Negre JM, Pérez-Lozano P, Miñarro M and Ticó J R. (2012) Predicting orally disintegrating tablets formulations of ibuprofen tablets. An application of the new SeDeM-ODT expert system. *Eur J Pharm Biopharm*, 80, 638–48.

Bandari S, Mittapalli RK, Gannu R and Rao YM. (2008) Orodispersible tablets: An overview: *Asian J Pharm*, 2 (1) 2–11.

Behnke K, Sogaard J, Martin S, Bauml J, Ravindran AV and Agren H. (2003) Mirtazapine orally disintegrating tablet versus sertraline: A prospective onset of action study. *J Clin Psychopharmacol* 23, 358–64.

Berthoumieu D, Trannoy P, Cordoliani JF, François A, Hédin JM, et al. (2010) Tabletting study for ODT's. *Manufacturing Chemist* Nov, 24–7.

Brown D. (2003) Orally disintegrating tablets-taste over speed. *Drug Del Tech* 3, 58–61.

Dobetti L. *Fast disintegrating tablets*. US Patent 2003; 6: 596,311

Dollo G, Chevanne F, Le Corre P, Chemtob C and Le Verge R. (1999) Bioavailability of phloroglucinol in man. *J Pharm Belg* 54, 75–82.

European Pharmacopeia (2011a), 7th ed., vol. 7.2, Council of Europe, Strasbourg (France), 01/2008:0478.

European Pharmacopeia (2011b), 7th ed., vol. 7.2, Council of Europe, Strasbourg (France), 04/2011: 20901.

European Pharmacopeia (2011c), 7th ed., vol. 7.2, Council of Europe, Strasbourg (France), 01/2008: 20908.

European Pharmacopeia (2011d), 7th ed., vol. 7.2, Council of Europe, Strasbourg (France), 01/2010: 20907.

Fernandes Tavares DF, Espada García JI, Martín Sabroso C, Gil Alegre ME and Torres Clarke A, Brewer F, Johnson ES, Mallard N, Hartig F and Taylor S. (2003) A new formulation of selegiline: Improved bioavailability and selectivity for MAO-B inhibition. *J Neural Transm* 110, 124–5.

Fu Y, Yang S, Jeong SH, Kimura S and Park K. (2004) Orally fast disintegrating tablets: Developments, technologies, taste-masking and clinical studies. *Crit Rev Ther Drug Carrier Sys* 21, 433–76.

Habib W, Khankari RK and Hontz J. (2000) Fast-dissolve drug delivery systems. *Crit Rev Ther Drug Carrier Sys* 17, 61–72.

Gafitanu E, Dumistracel I and Antochi S. (1991) Formulations and bioavailability of propyphenazone in lyophilized tablets. *Rev Med Chir Soc Med Nat Iasi* 95, 127–8.

García Montoya E, Suñé Negre M, Pérez Lozano P, Miñarro Carmona M, Roig Carreras M and Ticó Grau JR. (2010) Metodología de preformulación galénica para la caracterización de sustancias en relación a su viabilidad para la compresión: Diagrama SeDeM. *Farmespaña Industrial*, enero/feb 58–62.

Guidance for Industry: Orally Disintegrating Tablets: FDA. Dec 2008.

Jaccard TT and Leyder J. (1985) Une nouvelle forme galenique le lyoc. *Ann Pharm Fr* 43, 123–31.

Lindgren S and Janzon L. (1993) Dysphagia: Prevalence of swallowing complaints and clinical finding. *Med Clin North Am*, 77, 3–5.

Pérez P, Suñé-Negre JM, Miñarro M, Roig M, Fuster R, et al. (2006) A new expert systems (SeDeM Diagram) for control batch powder formulation and preformulation drug products. *Eur J Pharm Biopharm* 64, 351–9.

Sastry SV, Nyshadham JR and Fix JA. (2000) Recent technological advances in oral drug delivery: A review. *Pharm Sci Technol Today*, 3, 138–45.

Seager H. (1998) Drug-delivery products and the Zydis fast-dissolving dosage form. *J Pharm Pharmacol* 50, 375–82.

Suárez AI. (2009) Comprimidos bucodispersables: ventajas terapéuticas y tecnológicas de elaboración. *Ars Pharmaceutica*, 50–3, 153–67.

Suñé Negre JM, Roig Carreras M, Fuster García R, Hernández Pérez C, Ruhí Roura R, et al. (2005) Nueva metodología de preformulación galénica para la caracterización de sustancias en relación a su viabilidad para la compresión: Diagrama SeDeM, *Cien Tecnol Pharm* 3 125–36.

Suñé Negre JM, Pérez Lozano P, Miñarro Carmona M, Roig Carreras M, Fuster García R, et al. (2008) Application of the SeDeM Diagram and new mathematical equation in the Design of Direct Compression Tablet Formulation. Eur J Pharm Biopharm, 1029–39.

Suñé Negre M, Pérez Lozano P, Miñarro Carmona M, Roig Carreras M, Fuster García R, et al. (2011) Optimization of parameters of the SeDeM Diagram Expert System: Hausner index (IH) and relative humidity (%RH). *Eur J Pharm Biopharm* 79, 464–72. *http://www.ncbi.nlm.nih.gov/pubmed/21501683?dopt=Abstract*

USP 32/NF 27 (2009a), *The United States Pharmacopeia, 32ª rev and The National Formulary, 27th ed.* United States Pharmacopoeial Convention, Inc. (Ed) Rockville; <USP Monographs: 711>.

USP 32/NF 27 (2009b), *The United States Pharmacopeia, 32ª rev and The National Formulary, 27th ed.* United States Pharmacopoeial Convention, Inc. (Ed) Rockville; <USP Monographs: 701>, p. 266.

USP 32/NF 27 (2009c), *The United States Pharmacopeia, 32ª rev and The National Formulary, 27th ed.* United States Pharmacopoeial Convention, Inc. (Ed) Rockville; <USP Monographs: Ibuprofen Tablets>.

USP 32/NF 27 (2009d), *The United States Pharmacopeia, 32ª rev and The National Formulary, 27th ed.* United States Pharmacopoeial Convention, Inc. (Ed) Rockville; <USP Monographs: 1217: Tablet Breaking Force>.

USP 32/NF 27 (2009e), *The United States Pharmacopeia, 32ª rev and The National Formulary, 27th ed.* United States Pharmacopoeial Convention, Inc. (Ed) Rockville; <USP Monographs: 1216: Tablet Friability>.

Published by Woodhead Publishing Limited, 2013

7

3-D cellular automata in computer-aided design of pharmaceutical formulations: mathematical concept and F-CAD software

Maxim Puchkov, University of Basel, Switzerland and Center for Innovation in Computer-Aided Pharmaceutics (CINCAP GmbH), Switzerland, David Tschirky, University of Basel, Switzerland and Hans Leuenberger, University of Basel, Switzerland, Institute for Innovation in Industrial Pharmacy (Ifiip GmbH), Switzerland and Center for Innovation in Computer-Aided Pharmaceutics (CINCAP GmbH), Switzerland

DOI: 10.1533/9781908818508.155

Abstract: Development of modern pharmaceutical drug formulations is a challenge; it is time and resource expensive. There is a lot of research carried out to facilitate this work from the modeling point of view. This chapter presents a tool for an *in silico* design and development of pharmaceutical solid dosage forms taking into account process technology, composition, and shape of final product in development as a whole. This flexibility is offered by a new approach to model heterogeneous multiparticulate systems (such as pharmaceutical formulations): the cellular automata. In this chapter we present basic underlining principles of cellular automata; their applications in modeling of different physico-chemical processes related to pharmaceutical R&D, along with developed software package F-CAD (Formulation Computer-Aided Design). The functioning of F-CAD software is discussed with examples of base unit operations (e.g. wet granulation) and simulated drug release profiles.

Key words: Cellular automata, F-CAD, computer-aided formulation design, simulation of drug release, simulation of granulation, root-cause finding.

7.1 Introduction

7.1.1 The need to reduce time to market and to realize cost savings in pharmaceutical R and D

The complex task to introduce a new product onto the market

Only one out of 10 000 molecules extensively tested in the discovery phase reaches the market. Between the discovery of an interesting drug substance and the introduction of the final marketed dosage form of the successful drug substance, a complexity of activities and tests are required. Financial expenditure is estimated to be approximately US$1 billion for a company to introduce a new medication to the market. This expenditure also has to cover the costs of the interesting drug substances that failed during development and did not reach patients. This limits companies to reduce the price of their medications on the market in order to be able to continue R and D activities. Thus, if the costs of R and D could be reduced, all healthcare systems could benefit. If time to market could be reduced, then substantial savings could be achieved. Let us assume that a new, successful medication may contribute US$365 million to the sales volume of a company in its first year on the market. Thus, each day earlier on the market could mean US$1 million more in sales. In the case of a new approach using e-Development (Leuenberger et al., 2009), such improvements are no longer a distant possibility from a commercial point of view. This chapter describes such a new approach in the area of development and manufacture of solid dosage forms.

Published by Woodhead Publishing Limited, 2013

7.1.2 The classical approach in pharmaceutical R and D and its deficiencies

In the classical approach, a substantial slowdown concerning 'time to market' is linked intrinsically to the workflow and sequential activities. As a result of a lack of connectivity, problems often occur at the interfaces between the different departments involved. These different groups in research, early development, pilot plant manufacturing and scale-up, or large-scale manufacturing, usually have very different cultures. For this reason, a product manager is required to follow a product from the beginning, starting with R and D through to large-scale manufacturing of the final marketed dosage form. In general, for early tests in the preclinical and first clinical phases, a preliminary 'service dosage form' is prepared, usually a hard gelatine capsule formulation. Such a 'service dosage form' may be very different from the final marketed form, which is in general ready at the end of clinical phase 2 or at the beginning of clinical phase 3. Such an approach has many risks. The final marketed dosage form must be bioequivalent to its earlier 'service dosage form', which was far from optimal because of a lack of development time and resources allocated. Unfortunately, it is not uncommon that expensive 'repair actions' are required for development of the final marketed dosage form to achieve bioequivalence. What happens if the early 'service' dosage form was far from optimal? In such a case, the final marketed dosage form must be corrected to the quality of the dosage form tested in clinical phase 2. Thus, the market dosage form may not have the optimal bioavailability. Such an effect creates headaches for companies manufacturing generics. To show bioequivalence, these companies may need to reduce the bioavailability of their product to comply with the originator. Unfortunately, only in rare and extreme situations does non-robustness of an early dosage form become evident at an early clinical phase (see Leuenberger and Lanz, 2005; von Orelli and Leuenberger, 2004). The fact that early 'service' dosage forms are often poor quality is linked to the company having many drug candidate substances in the preclinical phase (approximately 12 or more) in simultaneous development. There are not enough resources and time slots for doing additional expensive laboratory work in order to develop robust formulations for all the proposed API for the first clinical trials. Thus, it is not surprising that the early dosage forms are far from six-sigma quality. This problem becomes accented because of regulatory issues, as the formulation cannot be changed during the forthcoming clinical trials.

7.1.3 Can a company afford in an early phase to develop a robust dosage form of six-sigma quality ready for the market?

It has been generally accepted that the quality of pharmaceutical products has a quality of approximately two sigma. A 'snapshot-view', i.e. single batch assessment of two sigma quality, corresponds to ca. 4.5% defectives. In a sequence of batch productions over a longer period of time, the percentage of defectives of the sum of batches increases to 20%. This higher value is because of drift of individual results as a consequence of measurements over an extensive time period. The resulting poor quality has triggered actions by regulatory authorities and has boosted FDA's PAT (Process Analytical Technology) and Quality by Design (QbD) initiatives. The PAT initiative has prompted the installation of additional in-process control units in manufacturing departments for optimizing quality. Several pharmaceutical companies in Switzerland and Germany have introduced at-line, on-line or in-line near infrared (NIR) spectroscopy control tools for nearly all process-steps such as raw material identification, blending, drying, and tableting. It is interesting that the PAT initiative did not have the same visible effect on R and D departments with their task to build-in and not to test-in the quality, but to implement according to ICH Q8.

The aim of pharmaceutical development is to design a quality product. The design space is proposed by the applicant and is subject to regulatory issues. In this context the following *key question* arises: Is it possible to *increase the quality* of a product *and to reduce simultaneously the costs* in pharmaceutical development?

It is well known that quality $Q(\mu, t)$ is a function of resources μ and time t. $Q(\mu,t)$ can be expressed as an exponential asymptotic function of the following nature:

$$Q(t) = Q_{opt}\,(1 - \exp\,[-\mu\, t])$$

with Q_{opt} = optimal quality for $t \rightarrow \infty$, μ = amount of means, i.e. tools, resources, etc. Depending on μ and time t, the 'learning'/'optimization' process shows in the beginning a fast increase and then levels off. For this reason, the so-called 20%/80% rule became popular in the pharmaceutical industry. The idea of the 20%/80% rule is to obtain 80% of the optimal quality with only 20% of time and resources invested. In a simplified manner, this means, in practice, that one person takes care of five projects simultaneously, dedicating 20% of their time and resources to each project. The resulting quality of the product corresponds to a sigma value

Published by Woodhead Publishing Limited, 2013

of 2.3 if calculated with 20% investments, which is very close to the reported value for pharmaceutical production. Even if the factor [μ t] is increased by a factor of 5, i.e. that one person dedicates 100% of their time to each project, a six-sigma value cannot be obtained. Such an approach would require an increase in the work force by five times, which is impossible. Therefore, the search for new tools and means is mandatory.

The authors of this chapter are convinced that it is possible to obtain a six-sigma value within the framework of an e-Development concept. Such an approach allows development of a market-ready and robust six-sigma quality tablet formulation in the early phase ready for clinical phase 1, as only a very few laboratory experiments are needed for validation. Such an approach would be the realization of a truly 'Right, First Time' concept (Leuenberger et al., 2010), which could lead to substantial savings and a significant reduction of time to market.

The concept of e-Development or computer-aided design (CAD) of the tablet or other pharmaceutical formulations is versatile, as it covers a vast amount of medical and engineering topics. Generally speaking, pharmaceutical technology is science on the convergence of different scientific disciplines, e.g. mechanical engineering and medicine, physical chemistry and anatomy, etc. In this respect, rigorous and well-studied methodologies are necessary for successful adjunction of the mentioned problems into a complete, systemically studied development concept.

The application of computer-aided approaches for system-based design of the robust dosage forms is very appealing. However, it has to be kept in mind that solid dosage forms have a number of fundamental problems, arising from particulate property of matter. Indeed, the behavior of powders is strictly stochastic, often showing chaotic and critical patterns. Keeping this in mind, we have to look for computer-based methods which deal with non-deterministic and probabilistic performance and confine those within defined engineering scope.

Modeling of powder flow, drug dissolution behavior, compaction, and disintegration of solid dosage forms is predicted to solve the aforementioned tasks. In this chapter we provide an overview of a single mathematical method for modeling of all typical unit operations encountered in the standard course of the dosage from development – the cellular automata.

7.1.4 Artificial intelligence in formulation development

To understand the need for newer methods in mathematical modeling of stochastic phenomena, like power behavior, it is important to review the main modeling trends of the past. One of the main trends in the second half of the last century was development of artificial intelligence-based modeling methods to help with design of pharmaceutical dosage forms.

Artificial intelligence can capture the knowledge of a formulation expert, document it and make it available and user-friendly. Turban compared artificial intelligence (AI) and – as he called it – natural intelligence (NI) of experts as follows (Turban, 1995):

- NI depends on persons, which results in a dependency on personnel changes,
- NI is difficult to transfer, whereas AI can be moved from one computer to another,
- AI can reduce costs,
- AI is consistent, decisions are traceable and can easily be documented,
- AI is not creative,
- NI uses a wider context of experience to solve problems.

Formulation strategies are often based on trial-and-error strategies and experience, whereas modeling and simulations represent attempts of rational approaches to formulation development. Attempts for a rational approach in formulation design have been numerous over decades, manly focusing on the expert system design and development.

Expert systems

Expert system (ES) is a versatile term, as ES are used in many disciplines. However, there are several common definitions:

- 'Computer program that draws upon the knowledge of human experts captured in a knowledge base to solve problems that normally require human expertise' (Partridge and Hussain, 1994).
- 'The label "expert system" is broadly speaking, given to a computer program intended to make reasoned judgements or give assistance on a complex area in which human skills are fallible or scarce' (Lauritzen and Spiegelhalter, 1988).
- '. . . knowledge-based system that emulates expert thought to solve significant problems in a particular domain of expertise' (Sell, 1985).

Because of the versatility of the definition of ES and other knowledge-based approaches, there are many ways of designing such systems. It is interesting to look at an example of such development at the University of Basel,

Published by Woodhead Publishing Limited, 2013

Institute of Pharmaceutical Technology. Because of the wideness of the term, it was initially decided at the University of Basel to have a close look at ES and to develop a knowledge-based ES, which takes into account the effect of percolation thresholds. This initial idea is still reflected in the title of the PhD thesis of Krausbauer 'Contributions to a science based expert system for solid dosage form design' (Krausbauer 2009). During this PhD thesis work, it became clear that the topic goes beyond the classical definition of the ES as a result of applying the cellular automata (CA) technique, which is capable of detecting percolation thresholds. This phenomenon was internally discussed by the team supporting the thesis of E. Krausbauer, consisting of G. Betz, M. Puchkov, and H. Leuenberger as head of the Institute of Pharmaceutical Technology. The application of CA to detect percolation thresholds was studied independently of the mentioned thesis by M. Puchkov (at that time, part-time post-doc of Mendeleyev University of Chemical Technology of Russia, Cybernetics Department). During discussions with the team it became evident that the initial idea from M. Puchkov to apply CA for simulating the drug dissolution profile could become an important tool for formulation design. Thanks to the effort of E. Krausbauer (Krausbauer, 2009) and his collaboration as team worker, development of the original ES led to the design of a new approach for creating a novel science-based ES based on first principles.

Knowledge-based information systems, often taken as a synonym for ES, are usually composed of an interface, an inference engine, and a knowledge base. The inference engine extracts knowledge from the data base, manipulates it, and creates new information, i.e. it simulates the process which should solve the problem given to the computer. Knowledge representation is mainly done with production rules. They express relationships between pieces of information with conditional statements. The most simple production rule is a list of IF clauses ended by a THEN clause:

IF (condition) THEN (action)

A more complicated form would be:

IF (condition 1) AND (condition 2) OR (condition 3) THEN (action)
UNLESS (exception)
BECAUSE (reason)

The limitation of production rules is that complex knowledge may require a large number of rules, which can be difficult to manage for the developer and for the end-user. Also, production rules are often unsuited to representing many types of knowledge (Rowe and Roberts 1998).

Common methods are also frames, semantic networks, decision trees/tables, and objects. The reader will find detailed information about these methods in *Intelligent Software for Product Formulation* by Rowe and Roberts (1998).

All these methods are restricted to sequential processing of knowledge. A different approach is that of neural networks. As the name implies, artificial neural networks are inspired by the functionality of the human brain. The artificial neuron takes one or more inputs – each multiplied with a weight factor – and potentially creates an output which is forwarded to another neuron. Whether or not an output is generated depends on the inputs which need to exceed a defined threshold. The threshold activation is computed by transformation functions which can be linear or non-linear. Compared to expert systems, neural networks need short development time, but need to be trained. The training consists of linking inputs and outputs and adapting weight values until inputs give a result close to that which had been determined experimentally.

Systems for solid dosage form design

Following extensive work by Rowe and Ronald, which outlines in detail the existing and developed software to aid in drug formulation development (Rowe and Ronald, 1998), a selected few are described below.

- Cadila System

Developed at Cadila Laboratories (Ahmedabad, India), this software aims to formulate tablets based on their physical (e.g. solubility), chemical (e.g. functional groups), and biologically interrelated (e.g. dissolution rate) properties (Ramani and Patel, 1992). Knowledge is stored as decision tablets with derived production rules. The output is a selection and proportions of different compounds which should satisfy the requirements of the user.

- Galenical Development System

This system was developed in Heidelberg in the 1990s. It was designed to assist in development of the following dosage forms: aerosols, tablets, capsules, i.v. injections, and others. The starting points are the physical and chemical properties of the API. Knowledge is stored as objects, frames, and production rules. The output is a formulation with production method, recommended packaging, and predicted product properties (Stricker, 1994).

■ Capsugel System

The system was developed at the School of Pharmacy, University of London (UK) in collaboration with Capsugel and the Universities of Kyoto (Japan) and Maryland (USA). It helps to design formulations of hard gelatine capsules (Lai, 1996). The system uses decision trees and production rules for knowledge representation. The output is a recommendation of a formulation with any necessary powder processing and filling conditions. It also provides recommended tests to validate the formulation and a documentation of the decision process. The broadness of its knowledge base is unique, with information on a large number of excipients, literature references, and knowledge from an international expert group.

■ CAD/Chem Formulation Design and Optimisation Program

This Windows-based computer package was developed by AI Ware Inc. (Cleveland, Ohio). It is based on neural networks, and relies on experimental results provided by the user which cover both sides of a cause-and-effect relationship. Ingredient and process conditions, as well as properties (experimentally measured), are needed as input data. Models always need to be validated, improved, and optimized during the development process of a solid dosage form. The output is a recommendation of the formulation composition.

■ DDDplus™ (Dose Disintegration and Dissolution Plus)

This software models and simulates dissolution profiles of solid dosage forms such as powders, tablets, and capsules. The aim is to save lab work, guide decision making, and evaluate formulations. The simulation is based on numerical integration of a set of differential equations that coordinate physical actions (particle size changes, changes in microclimate, and medium pH) that occur during dissolution. For successful simulation, a large number of input data are required. A few are listed here:

- Compression force,
- Tablet diameter,
- Porosity,
- pKa(s), solubility factor, mass transfer coefficient, shape factor, diffusion coefficient, particle density, particle size distribution, etc. of every component of the formulation,
- Type and composition of the medium,
- Type of the apparatus, stirring speed, initial pH, medium viscosity.

The output is a parameter sensitivity analysis and virtual trials with simulated dissolution profiles for all ingredients as well as calculation of pH changes. In summary, DDDplus™ is the first and only attempt at a CAD system, but based on differential calculus, i.e. it calculates but it does not assess.

As can be seen from this short overview of existing software tools, the integral approach is still missing. Different methods used in construction of the expert systems prevent any compatibility between the software packages. There is a clear need for a more consistent approach to designing and assessing the performance of a pharmaceutical formulation. One of the candidates for such a role is cellular automata.

7.2 Drug dissolution simulation model with cellular automata

7.2.1 Application of cellular automata for pharmaceutical formulation design

The cellular automaton was first proposed by von Newmann in the late 1940s. Systematic studies were done by Wolfram in 1980s and resulted in an extensive overview of the available types of cellular automata as described in *A New Kind of Science* (Wolfram, 2002). In *Cellular Automata of Physical Systems* (Chopard and Droz, 1998), an extensive overview is given of application of cellular automata for modeling different physical and chemical phenomena. CA is generally used for modeling many natural phenomena (Wolfram, 2002), as they are often evolutionary, i.e. the development of a system evolves from a certain operation of a previous generation. What makes CA potent for dissolution calculation is its ability to take into an account local interactions between domains with different properties. Apparently simple rules can result in complex structures. In this respect it is important to note that the evolutionary systems are often described by the basic form of the differential equation for evolutionary systems:

$$\frac{dN}{dt} = -kN$$

where t is the time, k is the rate constant, and N is the target variable. By separating the variables and integrating this equation we obtain the following form of the exponential functions:

Published by Woodhead Publishing Limited, 2013

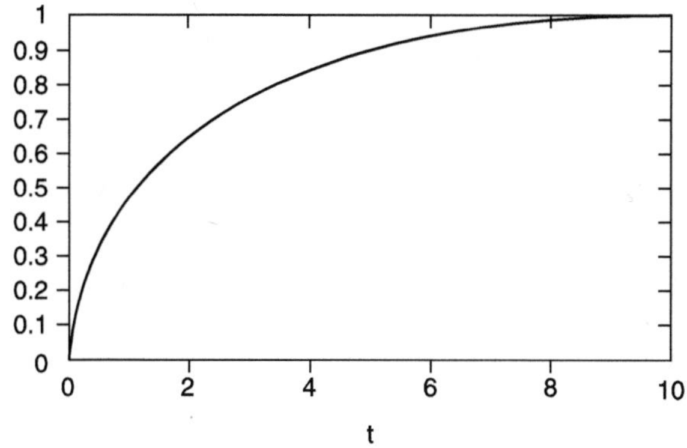

Figure 7.1 Generalized plot of equation in a form $N/N_0 = (1 - e^{-kt})$, where t is time

$$N = N_0\,(1 - e^{-kt})$$

The chart of the resulting function represents very closely the typical release profile from tablet formulation (see Figure 7.1).

Such similarity between the evolutionary equation and a typical release profile is not unexpected. Indeed, the release speed on the drug from a tablet formulation is dependent on the amount of the drug released and other associated parameters which regulate the value of the rate constant k. It is evident that the release kinetic is an evolutionary system and can be defined in space and time. This definition is also common to the cellular automata.

Chopard defined cellular automata as follows: 'Cellular automata (often termed CA) are an idealization of a physical system in which space and time are discrete, and the physical quantities take only a finite set of values'. In other words, CA provide discrete models of equally sized cells, arranged in a regular grid, each in one of a finite number of states. After every time step (so-called iteration or generation), the new state of a cell is determined by its previous state and the states of the neighboring cells. Cells can be classified in different cell types, although on every type a finite number of rules are applied, i.e. every cell of the same type follows the same rules, dependent on the types and states of the neighboring cells. The rules are always applied to all cells, which results in a new generation of cells. The neighborhood can be defined in different ways and there are several types of neighborhood known. Two common neighborhoods (von Newmann and Moore) are shown in Figure 7.2.

The blank cells do not affect the state of the black cell in the next generation, only the grey cells and the state of the black cell itself do.

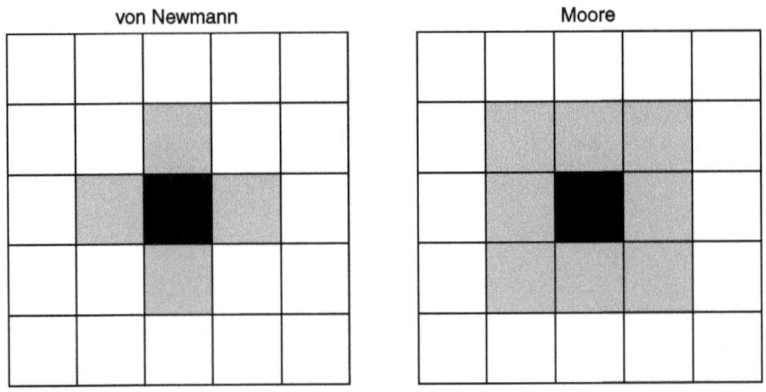

Figure 7.2 von Newmann and Moore neighborhood

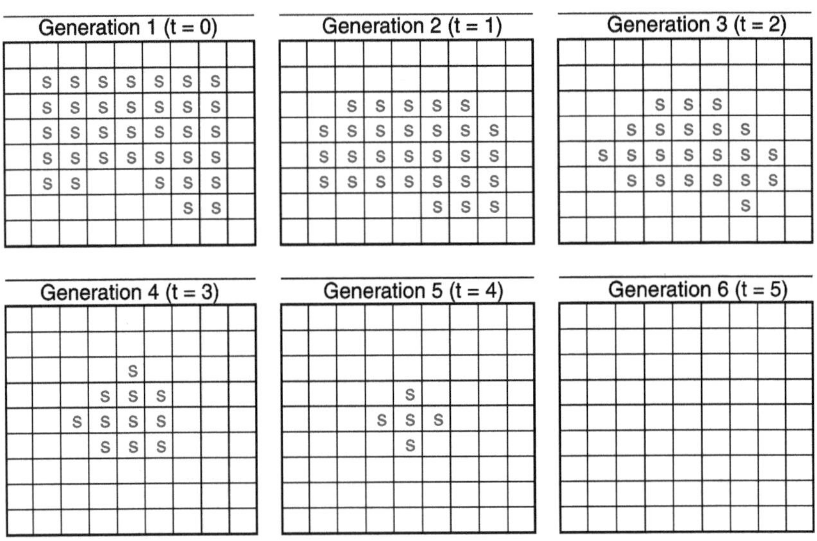

Figure 7.3 Example of 2-D cellular automata, a solid gets dissolved by liquid

Figure 7.3 visualizes 2-D CA with a simplified example of a solid substance being dissolved in a liquid dissolution medium. The rule set is simple: cells of the solid type (s) are changed into a liquid cell (blue) if they are surrounded by four or more liquid cells in the Moore neighborhood. This is a 2-D example of CA with only one rule and two cell types. The more rules, the more types and the more dimensions, the more complex (also natural) behavior can be simulated without changing the complexity of the rules which are kept simple and are always applied on all cells.

Published by Woodhead Publishing Limited, 2013

Mathematically, the dissolution of a solid in dissolution medium can be expressed using the Noyes-Whitney equation:

$$\frac{dC}{dt} = K\,(C_s - C)$$

where C is the concentration of the solute at time t, C_s is the solubility on the equilibrium at experimental temperature and K is a first-order proportionality constant.

The Noyes-Whitney equation in differential form has a form of Fick's second law of diffusion and can be represented in the 3-D domain as follows:

$$\frac{\partial\phi}{\partial t} = D\,\nabla^2\phi$$

where ∇^2 is $\left(\frac{\partial^2}{\partial x^2}+\frac{\partial^2}{\partial y^2}+\frac{\partial^2}{\partial z^2}\right)$, ϕ is the concentration, t is time, and D is the diffusion coefficient.

The translation of this equation into CA rules for dissolution simulation can be described using the finite differences method for computing the numerical solutions of the systems of differential equations. To demonstrate this, Yang et al. used the 1D heat equation (Yang and Young, 2012):

$$\frac{\delta T}{\delta t} = \kappa\frac{\delta^2 T}{\delta x^2}$$

where T is temperature and κ is the thermal diffusivity. This equation can be discretized with central difference for spatial derivative and forward scheme for time derivatives, which results in

$$T_i^{n+1} - T_i^n = \frac{\kappa\Delta t}{(\Delta x)^2}\left(T_{i+1}^n - 2T_i^n + 2T_{i-1}^n\right)$$

where *i* and *n* are the spatial and time indices. If time steps and spatial discretization are chosen such that $\frac{\kappa\Delta t}{(\Delta x)^2} = 1$, the resulting equation is:

$$T_i^{t+1} = (T_{i+1}^t + T_i^t + T_{i-1}^t) - 2T_i^t$$

which is Wolfram's 1D cellular automata with rule 182 (10110110) (Figure 7.4).

The transformation to the CA rules from the forward finite difference scheme can be presented as shown in Figure 7.5.

The target value for the differential function at T_i^{t+1} is the sum of the function values at previous steps (i.e. black-grey squares) minus $2T_i^t$. This

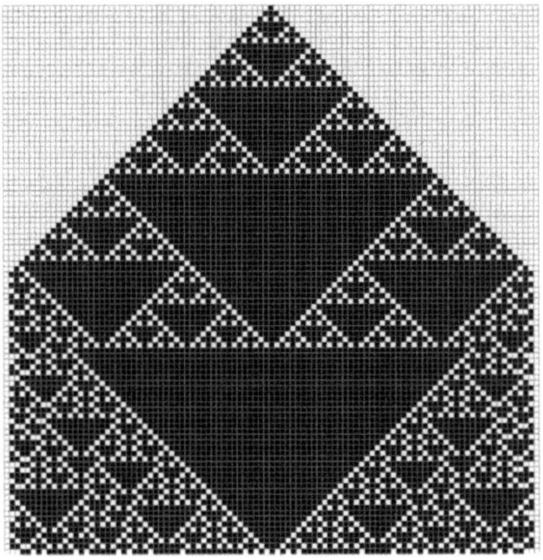

Figure 7.4 Evolution of rule 182 cellular automata

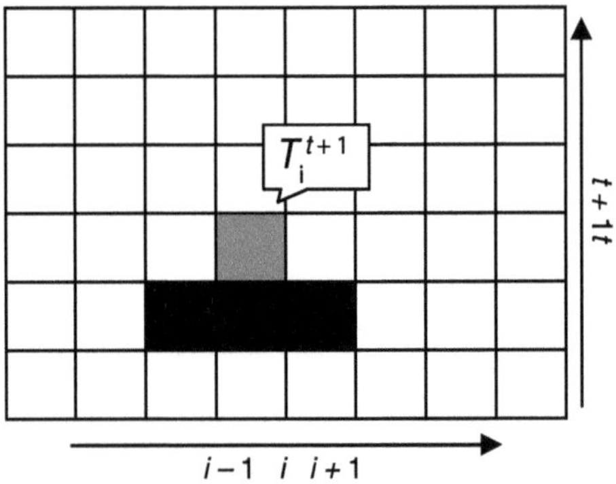

Figure 7.5 Finite-difference 4-dot forward schema to solve 1D diffusion equation (i indicates spatial position and *t* is time)

approach is known as the forward 4-dot scheme for numerical solution of differential equations.

Let us consider the following CA cell development based on rule 182. The successive iteration (or value of the grey cell) can be calculated from previous states of cells (black squares). In this respect we can see eight combinations as follows:

Published by Woodhead Publishing Limited, 2013

```
if ((cell[i-1,t]=1) and (cell[i-0,t]=1) and (cell[i+1,t]=1)) then cell
  [i,t+1]=1
if ((cell[i-1,t]=1) and (cell[i-0,t]=1) and (cell[i+1,t]=0)) then
  cell[i,t+1]=0
if ((cell[i-1,t]=1) and (cell[i-0,t]=0) and (cell[i+1,t]=1)) then
  cell[i,t+1]=1
if ((cell[i-1,t]=1) and (cell[i-0,t]=0) and (cell[i+1,t]=0))
  then cell[i,t+1]=1
if ((cell[i-1,t]=0) and (cell[i-0,t]=1) and (cell[i+1,t]=1)) then
  cell[i,t+1]=0
if ((cell[i-1,t]=0) and (cell[i-0,t]=1) and (cell[i+1,t]=0)) then
  cell[i,t+1]=1
if ((cell[i-1,t]=0) and (cell[i-0,t]=0) and (cell[i+1,t]=1)) then
  cell[i,t+1]=1
if ((cell[i-1,t]=0) and (cell[i-0,t]=0) and (cell[i+1,t]=0)) then
  cell[i,t+1]=0
```

Graphically this pseudo-code can be presented as shown in Figure 7.6.

The resulting numerical solutions of the diffusion equation through rule 182 might be presented in the form of a bell-shaped curve or cumulative curve vs. time. The resulting curves are shown in Figure 7.7.

As can be seen from Figure 7.7, numerical solutions with CA of classical physicochemical equations are possible and yield results very close to the analytical solution. As an advantage, such CA-based solutions have easy to handle boundary conditions, native to CA handling of localities, and respecting conservation laws.

Because of the high flexibility of CA-based models of physicochemical phenomena, the CA-based algorithm is very promising and convenient as the basic model for formulation design and modeling. The CA-based models were adapted by M. Puchkov and H. Leuenberger assisted by E. Krausbauer during his PhD work (Krausbauer, 2009) for use as a simulation engine of the release profiles from solid dosage forms.

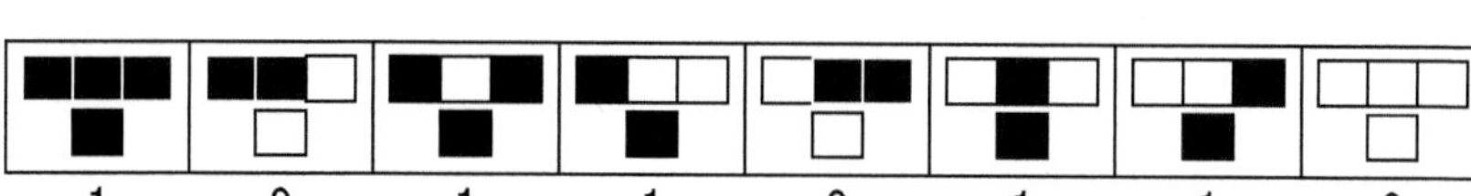

Figure 7.6 Graphical representation of rule 182 and its binary coding

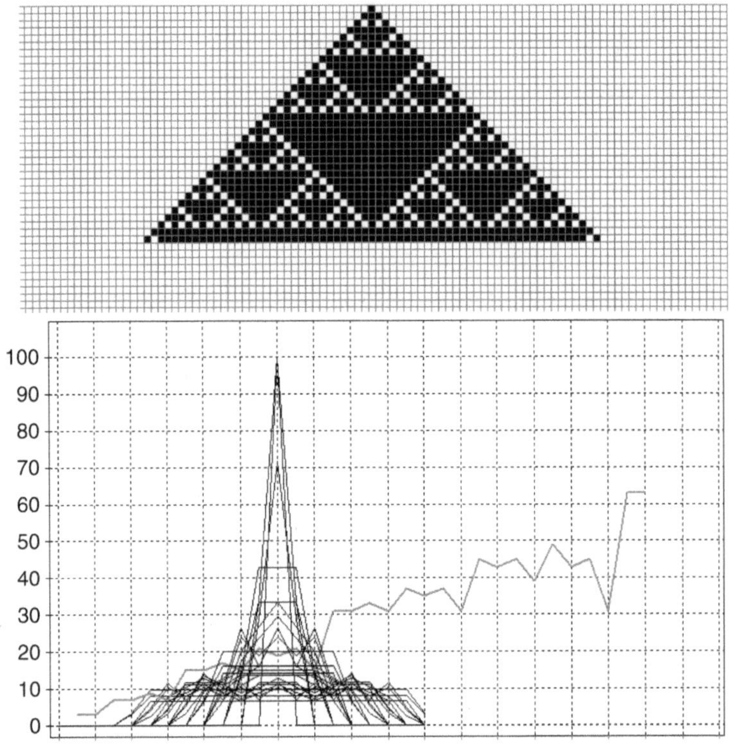

Figure 7.7 **Numerical solution of the diffusion equation through 1D cellular automata applied rule 182. The upper figure depicts 32 iterations of rule 182. The lower figure shows 32 bell-shaped curves of the concentration vs. position and the diagonal line shows the cumulative function of concentration vs. time**

7.2.2 Cellular automata model for tablet compaction

Despite dissolution profile calculation being the main goal for simulations, the particle arrangement algorithm is another essential part of the whole system. Unlike natural compression, where the powder is first loaded into a die and then compacted due to the volumetric shrinkage, the particles are 'grown' to the target mass and size distribution within a final, desired, and rigid tablet volume.

This processing is illustrated step by step in Figure 7.8.

Published by Woodhead Publishing Limited, 2013

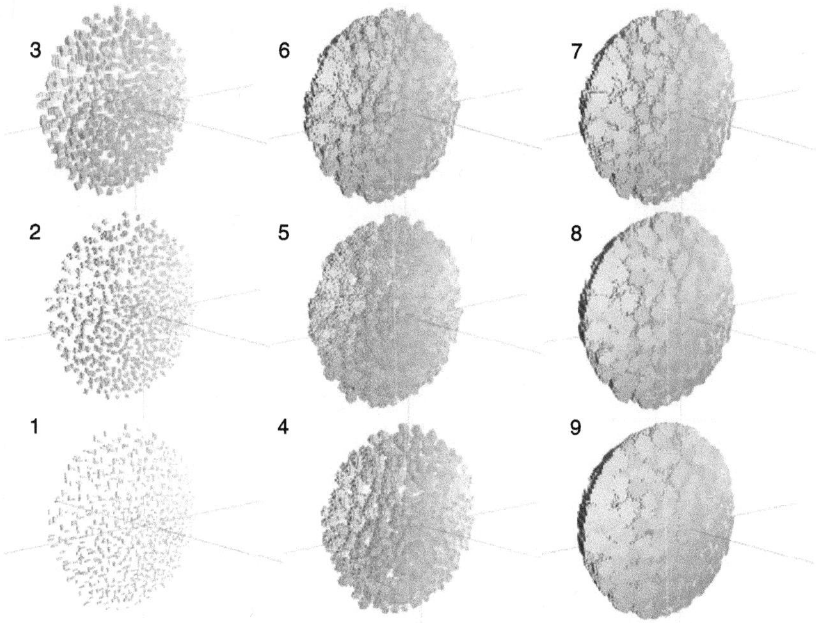

Figure 7.8 Growth of particles in a simulated tablet: bottom left – seeds; bottom right – grown particles after ninth iteration

The 'growth' process starts at 'seeding' the initial germ-particles of three individual cells in the centers of the future particles. The locations of the center particles are determined by the sphere packing algorithm (Figure 7.12). The initial centers will remain the barycenters of the developed particles. Spatial shift might occur because of constraints that force the particles to rearrange their locations and shapes. Once the centers are positioned, the subsequent 'growth' process is governed by CA rules which transform the initial seeds into spherical objects. At this point growth is continued until the particle does not meet the boundary or another growing particle. At this event, diametrical growth is stopped, but the particle is trying to allocate the gained mass at the nearest empty place, i.e. the particle deforms.

This approach allows simulation of a higher tablet density in the vicinity of contact surfaces, in a similar way as happens in reality during the compaction process. Figure 7.9 shows the development of the solid structure rendered for visualization purposes at lower resolution, as a visualization of degradation of the porous network down to individual porous domains.

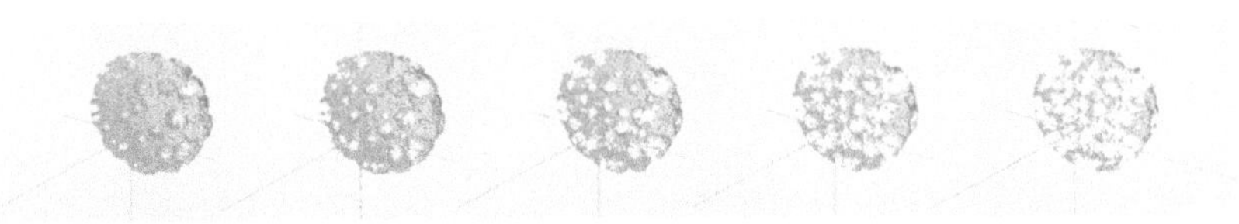

Figure 7.9 Left to right: degradation of a porous network (pores depicted as pink) during growth of solid particles (solids are transparent)

The overall efficiency of such an inverted approach to compaction simulation is delivering very realistic and robust results when applied to hundreds of millions of cells as shown in the following example. The renderings from computer memory for tablets where the active ingredient was removed are shown in Figure 7.10. On the left of each photo the real tablet with washed out API (caffeine) is shown (Bonny, 1994), whereas on the right the corresponding result of a CA-based growth mechanism of particle arrangement and compaction simulation is shown. The simulation was performed for three different size fractions of the API, which were visually compared with their real counterparts (see Figure 7.10).

The particle size distribution of the simulated granules or particles varies during the growth steps. The resulting distribution function resembles the realistic figures (see Figure 7.11).

It could be expected that the size distribution function would be not very different to a delta function because of homogeneous time steps and equal rules application during the growth process; however, the heterogeneous and iteration-dependent constraints (walls and neighboring particles) change the distribution function to Gaussian or similar type.

7.2.3 Creating a virtual tablet

The composition of the virtual tablet is set up together with the particle arrangement and compaction. This approach allows us to include effects of unit operations on the formulation. However, the first step is to define the components of the test formulation. All that is needed is the true density value for each component, a user-defined color for visual representation, a name, and a type of the component. Depending on the type selected for a particular ingredient, different rule sets can be applied to the cell component. Different cell types allow us to model a vast variety

Published by Woodhead Publishing Limited, 2013

(a)

(b)

(c)

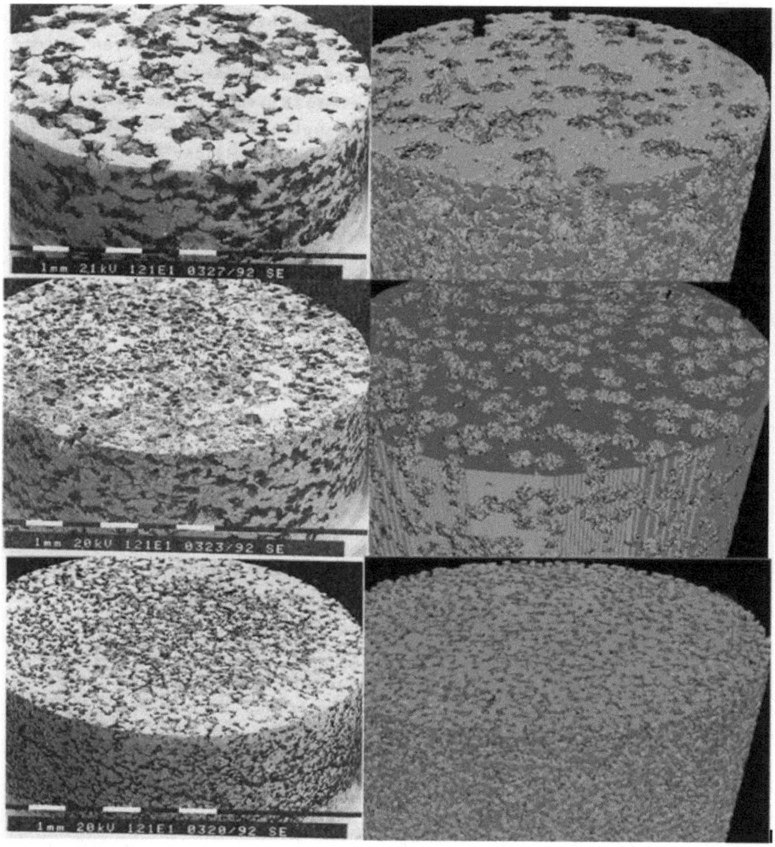

Figure 7.10 Computer-generated tablet (left) and real tablet with leached out API (caffeine) (Bonny, 1994). (a) Caffeine 500–710 μm, (b) caffeine 250–355 μm, (c) caffeine 125–180 μm

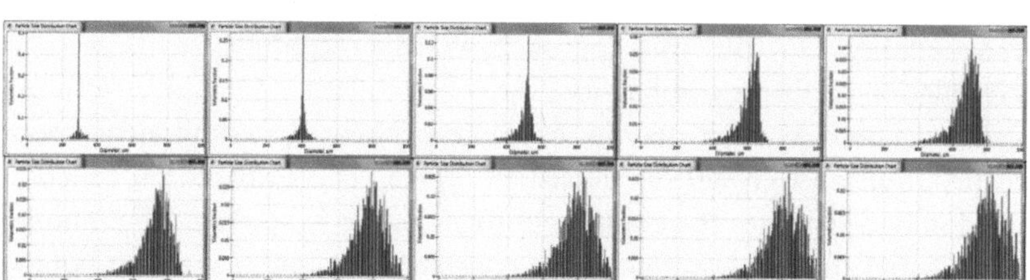

Figure 7.11 Particle size distribution of individual particles in a compact with respect to growth iteration (top left: initial set, bottom right: after tenth iteration)

Table 7.1 Available compound types in F-CAD

Type #	Description of compound properties
0	Pore
1–9	API
10–19	Non-swelling, soluble fillers
20–29	Non-swelling, soluble binders
30–39	Non-swelling or negligibly swelling non-soluble fillers (MCC, etc.) absorbing water
40–49	Hydrophilic swelling matrices (e.g. HPMC)
50–59	Spherical disintegrants, swelling e.g. starches
70–79	Hydrophobic ingredients (glidants, etc.)
200	Dissolution media

of different phenomena and behaviors of ingredients, retaining high flexibility and simplicity. The type depends on the properties of the substance. In Table 7.1 we show the selected types and their functional descriptions, which are used in our simulations. Each type is associated with its own rule set (Table 7.4) for the dissolution calculation with CA.

As a second step (after components definition), the created tablet shape (0) is loaded into the PAC module. The discretized tablet shape in terms of CA-modeling is the constrained mesh where the CA will be defined. We will not describe in detail how the meshing and discretization of the smooth arbitrary geometry can be realized; however, it is important to note that there are several possible ways. The one we use in our simulations is based on the ray-casting method.

Filling of the components into the tablet in accordance with their individual concentrations and particle sizes finishes creation of the virtual tablet. However, it must be noted that this step allows very wide functionality, i.e. with this approach we can introduce such effects as granulation or direct compaction, etc.

We define two main operations while packing the components: seed distribution and growth as described above. The distribution function randomly distributes the compound for which it is applied. The number of cells to distribute is a function of concentration and true density of the component. At that moment it is noted that all components are defined in volumetric fractions. The software distributes the number of cells needed to reach this mass. As an example, Figure 7.13 shows the top view of a virtual tablet of pure caffeine with porosity of approximately

Published by Woodhead Publishing Limited, 2013

10% v/v encased in intrinsic dissolution constraints. The circular layer simulates an insoluble compound, which enables an intrinsic dissolution simulation by blocking the contact of the virtual liquid with dissolvable solid of the tablet. The same tablet is shown in Figure 7.14, but this is the lateral view.

If the distributed particles have a diameter bigger than unity, the 'seed' coordinates have to be arranged in such a way that imaginary spheres of the same diameter are densely packed. In this case the spheres are also distributed randomly, but only in positions where spheres do not overlap with one another (see Figure 7.12). Such an approach allows even distribution of the 'nucleation' or starter centers (the seeds) for further evolutionary growth of the particles or granules.

Particle growing enables allocation of particles or granulates in 3-D tablet models. To achieve this, 'seeds' are placed into matrix cells positioned at the center of each particle. A seed is composed of three cells and is randomly oriented. Each particle in the matrix grows out of its own seed. The growing process is achieved by transforming each 'empty' cell in the Moore neighborhood of seed cells into a particle cell according to the target rule. In the same way, each newly created particle cell extends by transforming empty neighboring cells into particle cells.

After a certain number of growing steps, particles will meet each other, i.e. they will share neighboring cells. In this case, particles will grow around occupied cells up to a certain extent. The resulting effect is a deformation aspect of particles, similar to real compacts. In order to

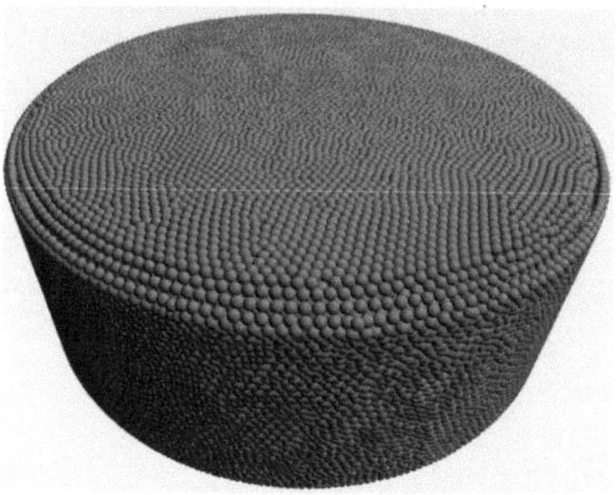

Figure 7.12 Packing of virtual 'placeholder' spheres to find central positions from seeds for further growth of the granules or larger particles of formulation components

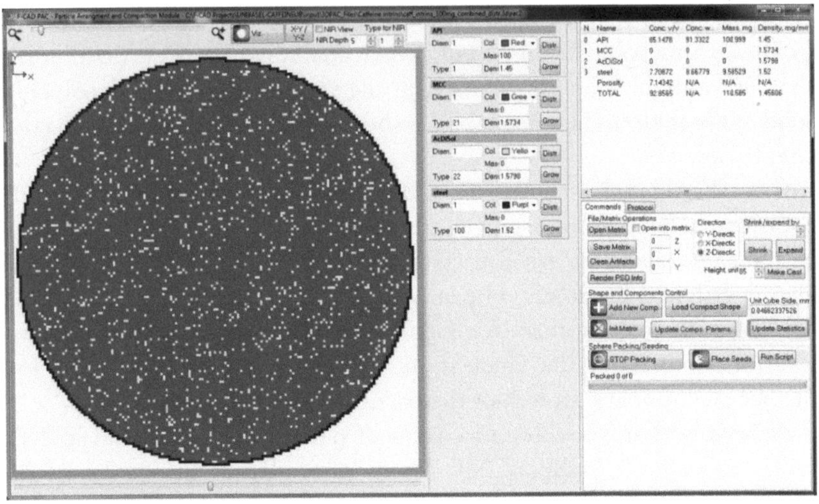

Figure 7.13 Interface of the PAC module with top view of a tablet filled with distributed API cells and surrounded by a steel mantle

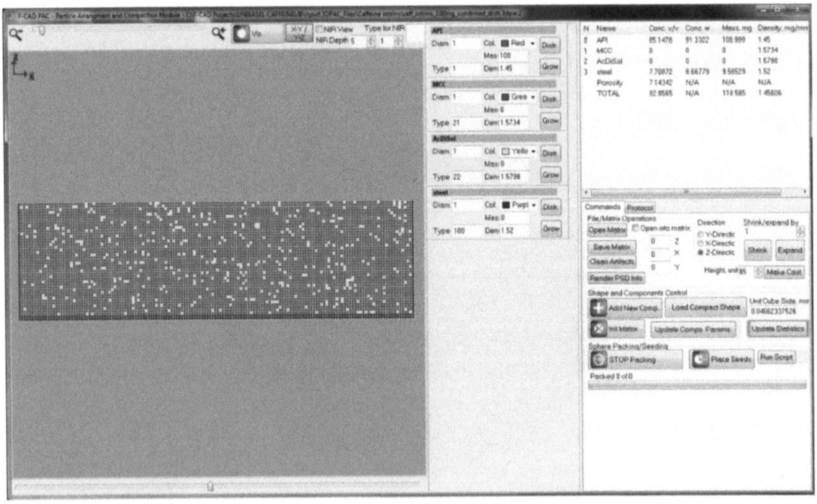

Figure 7.14 Interface of the PAC module with side view of a tablet filled with distributed API cells and surrounded by a steel mantle

Published by Woodhead Publishing Limited, 2013

respect the difference of hardness between components, the deformation potential of in silico particles should be calibrated.

The growing algorithm will stop when the volumetric ratio of each component is obtained and/or when the desired tablet porosity is reached. The result obtained with the particle growing algorithm is a discrete compacted mixture of ingredients ready for in silico dissolution in the cubic matrix.

As was already noted, the growing process is based on cellular automata. To illustrate the growth of one seed, Figure 7.15 shows the growth of a seed with an arbitrary-selected rule set. This rule set is growing a sphere-like particle out of the starting seed in four iterations.

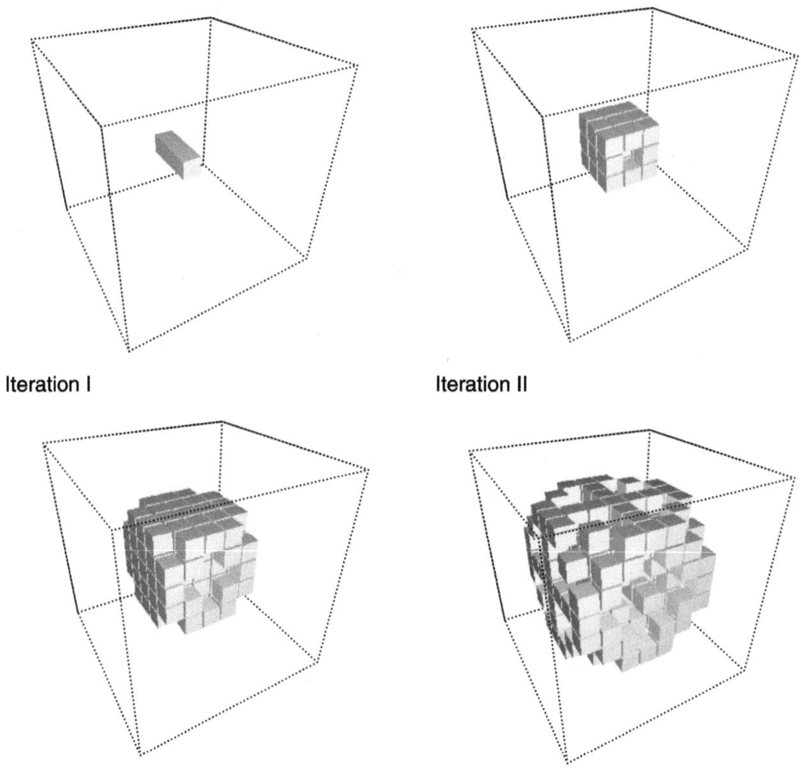

Figure 7.15 Iterations of 3-D CA for 'growing' one particle from a seed (Iteration I–IV)

The software realization of the growing procedure is similar to the one in Figure 7.15, but with a different rule set. As visualization, a screenshot of a PAC module interface, with the lateral cross-section of a tablet (a) and the calculated particle size distribution (b) is shown in Figure 7.16.

The resulting particle size distribution is calculated as follows: every seed has its own identity. This identity is passed on to the cubes which arise out of one seed during the growing process (the ‘offspring’). The volumes of the cubes with the same identity are added and the diameter of a sphere with this volume is then taken into an account for particle size distribution. This process is done for all particles. Table 7.2 shows the growing of micro-crystalline cellulose (MCC)-simulating seeds in a virtual tablet (Figures A^1–D^1 and A^2–D^2) and the associated particle size distributions (Figures a–d). Figure (a) in Table 7.2 shows only one peak in the particle size distribution plot, because all seeds are composed of three unit cubes which makes them all the same size. Figures A^2–D^2 are graphic visualizations of virtual tablets which are similar to the tablets shown in Figures A^1–D^1.

The evolution of the particle size distribution from a single delta function (the starting peak) into a bell-shaped curve could be explained by distribution of possibilities to grow for all particles. This is indeed a stochastic process and we can observe an interesting transition from an

(a)

(b)

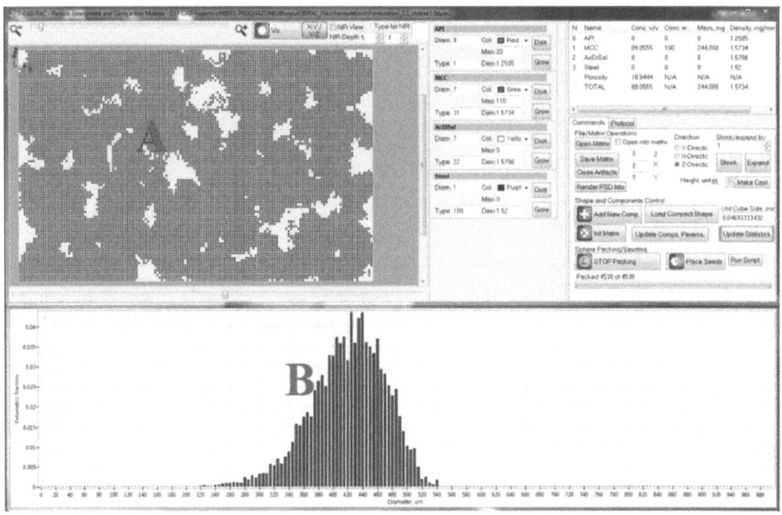

Figure 7.16 **Interface of the PAC module with lateral view of a tablet and particle size distribution plot**

Published by Woodhead Publishing Limited, 2013

Table 7.2 **Visualization of growth iterations of a single component**

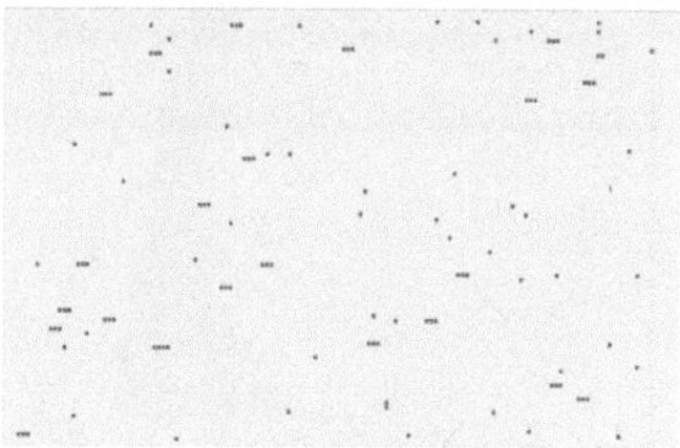

Figure A¹: MCC seeds in a lateral view on a simulated tablet

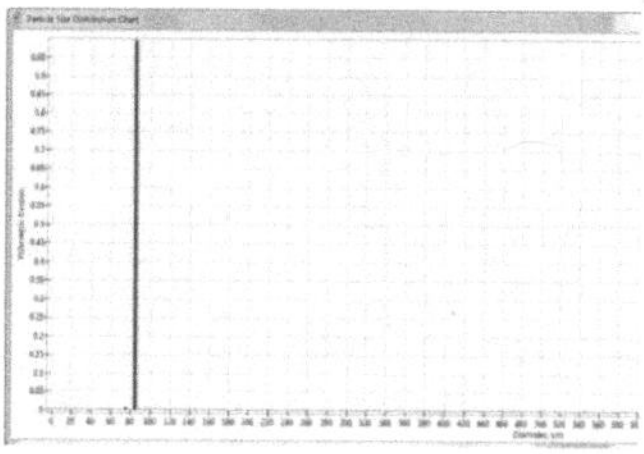

Figure a: Particle size distribution of MCC seeds v

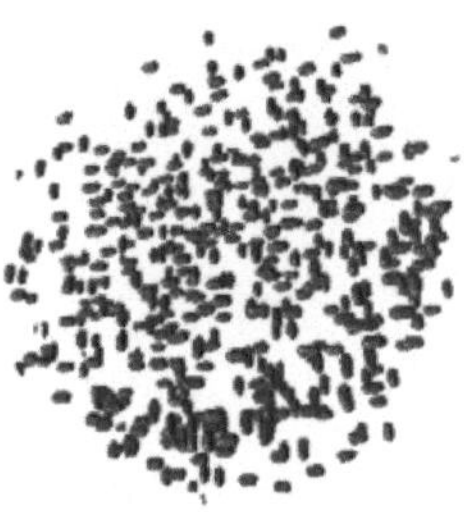

Figure A² : 3D visualization of MCC seeds

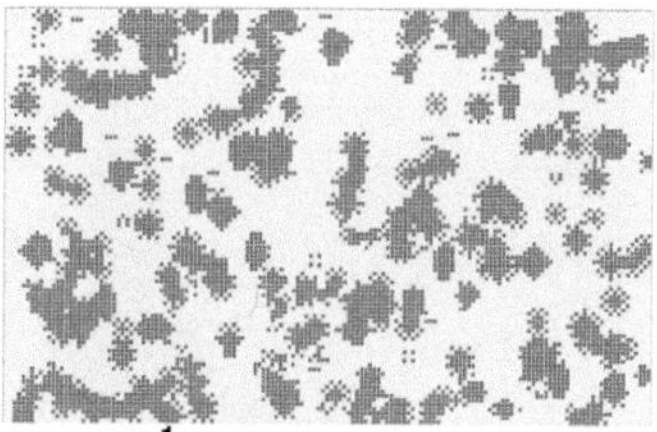

Figure B¹ : MCC particles growing step 4 in a lateral view on a simulated tablet

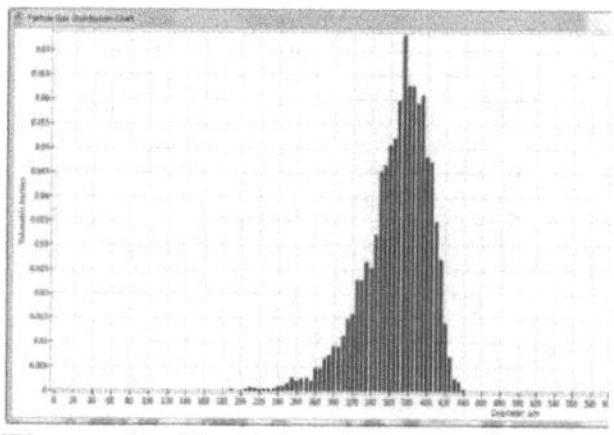

Figure b: Particle size distribution of MCC particles after growing step 4

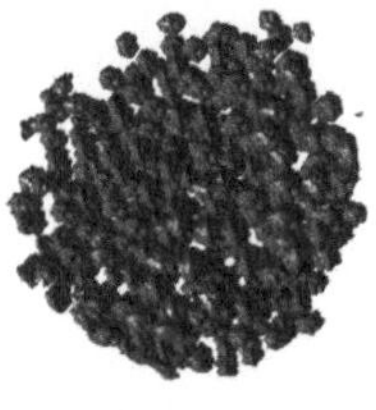

Figure B² : 3D visualization of MCC particles

(continued)

Table 7.2 **Visualization of growth iterations of a single component (*continued*)**

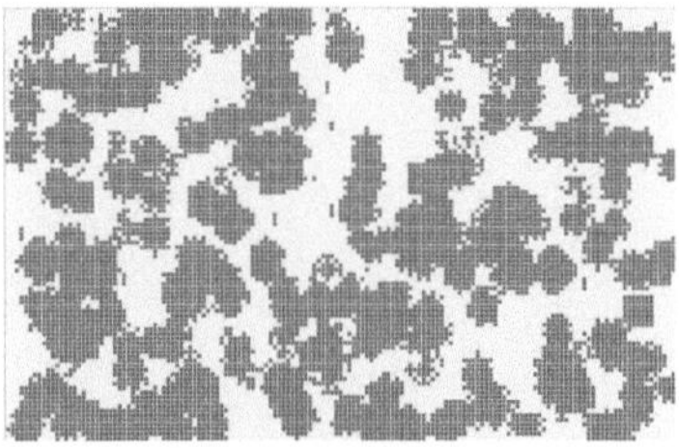 Figure C^1: MCC particles growing step 5 in a lateral view on a simulated tablet 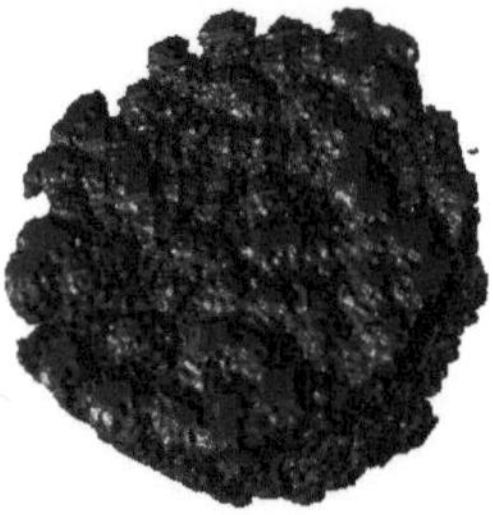 Figure C^2 : 3D visualization of MCC particles	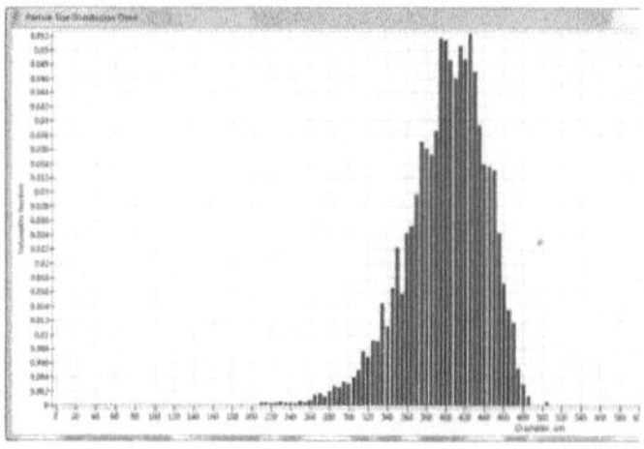 Figure c : Particle size distribution of MCC particles after growing step 5

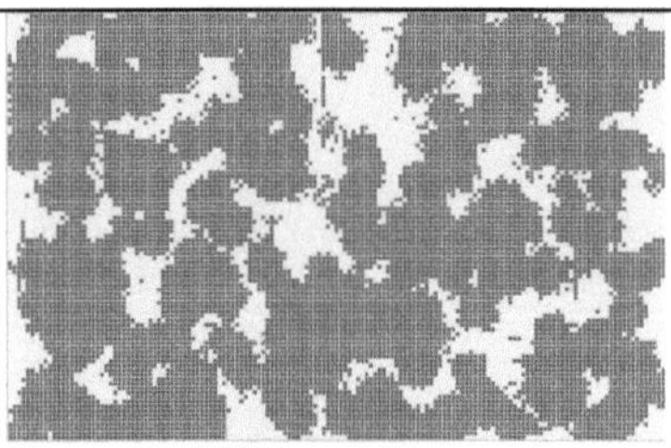 Figure D^1 : MCC particles growing step 6 in a lateral view on a simulated tablet 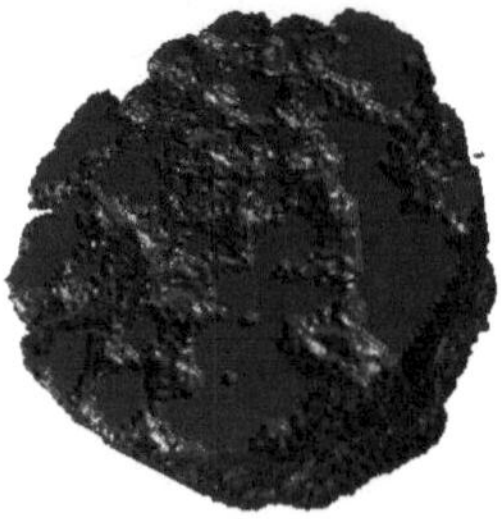 Figure D^2 : 3D visualization of MCC particles	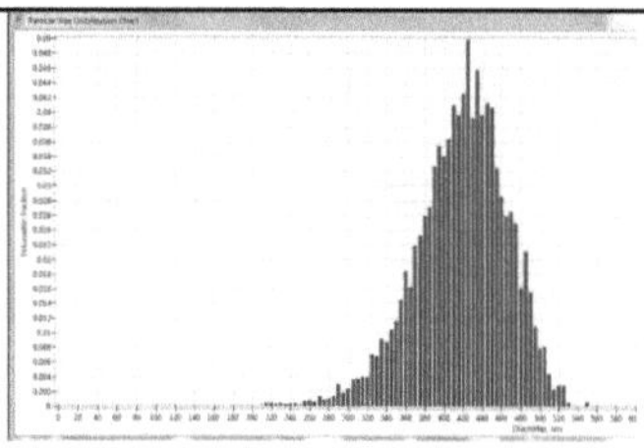 Figure d: Particle size distribution of MCC particles after growing step 6

Published by Woodhead Publishing Limited, 2013

ordered system at initial conditions into a fully random and chaotic arrangement.

As an intermediate conclusion it is important to say that CA-based methods for creating virtual tablets are extremely flexible and allow modeling of arbitrary tablet geometries, including multiple layer tablets, dry coated tablets, etc.

7.2.4 Dissolution profile calculation with cellular automata

Generation of the release profile from a virtual tablet is a separate task and is fully based on the CA rules. The calculation matrix – where the virtual tablet is defined – is finite and cubic, as well as the grid which forms the smallest units of the matrix: the unit cubes. Time is also discrete in CA, one time unit corresponds to one update of the whole system which leads to the next generation matrix. The unit cubes have different types with different properties, which are represented in rule sets. The available types are listed in Table 7.1, and correspond to the behavior of different components in a real formulation.

For a better understanding, the meaning of cell types and their corresponding rules are described in the following figures. In Table 7.3 the cell types are generalized for better understanding of the typical rule sets used to calculate the release profiles which are showing the possibility and the performance of the model. The symbols and number-coding in Table 7.3 are further used in visualization figures in Table 7.4.

Table 7.3 F-CAD cell types

Symbol	Representing cell type
0	Dissolution medium
2	Pore
5	API
6	Hydrophobic offspring cell
3	Swellable compound cell
D	Disintegrating compound cell

Table 7.4 Basic CA-update rules for different types of the components

Pores

The property of pore cells is regulated with $C1_{pore}$. To mimic the pores being wetted with a certain speed, pore cells are given a value (C1) which defines how many calculation steps are necessary to change a pore cell with contact to a liquid cell in the Moore neighborhood into a liquid cell. The higher the value of $C1_{pore}$, the more iteration will be needed to change the type of a pore cell. One could also say, the more hydrophobic the substances comprising a tablet formulation are, the slower will be the wetting process and the higher $C1_{pore}$ needs to be for an accurate simulation. In this case the primary constant C1 is the measure for hydrophobicity of the API or other ingredients.

As illustrated in Figures A–D, every liquid cell in the Moore neighborhood of a pore cell subtracts one unit from $C1_{pore}$ value until $C1_{pore}=0$ and the cell changes its state to that of a liquid cell.

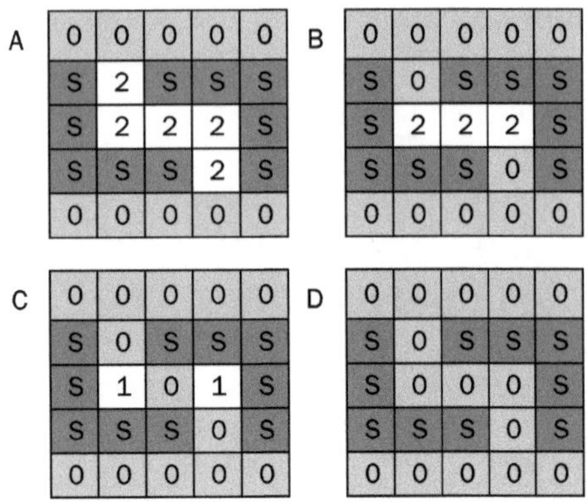

Active pharmaceutical ingredient (API)

The solubilization property of a non-hydrophobic API cell is characterized with $C1_{API}$, no C2 is necessary. $C1_{API}$ defines the number of iterations necessary to change the solid state of the cell to a liquid state. As for the pore cells, every liquid cell in the Moore neighborhood subtracts one unit from $C1_{API}$ at every iteration. As soon as an API cell changes its state from

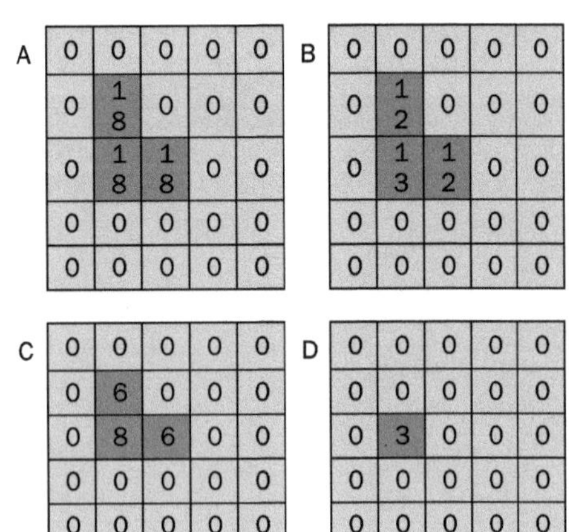

Published by Woodhead Publishing Limited, 2013

solid to liquid, one unit is added to the dissolution counter, which corresponds to the amount of drug dissolved in the experimental dissolution test during the same time interval. In the example on the right-hand side, an API particle getting dissolved is shown. Two units would be added to the dissolution counter before step D.

Hydrophobic API (hAPI)

The difference to API cells is that a hAPI cell is given a $C2_{hAPI}$. Hydrophobicity is imitated by giving the pore cells in the Moore neighborhood of an API cell a new $C1_{pore}$. $C1_{pore}$ is calculated by dividing $C1_{hAPI}$ by $C2_{API}$. In the example on the right-hand side, a hAPI cell with $C1_{hAPI}=18$ is surrounded by pore cells (p) and solid cells (S). $C2_{hAPI}$ is 3. As a consequence, pore cells in the Moore neighborhood receive a $C1_{pore}$ of 6. This step is not the end of the first iteration, but step 1.2 (Table 7.5). The end of generation one is shown in Figure C.

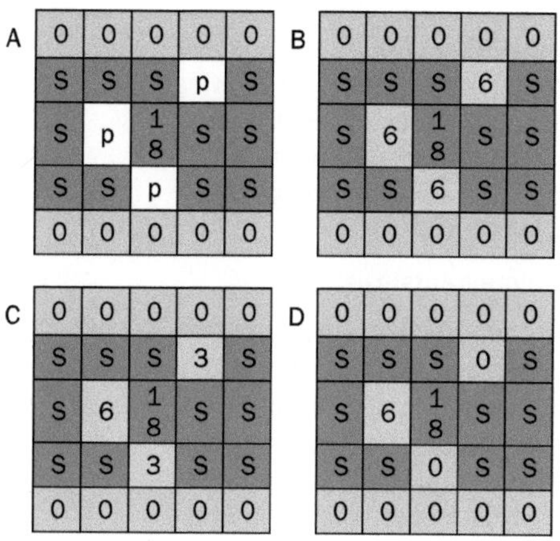

Swelling compound (Sw)

This cell type is used to simulate compounds getting more voluminous when coming into contact with water. Liquid cells in the Moore neighborhood are given (similar to hAPI cell type) a C1, which is calculated by dividing $C1_{Sw}$ by $C2_{Sw}$. The smaller $C2_{Sw}$, the higher is the expansion capacity of Sw cells. In Figures A–D, 2 generations are shown,

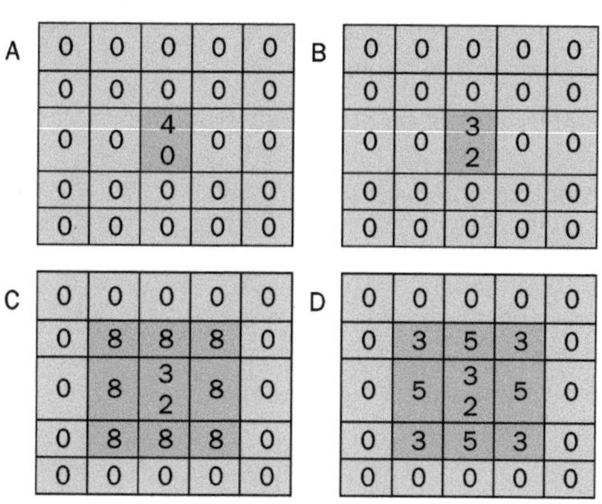

(*continued*)

Table 7.4 **Basic CA-update rules for different types of the components (*continued*)**

whereas the initial $C1_{Sw}=40$, $C2_{Sw}=3$. Figure A shows the initial state, Figure B shows the decrement of $C1_{Sw}$ (step 2 in Table 7.5), and Figure C shows the matrix after step 3. Figure D shows the matrix after step 2 of the second iteration.

This procedure enables simulation of complex swelling behavior with particles growing to a certain extent and then remaining in equilibrium between swelling and getting dissolved.

Disintegrants (Dis)

The approach of disintegration simulation as it is described here was a first attempt to simulate a quick exposure of API cells to liquid as is the case for disintegrating formulations.

The constants of Dis cells are both zero. This results in an immediate change of state after the first iteration as seen in Figures A and B. This change happens no matter whether or not the Dis cell has contact with any other liquid cell.

In the illustration pore cells are given a $C1_{pore}$ of 2, the solid cells are not given any attention.

This simplified disintegration rule set has limited usage and has to be expanded by movement of the cells during the simulation.

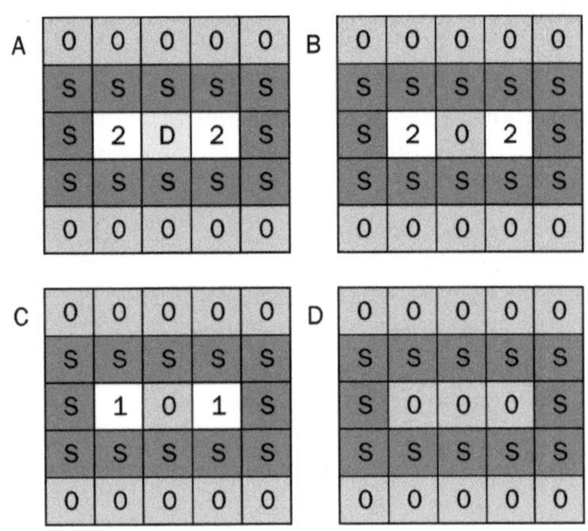

Published by Woodhead Publishing Limited, 2013

Fillers absorbing water (e.g. MCC)

In the case of sorption fillers or similar formulation components, the liquid in the neighborhood will be converted into pore until the sorbent cell is completely saturated (regulated by the C2 value). Once the saturation event is triggered, the filler is no longer changing the state of the liquid cells, hence allowing the liquid cell to dissolve adjacent API or other component cells.

Figure B shows the conversion of liquid cells into pore cells. During the same iteration, the value decrement is done (Figure C). If the sorbent cell F is not yet saturated, liquid cells in the Moore neighborhood will again be changed into pore cells (Figure D).

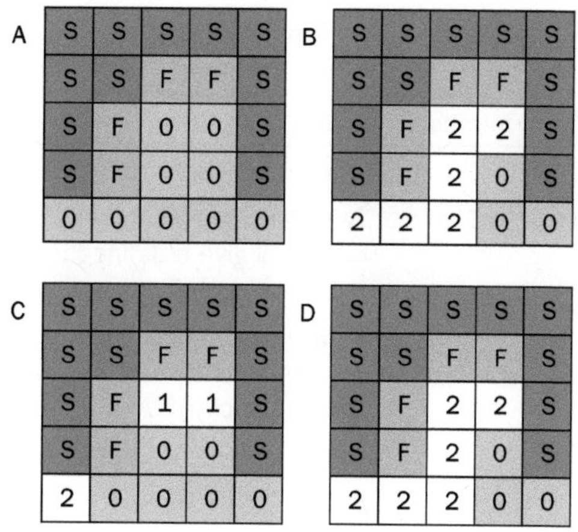

As can be seen from Table 7.4, the rule sets are dependent on the primary and secondary constants, introduced into these CA-based dissolution models. Technically speaking, every cell contains two constants: the Primary Constant (C1) and the Secondary Constant (C2). The definition of the constant is as follows: C1 and C2 are constant for every unique substance for time = 0. For any successive time step those values are subject to change during the calculation according to the rules in Table 7.4. Each cell type and subtype has its own constants, which need to be calibrated prior to tablet dissolution simulation. The calibration is best done by comparing experimental dissolution profiles to in silico generated dissolution profiles for a tablet with equal shape and porosity. The constants C1 and C2 are adapted until the simulated profile best fits the experimental one. C1 indicates the number of iterations needed to change the state of a cell from solid to liquid. The lower the value for C1, the fewer iterations are required. The physical meaning of C1 is reciprocal solubility per unit of time. C2 does not influence the state of a solid cell itself, but has several different functions which depend on the cell type and are explained and illustrated in Table 7.4.

Table 7.5 Calculation cycle of F-CAD dissolution calculation

Step number	Action
1.0	Initial updates
1.1	Type 30 value increases, i.e. all cells with type 30–39 (e.g. MCC) will give a defined value to liquid cells in their Moore neighborhood. Examples are given later in this section
1.2	Pore hydrophobization, i.e. pore cells neighboring a hydrophobic API cell are given a defined value to simulated hydrophobicity of API. An example is given later in this section
2	Value decrements, i.e. liquid cells subtract one unit from any solid cell in their Moore neighborhood
3	Swelling propagation. An example of the behavior of a swelling compound is given later in this section
4	Final update of the matrix, i.e. all cells with a C1 of zero are changed into a liquid cell with the associated properties. Also the number of API cells which changed their state due to virtual solubilization is added to the 'dissolution' counter

The calculation cycle, i.e. the sequence in which the rules are applied on the system, is the same for all dissolution calculations and is structured as shown in Table 7.5.

The release profile of the API is calculated for each time point in accordance with an initial set of conditions. The rules for CA matrix described in Table 7.4 are applied at each iteration step, and the statistics of CA cell count are collected. The amount of drug released is calculated in accordance with the number of cells which have changed their state from solid to liquid.

Release kinetics could be significantly altered by the particles located right on the surface, i.e. in direct contact with dissolution media. This effect is taken into account by the CA model and is illustrated in Figure 7.17. The enlargement section of the simulated release profile shows the release of the drug which is located directly on the surface of the compact. Usually, these effects are overlooked for immediate release formulations due to sampling times resolution; however, extended release formulations with hydrophilic matrixes have often displayed an initial 'burst' effect which is governed by a fast penetration of a dissolution medium into the surface layer of a compact.

Another important property of a pharmaceutical compact is its shape. The shape adjustments are often required not only because of marketing

Published by Woodhead Publishing Limited, 2013

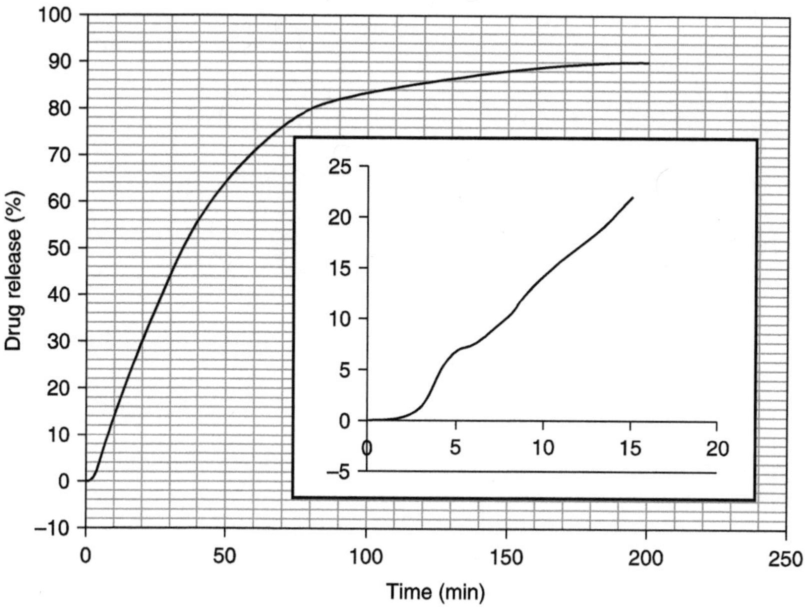

Figure 7.17 **Arbitrary simulated formulation release profile with an enlargement of the first 15 minutes. The 'drug on surface' effect is expressed on the fifth minute of the release curve**

issues, but also coating necessity, etc. However, a formulation might be sensitive to the shape alterations; hence changes in the release profiles are expected. The CA-based models of drug release emulation are capable of displaying the shape effect on the release profile. The calculated release profiles for identical formulations and identical compact volumes and porosities are shown in Figure 7.18. This property of the CA-based release models is very helpful for research work on geometrically controlled drug delivery devices and formulations.

It is well known that different unit operations such as direct compaction, or wet granulation, result in differences in particle sizes and different particle arrangements, which need to be taken into an account while doing simulations and modeling. Direct compaction assumes intermixed particles of API and excipient to form a compact, the wet- or dry-granulation process clearly specifies the inner and outer phases. In order to simulate granular arrangement of particles and corresponding release-profile changes, the 'Swiss cheese' procedure could be used. Following its

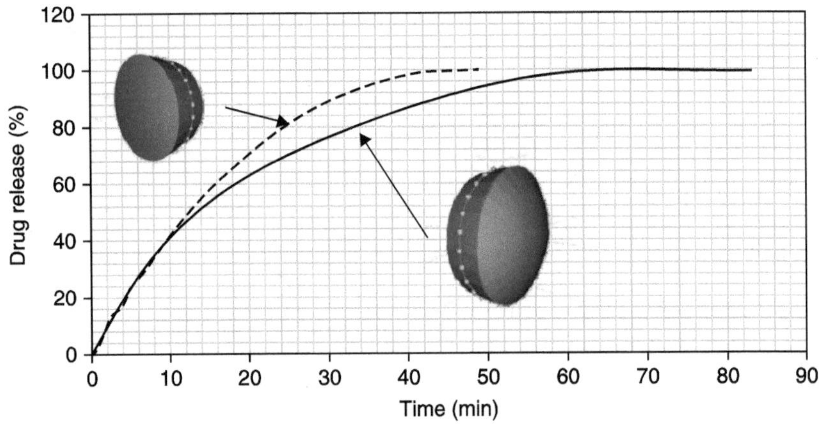

Figure 7.18 **F-CAD-generated release curves for identical formulations, identical porosities, masses, and compact volumes. The difference is the shape of the two compacts: flat round vs. round concave**

name, the 'Swiss cheese' structure is developed by growing only granules until a specified or desired size distribution. Once the granules are created, the remaining space is filled completely with auxiliary (starting) material (keeping its initial size) and the larger-sized granular material is removed. The remaining structure very much resembles Swiss cheese, hence its name.

The holes in the 'cheese' are filled with a composition of the inner phase and the auxiliary material is exchanged with a composition of the outer phase of the tablet formulation. Figure 7.19 shows the drug release profiles of a relatively well soluble drug substance in two identical compositions, where the only difference in the formulations is of the unit operations involved: one simulates direct compaction and the other is granulated. This example shows that release curves could show significant differences depending on the unit operation employed, and gives a good approximation for investigation of the unit operation influence on the final release profile of the drug.

As it can be seen from Tables 7.3 and 7.4, the number of basic CA types used for modeling the dissolution behavior of tablet formulation is not extensive. However, those types and the rules with those types calculated during the CA-update cycle allows modeling of a very large number of phenomena which occur during dissolution of a tablet formulation.

Published by Woodhead Publishing Limited, 2013

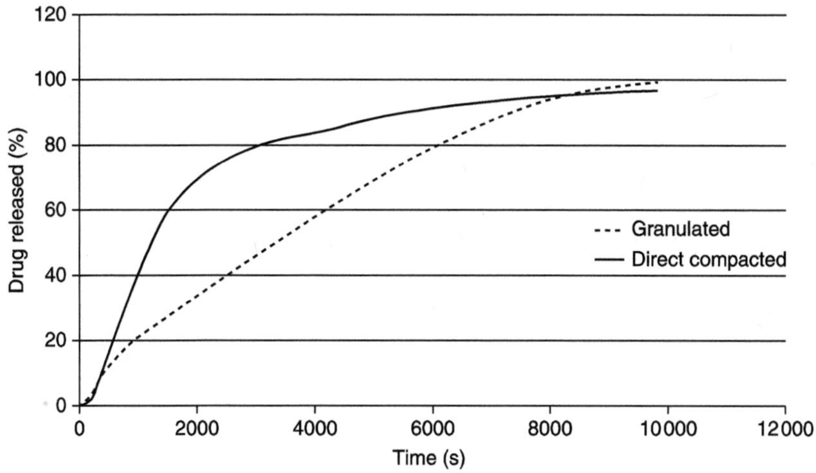

Figure 7.19 Release profiles generated for two different unit operations: direct compaction and wet granulation. Both are simulated curves, the formulation compositions are identical

To illustrate the modeling of solid dosage forms with cellular automata, several laboratory experiments with model drug (caffeine and proquazone) formulations were carried out. As an initial step the intrinsic dissolution rate (IDR) profiles were acquired. The usual purpose of those experiments, where pure API is compacted into a tablet with constrained surface, is to measure the dissolution kinetics of the API in the target buffer and to obtain the calibration value of C1. The value for C1 is obtained either by manual fitting until the experimental and simulated curves match or by applying optimization algorithms such as the Nelder-Mead simplex-based method. The machine-assisted C1 search is recommended in cases where the formulation for IDR-profile determination is necessary, e.g. low compressibility or compatibility of the target API. Simplex-based methods are capable of finding two or more optimal parameters, i.e. in this case the C1 for both API and the excipients could be found. As a disadvantage of this method, the 'entrapment' of simplex in local extremuma should be noted.

Figure 7.20 illustrates the two IDR-profiles: one is the average of the caffeine release profile (including the error bars) and the other one is the simulated curve of the same formulation with the same geometry constraints (see Figure 7.14). The two curves are practically indistinguishable from each other, which is shown as complete overlap

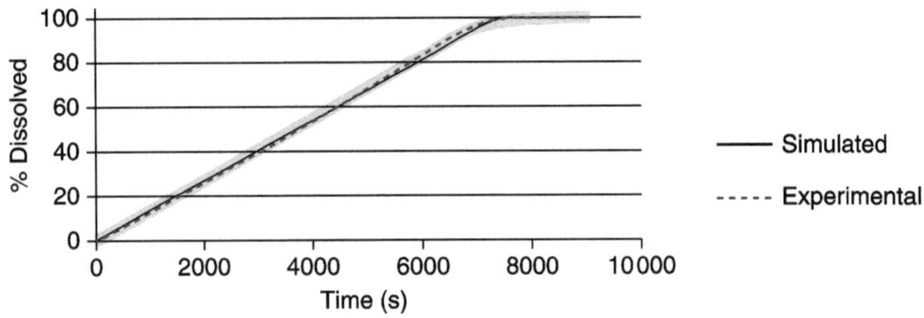

Figure 7.20 Experimental and simulated intrinsic dissolution profile of caffeine

of the curves. It has to be kept in mind that the CA-based calculation methods are not based on the fitting approach; therefore, to obtain the simulated release curve the time step has to be defined. In the presented curves the time step was set to 1 s, i.e. each update cycle of the whole calculation matrix corresponds to 1 s of real dissolution time. In such a case, it is very advantageous to use massively parallel software realizations of the CA-based dissolution algorithms. As a performance example, the parallel version of CA-based proquazone IDR-profile (Figure 7.25) was calculated for 300 000 s (approx. 3.5 days) in only 10 min.

In comparison to models based on fitted equations, the CA-based approach significantly widens the possibilities of modeling different phenomena occurring during the dissolution runs. As an example, we would like to show the influence of the size of the granules on release profile (see Figure 7.21). The experimental release curves (line with error bars) were obtained by compacting 7 mm tablets of granulated caffeine (approximately 450 μm). In this respect the deviation from the average curve is explained by random arrangement of the granules in the tablet, causing the fluctuations during the release. On the same figure, six simulated release curves are shown. The six virtual tablets were made to mimic the particles' size distribution of the real caffeine granulate. As can be seen, each simulated curve yields a different profile. This is because of the random arrangement of the granules each time the virtual tablet is constructed. It can be seen that the simulated curves very closely describe the variability of the experimentally acquired release profiles. In this particular example, the CA-based drug release model is capable of root case finding for out-of-specification problems, i.e. formulation-induced release profile variability.

Published by Woodhead Publishing Limited, 2013

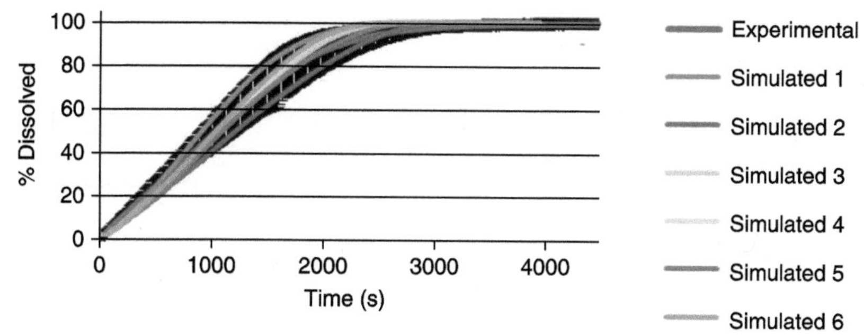

Figure 7.21 **Experimental and simulated intrinsic dissolution profile of granulated caffeine**

The task of exploring the phenomena observed during the drug dissolution could be fascinating, while studied with CA models. One such example is presented in Figure 7.22.

Here the release curve of the pure caffeine tablet without constraints was studied. It can be seen that the release rate at approximately 900 s is changing. This change was consistent for all six tablets dissolved, and yielded low variability as shown by the error bars. The visual inspection of the tablet behavior in the dissolution bath (USP 2) was possible throughout the whole dissolution. It has been observed that the tablets after 900 s of dissolution were falling apart, thus yielding a higher solid–liquid interface area. According to the Noyes-Whitney equation, such an event should increase the rate of the dissolution, which was successfully observed in Figure 7.22.

In order to prove this hypothesis, the virtual tablets were constructed with higher porosity at the core of the tablet. When the outer, denser layer was completely dissolved, the inner part of the virtual tablet yielded a higher dissolution rate as its contact surface to the cells of type 200 (dissolution media, see Table 7.3) was increased. The resulting simulated approximation is very close to the experimentally obtained release curve.

It has to be kept in mind that the ability of the CA-based model to calculate the release profile features is only possible if the mechanism of the drug release from a tablet formulation is understood. On the other hand, modeling with CA allows us to find the explanation for observed phenomena and a proof of the proposed explanation.

The few examples above concerned tablets compacted of pure API (caffeine). However, it is uncommon to have such formulations in reality for a multitude of reasons. In general, the tablet formulations contain 5–60% w/w of excipients which serve different functions: from

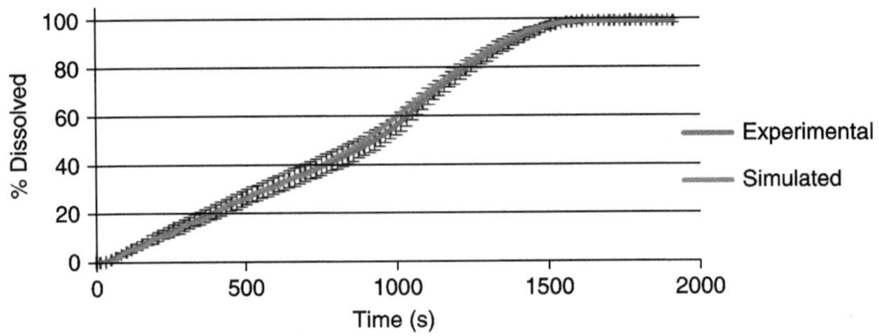

Figure 7.22 **Experimental and simulated dissolution profile of pure caffeine tablets**

compatibility and compressibility enhancement to release profile modifications, etc. It is indeed of interest to calculate and to study the influence of excipients on release rate of a tablet or capsule formulation.

The results of such a study are presented in Figure 7.23, depicting the release profile from caffeine tablet formulation with 54% v/v of MCC. In this formulation MCC plays the role of a disintegrant, forcing the caffeine crystals to expose a higher surface to the dissolution media. The simulated MCC function introduced such action to the vicinity of API cells. Similar to reality, such action forced an accelerated release from the CA-based tablet model. The resulting curves (simulated 1a and simulated 1b) closely approximate the experimental release profile of the tablet formulations with MCC.

In the next example, the disintegration action of MCC is enhanced by adding 2.5% v/v of crosscarmellose sodium (Ac-Di-Sol) to the formulation with MCC (see Figure 7.24). The synergistic effect of Ac-Di-Sol and MCC yields a higher release rate of caffeine as can be seen from Figure 7.24. The imprecise simulation of the experimental release curve (simulated 1, synergistic effect of the disintegration is off) is shown for comparison with curve 'simulated 2', where the synergistic effect of the MCC and Ac-Di-Sol on the release rate is used. In this case the synergy between those two components was taken into account by reducing the primary constants for both excipients to 0, i.e. virtually 'disintegrating' the API cells in the vicinity of the excipient. The resulting simulation curve provides a very close approximation of the experimentally acquired release profile (see Figure 7.24).

Following the example with Ac-Di-Sol and MCC formulation, it must be kept in mind that successful simulation of the release profile is not

Published by Woodhead Publishing Limited, 2013

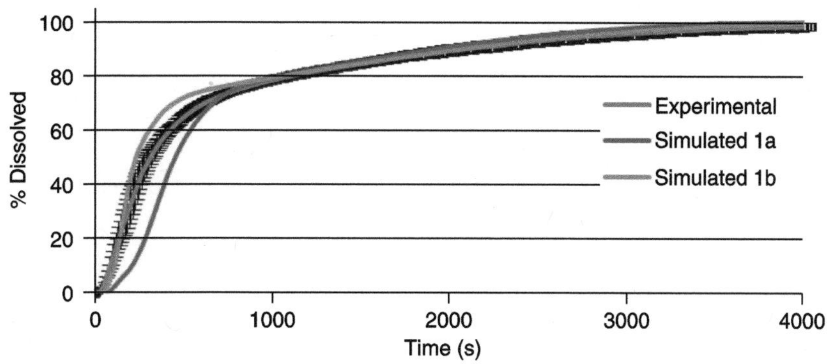

Figure 7.23 Experimental and simulated dissolution profiles of Formulation 1.4

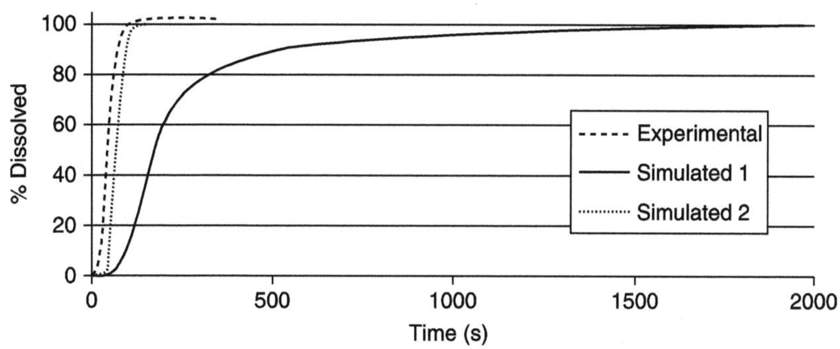

Figure 7.24 Experimental and simulated dissolution profiles of formulation with MCC and Ac-Di-Sol

possible without understanding the physicochemical nature of the studied phenomena.

The above-mentioned examples describe simulations of the formulations with well-soluble drug substances. In the following example the low-soluble drug Proquazone is used in the example of simulations for a more challenging formulation. The IDR profile of proquazone tablet is shown in Figure 7.25. The simulated curve represents the virtual tablet simulated release profile with constrained geometry. The primary API constant was found and was kept for additional simulation of the release profile where the virtual tablet was not subject to any geometry constraints, i.e. just a simulation of the pure API compacted tablet in dissolution media. As can be seen in Figure 7.26, the simulated curve closely describes the experimentally obtained release curve, keeping the primary API constant intact.

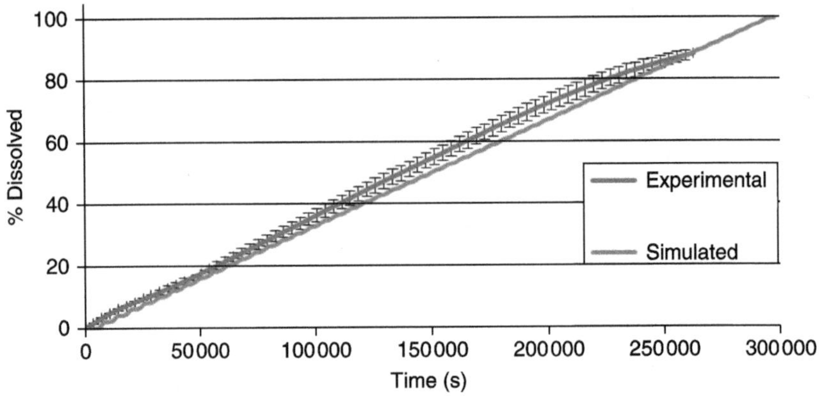

Figure 7.25 Experimental and simulated intrinsic dissolution profiles of proquazone

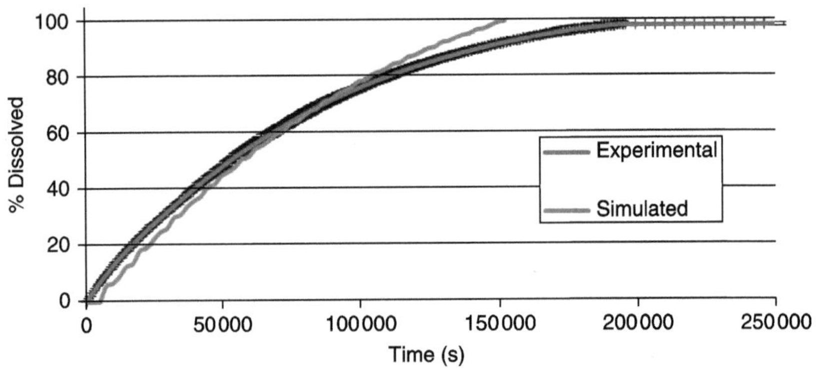

Figure 7.26 Experimental and simulated dissolution profiles of pure proquazone tablets

This example demonstrates that the influence of tablet geometry on the release rate of the tablet is significant, and this effect could be easily taken into account by CA-based dissolution models. It is also important to highlight that the actual solubility of the API (caffeine or proquazone) does not influence the performance of the calculation model.

As described above, the presented dissolution examples were calculated with the help of CA-based formulation design and modeling software: F-CAD developed by CINCAP GmbH, Switzerland. In order to complete the illustration of the modeling of a tablet formulation, the basic concepts of F-CAD are presented in the next section.

Published by Woodhead Publishing Limited, 2013

7.3 F-CAD: software package for CA-based formulation design

F-CAD (Formulation – Computer-Aided-Design) is a software package developed by CINCAP GmbH (Switzerland) to support efficient and reliable tablet formulation development. It is based on the mathematical concept of cellular automata, as described in previous sections. In this respect, F-CAD is not an expert system because it is not directly based on human expert knowledge but is a computer-aided design (CAD) tool.

In accordance with the previous sections and details on the CA-based compaction and dissolution models, the input data for F-CAD software are not extensive: only a few physicochemical properties of the compounds are needed. In fact the input data are split into two major parts: physicochemical and geometry-related parameters of pharmaceutical formulation. Physicochemical parameters describe components' solubility, water (or other solvent) sorption, swelling kinetics, and others. Geometry-related parameters span from individual component properties to granulate and tablet geometrical parameters, i.e. sizes, shape factors. Therefore, the software, by means of the mathematical model used, is capable of taking into account solubility, swellability, and particle size distribution of all compounds and any desired shape of a tablet. The software consists of several independent software modules which have been developed, upgraded and improved over the last decade. The aims in developing the F-CAD software were in agreement with the statements in the introduction section, i.e.:

- Enable a formulation design for the market with a minimum amount of drug substance and time,
- Explore formulations which could not be tested in vitro due to lack of API or other reasons,
- Minimize laboratory experiments, hence shortening time-to-market,
- Check for equivalence in case of excipient change,
- Save money by quality improvement,
- Apply root-cause analysis in case of 'out of specification' (OOS) problems.

7.3.1 F-CAD modules

The software consists of several independent software modules, all serving a different purpose during the design of a tablet. The modules are listed in chronological order as they were used during the general workflow:

- Tablet Designer (TD)

  This module enables tablet shape design with complex geometry. The output is a discrete tablet which is discretized and then transferred to the Particle Arrangement and Compaction module.
- Discretizator module

  This module enables transformation of the complex, arbitrary-shaped tablet into a discrete cubic grid (or 3-D matrix). This matrix serves as an input file for the Particle Arrangement and Compaction module.
- Particle Arrangement and Compaction module (PAC)

  Here, the virtual tablet is filled with particles and the complete composition of the formulation is entered. A growth algorithm is used to design different particle sizes and, in combination with seed distribution functionality, is allowed to mimic conditions after granulation.
- Dissolution Simulation (DS)
- To calculate the dissolution of a previously designed and packed tablet, the concept of cellular automata is used. The dissolution of every API cell is calculated using the generalized description of the solid–liquid interface (Puchkov and Leuenberger, 2011) which correlates to the Noyes-Whitney equation.

7.3.2 Tablet designer and discretization module

The virtual tablet was designed using the Tablet Designer module (Figure 7.27). With this module any arbitrary shape of tablet can be designed and further used with F-CAD. In addition, the software calculates the tablet volume and porosity if test compounds are filled into the matrix. The designed tablet is then transferred to the discretizer.

In the discretizer module the matrix gets rendered. This process is based on a ray-casting discretization algorithm. Technically speaking, rays penetrate the cubic matrix in x- and y-directions. The distance between the penetrating rays correlates with the matrix side length, divided by the number given in 'Cube size, units'. The ray cast finds the coordinates of intersection points of the ray with the tablet shape. The matrix around the tablet is filled with unit cubes, except for the tablet

Published by Woodhead Publishing Limited, 2013

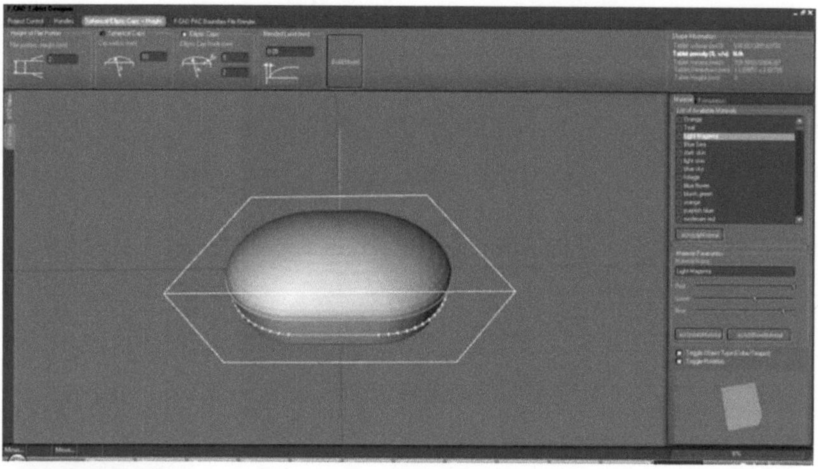

Figure 7.27 Interface tablet designer module

which forms a hollow space. After the process is done for the whole matrix, the matrix is inverted, finally producing a rendered tablet, filled with unit cubes.

The number in 'Cube size, units' defines the number of cubes at the edges of the cubic grid around the tablet (Figure 7.28). Like this, the size of the smallest unit (one particle) is specified. More cubes result in more cells which need to be calculated for every iteration of the dissolution calculation process. Thus, it is not always possible to simulate the dissolution of a virtual tablet which contains as many particles as a real tablet. Consequently there is a compromise to be made between precision of the calculation and speed.

7.3.3 F-CAD modes of operation (general schema)

A generalized task design and operation workflow consists of three main phases: 1. 3-D design of a tablet geometry in order to define the wall constraints; 2. packing the components into the hollow tablet; and 3. calibration for new API or direct calculation of the release profile if calibration constants C1 and C2 were defined.

In the case of a new active substance, calibration is mandatory. The calibration of an ingredient, API or an inactive excipient, is usually carried out with laboratory experiments for intrinsic dissolution rate (IDR) data.

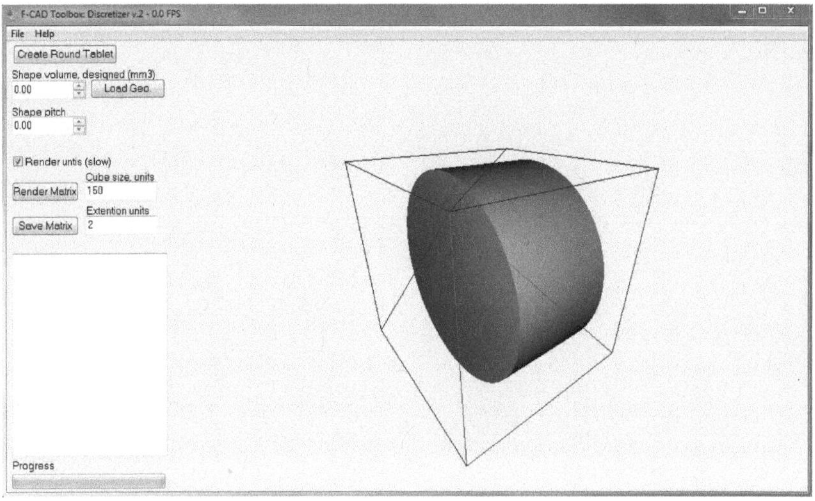

Figure 7.28 User interface of the discretizer module, showing a round, flat tablet

Attempts are made to simulate the IDR profile with F-CAD using the dissolution constants at first approximation. Where the resulting release profile deviates from the laboratory data, the optimization algorithm (Nelder-Mead simplex method) is used to find the solubility constant at which the experimental and calculated release profiles converge.

Release profile simulation is an iterative approach, i.e. the search for best and robust formulation is performed in a circle until the best satisfactory result is achieved. It is also important to do confirmation trials and it is necessary to recalibrate formulation excipients where there is low performance.

7.3.4 F-CAD input data

Generally, the required data set for successful development with F-CAD does not exceed the standard data on new or generic API. The API-related data include solubility and stability profiles at different pH ranges, true density, particle size distribution. In the case of known polymorphs, the same set of data should be readily available for different polymorphic modifications. For calibration purposes the intrinsic dissolution rates for an API of interest are required. The excipients used must be investigated also for their particle sizes, true densities and any effect on the API solubility. The latter is usually accomplished by studying the IDR

Published by Woodhead Publishing Limited, 2013

of binary mixtures between an excipient and an API of interest. For simplicity the IDR of a trial formulation consisting of the API and of excipients of interest, which need to be chemically compatible (Leuenberger, et al., 2010), is often tested at first. It is important to note that once being characterized an excipient can be further used with different APIs and excipient mixtures.

7.4 Conclusions

In this chapter we introduced the concept of a CAD-based approach to solid dosage formulation design and assessment. The studied concept is based on the 3-D cellular automata, which allows us a greater flexibility in modeling the performance of tablet formulations.

Besides flexibility, the 3-D CA offer deep, mechanistic understanding of physicochemical phenomena which take place during compaction and dissolution of solid dosage forms. However, it must be kept in mind that the versatility of formulations and processes requires more work on the model and additional effects in the form of rules should be continuously researched and introduced into the modeling concept.

The software realization of CA-based models is a feasible task and the first software product for accomplishing such a task was presented in this chapter. In general CA-based algorithms are best realized with massively parallel computation systems, which are currently receiving very strong attention.

The software discussed in this chapter, F-CAD, and its mathematical concept are very useful and helpful for fast and reliable formulation development. The overall concept was initially developed and programmed for seamless introduction into formulation R and D; the generally required initial data set is not extensive and is usually satisfied with routinely collected data for new or generic API. Introduction of an F-CAD system into a routine formulation development work would be beneficial as it speeds up time-to-market, cuts down the time and costs of extensive laboratory trials, and stores acquire knowledge and experience on API, excipients, and their interactions in a readily available compound library for further use.

7.5 Acknowledgments

The authors of this chapter would like to acknowledge Prof. Dr. Jörg Huwyler from University of Basel for his valuable comments and support of this work. We also acknowledge Swiss National Science Foundation for SCOPES programs and grants allowing international exchange of scientific contributors.

7.6 References

Bonny J. 1994 *Wirkstofffreisetzung aus MatrixRetardformen: Die Bedeutung der fraktalen Geometrie und der Perkolationstheorie.* Basel: University of Basel.

Chopard B and Droz M. 1998 *Cellular Automata of Physical Systems.* Cambridge University Press.

Krausbauer E. 2009 *Contributions to a science based expert system for solid dosage form design.* Dissertation, University of Basel: s.n.

Lai S. 1996 *Pharm Technol Eur* 8, 60–8.

Lauritzen S and Spiegelhalter D. 1988 Local Computations with Probabilities on Graphical Structures and their Application to Expert Systems. *J R Statist Soc* 2, 157–224.

Leuenberger H and Lanz M. 2005 Pharmaceutical powder technology — from art to science: the challenge of the FDA's Process Analytical Technology initiative. *Advanced Powder Technology,* 16(1), 3–25.

Leuenberger H, Leuenberger M and Puchkov M. 2009 Implementing virtual R&D reality in industry: in-silico design and testing of solid dosage forms. *Swiss Pharma,* 31(7–8), 18–24.

Leuenberger H, Leuenberger M and Puchkov M. 2010 Right First Time: Computer-aided scale-up for manufacturing solid dosage forms with a shorter time to market. *Swiss Pharma,* 32(7–8), 3–13.

Partridge D and Hussain K. 1994 *Knowledge-Based Information System.* s.l.:McGraw Hill.

Puchkov M and Leuenberger H. 2011 Computer-Aided Design of Pharmaceutical Formulations: F-CAD Software and a Mathematical Concept. *Glatt International Times*, August, 31, 2–6.

Ramani K and Patel M. 1992 An expert system for druf preformulation in a pharmaceutical company. *J Informs*, 101–8.

Rowe C and Ronald R. 1998 Artificial intelligence in pharmaceutical product formulation: knowledge-based and expert systems. *Research Focus* 4, 153–9.

Rowe R and Roberts R. 1998 *Intelligent Software for Product Formulation.* London: Taylor & Francis Ltd.

Sell P. 1985 Expert systems – a particular introduction. *Camelot Press.*

Stricker H. 1994 *Pharm Ind* 56, 641–7.

Turban E. 1995 *Decision Support Systems and Expert Systems.* 4. ed. s.l.:Englewood Cliffs.

von Orelli J and Leuenberger H. 2004 Search for technological reasons to develop a capsule or a tablet formulation with respect to wettability and dissolution. *Int J Pharm* 287, 135–45.

Published by Woodhead Publishing Limited, 2013

Wolfram S. 2002 *A New Kind of Science*. Champaign, IL: Wolfram Media.
Yang X and Young Y. 2012 *Cellular Automata, PDEs, and Pattern Formation*. [Online] Available at: *http://arxiv.org/abs/1003.1983*. [Accessed 31 May 2011].

8

OXPIRT: Ontology-based eXpert system for Production of a generic Immediate Release Tablet

Nopphadol Chalortham, Chiangmai University, Thailand, Taneth Ruangrajitpakorn, NECTEC, Thailand, Thepchai Supnithi, NECTEC, Thailand and Phuriwat Leesawat, Chiangmai University, Thailand

DOI: 10.1533/9781908818508.203

Abstract: We introduce an ontology based expert system for suggesting production of an immediately released tablet in generic version called OXPIRT. It was designed to assist pharmacists by providing a list of ingredients in formulation, a manufacturing process, a step-by-step instruction of laboratorial scale production for testing, and a validation in terms of pharmaceutical equivalence to the original drug. For practical usage and efficacy, the domain knowledge of an original drug and a generic drug production from a regulated guidebook and expired patents is represented in ontology format while the operational knowledge for calculating a formulation and suggesting a manufacturing process is given in the production rules. Experiments were conducted on four drugs to approve its capability, and we found that the system worked very well on recommending a generic table production in an actual situation.

Key words: generic drug formulation, immediate released tablet formulation, OXPIRT, expert system, ontology.

8.1 Introduction

Every drug newly invented by a brand name company is usually covered by patent protection (Christian, 2010). The drugs are commonly sold at expensive prices, which recoup costs of development. Without patent protection, a drug can be freely reformulated into a generic version by other drug companies. The drug can be sold at a relatively lower price as generic production does not involve investment in drug discovery, and profitability can be maintained at a lower cost to consumers. Additionally, generic manufacturers do not bear the full cost of proving the safety and efficacy of drugs through clinical trials as these trials have already been conducted by the original company. In Thailand, domestic drug companies are particularly focused on generic drug development as inventing new drugs requires import of expensive technology from aboard. In an annual survey, it was stated that the price of original drugs was over 110% more expensive in Thailand than generic drugs (Sirisinsuk and Katechoen, 2009). In universal agreement, generic drugs can be legally produced for drugs where: 1. the patent has expired; 2. the generic company certifies that the patents of the brand company are either invalid, unenforceable or will not be infringed; 3. for drugs which have never held patents; or 4. in countries where a patent(s) is/are not in force. In Thailand, a patent right is legally in force and its length is dependent on the country to which the patent belongs.

To reformulate an original drug, its patent is the most fundamental source for details. However, a drug patent generally contains implicit details for protecting the exact reproduction of inventions. These implicit details include an amount of excipients, a type of excipients, a crystal form of excipients and so forth. Such implicit details are a challenge to pharmacists who attempt to reformulate the original drug as they specifically require pharmaceutical expertise, case-based experience and it can be time-consuming to totally figure the missing information. Moreover, an approved generic drug in the market must be qualified in terms of a pharmaceutical equivalence between it and its original drug. Therefore, generic drug formulation and production is not a simple task in practice for inexperienced pharmacists.

In the world of information technology, computer applications have been developed to deal with such complicated tasks. In the pharmaceutical field, applications called expert systems are employed to suggest formulation and production of drugs. An expert system is a computer program which emulates pharmaceutical expertise to resolve significant problems in a particular drug production and formulation. Basically, an expert system deploys an inference engine to infer implicit details regarding explicit facts. To effectively infer a result, the facts held in an expert system are usually provided as domain knowledge.

In the pharmaceutical domain, domain knowledge in an expert system was firstly represented within the rule itself to execute an action once a condition had been met, namely a production rule. Later, domain knowledge was extracted alongside the rule to purely store relevant facts. For a decade, ontology has been brought to represent knowledge in many scientific domains (Davies, 2006). The advantages of ontology in knowledge representation are the capability of the knowledge sharing, the re-use of knowledge and the better engineering of a knowledge-based system with respect to acquisition, verification and maintenance (Lacy, 2004). Lately, ontology has been involved in representing domain knowledge for an expert system and it effectively reflects sharing a common understanding of the structure of information among software agents.

Previous expert systems in the pharmaceutical field were developed for recommending an original drug, and are not all applicable to generic drug production. Moreover, many pharmaceutical expert systems such as Capsugel (Bateman et al., 1996), Sanofi (Rowe, 1998) and Boots (Wood, 1991), are focused on only one or two relevant dosage forms such as capsule and cream. As tablet is certainly the most preferred dosage form, covering 70–80% of all medicines (Augsbuger and Hoag, 2008), it deserves the primary intention.

8.2 OXPIRT architecture

The Ontology-based eXpert system for Production of a generic Immediate Release Tablet (OXPIRT) is an expert system designed to specifically assist with reformulating and producing a generic immediate release tablet (Nopphadol, 2011). A knowledge base relevant to generic tablet production is designed and represented in an ontology called pharmaceutical tablet production ontology (PTPO) (Nopphadol, 2008), while a set of production rules is assigned to help with analysing the conclusion in each condition. In an application, an inference engine is applied to simulate the reasoning process to pursue a conclusion from implicit information. An overview of OXPIRT is illustrated in Figure 8.1.

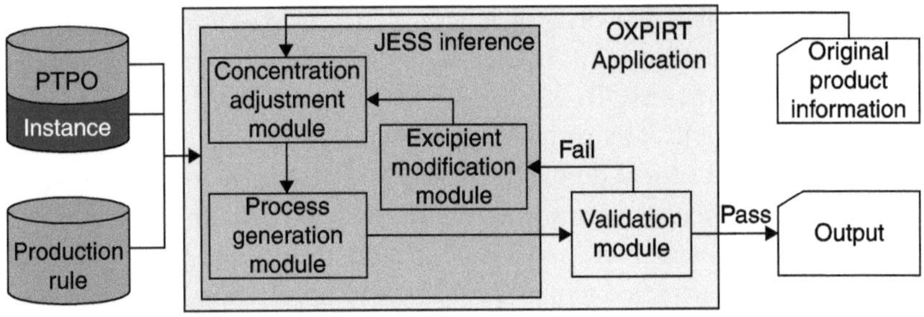

Figure 8.1 The OXPIRT process and its components

8.2.1 Pharmaceutical tablet production ontology

PTPO is knowledge relevant to generic tablet production represented in ontology knowledge representation (Nopphadol, 2008). The knowledge includes detail on the active pharmaceutical ingredient (API or main drug) and excipients, the possible role and range of concentration of an ingredient, manufacturing process, tablet property, original product information and so on. To make the knowledge systematically precise, a pharmaceutical expert manually gathers these details from the *Handbook of Pharmaceutical Excipients* (Rowe, 2005) and the expired patent of the original tablet, and designs PTPO according to its relation with each concept. Like other ontologies, the PTPO component consists of a class to represent a concept and a relation to represent a relationship between classes or class and its instance. These components, however, are not sufficient to cover the necessary knowledge of a generic tablet production; hence extra components, such as role of concept and special relations, are additionally designed to scope all knowledge mandatory to a generic tablet and herbal tablet production. In this work, PTPO was developed using the ontology editor tool Hozo (Kozaki, 2002).

PTPO class

A class in PTPO is designed to classify a concept or element relevant to tablet production. Each class is designed separately to represent particular concepts regarding tablet formulation and production, including maindrug, excipient, process, standard quality control (SQC), equivalent quality control (EQC) and caution. A list of these classes and their definitions is shown in Table 8.1.

Published by Woodhead Publishing Limited, 2013

Table 8.1 A list of the main classes designed for PTPO

Main class	Definition
maindrug	Represents active ingredient in a tablet formulation
excipient	Represents inactive substances that play a role in constructing a quality tablet, such as binding ingredients, accelerating the reaction, etc.
process	Represents a manufacturing process and an available action for tablet production
SQC	Represents a list of tablet-independent quality controls used for validating formulation based on *United States Pharmacopeia* standard
EQC	Represents a detail of pharmaceutical equivalence between a reference tablet and a tablet produced from a suggested formulation from OXPIRT
caution	Represents a list of problems that could possibly occur during the experimental process

Table 8.2 A list of relations designed for PTPO

Relation	Definition
is-a	Indicates hierarchical relation of each class
part-of (p/o)	Expresses a possessive hierarchy or a part–whole relation
attribute-of (a/o)	Links a class and its instance
precede	States a particular preceding order among classes
incompatiblewith	Clarifies an incompatibility between classes related to main drug and excipients

PTPO relation

A relation in PTPO is a representation of linking between the designed classes to create a relational structure within tablet production knowledge. Normally, three relations, 'is-a', 'part-of', and 'attribute-of', are assigned to general ontology, but these three relations are insufficient for PTPO as production of a qualified tablet involves other complicated and specific concerns, for example a particular orderliness of processes and an incompatibility among ingredients. Table 8.2 gives a list of relations and their definitions used in PTPO.

For only the 'part-of' relation, it is mandatory to assign a class constraint that limits the number of possible values for the class, called cardinality. A cardinality can be specified to a concrete number more than zero, number in range or least number. Ordinarily, it is used to minimize or state a number of a required class. In PTPO, the 'incompatiblewith' relation is additionally designed to prevent a selection of ingredients incompatible with each other that could cause inactivity of the API. For example, the Maillard reaction is a reaction in lactose that causes a tablet to change its colour and become inactive because of a malfunction in the main drug with ammonium functional group (Morales, 1997).

Taking classes and relations together, PTPO is crafted into a systematically related knowledge representation. Partial graphical detail of PTPO is illustrated in Figure 8.2. Classes are represented by a square shape and relations between classes are shown as lines. The TabletProduction class has four 'part-of' classes which are TabletFormulation class, Process class, ManufacturingProblem class and QualityControl class. For each 'part-of' class, cardinality is assigned differently: for instance, TabletProduction requires only one TabletFormulation as '1' is set for this 'part-of' class, whereas ManufacturingProblem may or may not be needed in TabletProduction as its cardinality is specified for '0. .', which means at least zero. Moreover, Process class has two sub-classes, DirectCompression and Granulation. These two classes are types of processes for manufacturing a tablet, therefore 'is-a' relation is defined to connect them with the Process class. Likewise, WetGranulation and DryGranulation are sub-classes of granulation and they are connected to Granulation class with 'is-a' relation. To complete DryGranulation class, there are four operations in sequence so they are listed with 'part-of' relation and linked to each other with 'precede' relation to specify a particular order for them.

Role of concept

A role of concept is applied in PTPO to indicate the role of ingredients in individual tablet formulation. It is possible that one ingredient can be used in a tablet formulation for several functions. However, each ingredient has a different range of available concentrations and amounts for each function. For instance, microcrystalline cellulose is an excipient that can function either as a disintegrant or as a binder when its concentration is between 5% and 15% and between 20% and 90% respectively (Rowe, 2005). Hence, a role of concept is applied to handle the boundary of this ingredient.

Published by Woodhead Publishing Limited, 2013

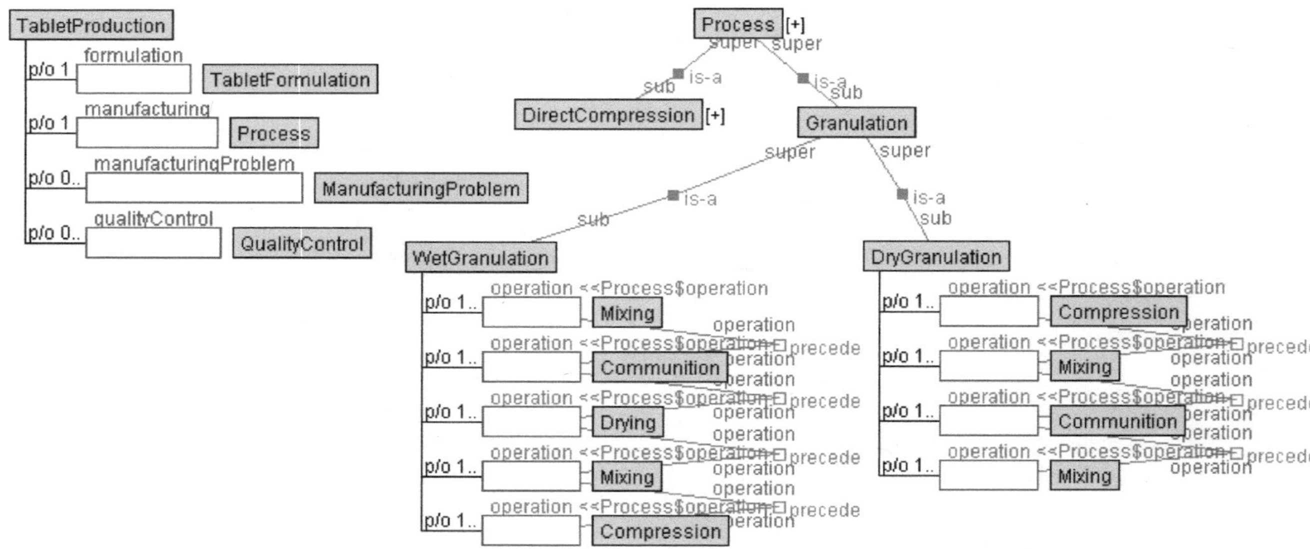

Figure 8.2 Graphical examples of PTPO

Instance in PTPO

Once PTPO is completely designed, an instance of each leaf node is attached by experts. Instances are collected in a database linked by 'attribute-of' relation of PTPO. They are data type to specify individuals to a certain integer or entity. However, some instances relevant to tablet formulation will be later assigned by a user based on each case. For example, dissolution profile and disintegration time are specifically different based on preformulation study of an original product, therefore case-by-case information will be entered by users through an OXPIRT user interface.

8.2.2 Tablet production rule

Tablet production rule (TPR) is a collection of operation knowledge gathered from experts on generic tablet reformulation based on different cases. The operation knowledge is designed for tablet formulation based on two types of information: 1. API preformulation study, such as physiochemical properties and 2. characteristics of an original tablet product, such as disintegration time and dissolution profile, gained from both its expired patent and laboratorial experiments. The components of production rules are in the form:

IF <condition(s)> THEN <action>

when the <condition(s)> is met, the <action> will be executed. To cover all purposes, three sets of rules are designed separately regarding 1. generic tablet production, 2. herbal tablet production and 3. improving non-equivalent formulation. TPR designed for OXPIRT is exemplified in Figure 8.3.

IF <solubility of drug is in type of 'slightly soluble'>

THEN <amount of lubricant at minimum level>

IF <hardness of original product is more than four kilograms>

THEN <amount of binder at maximum level>

Figure 8.3 Examples of OXPIRT production rules for generic tablet production

Published by Woodhead Publishing Limited, 2013

8.2.3 OXPIRT application

OXPIRT application requires a knowledge base from both PTPO and TPR. An inference engine called JESS (Friedman-Hill, 2003) is applied to reason and accomplish a reasonable conclusion. In OXPIRT, four modules are established as 1. concentration adjustment module, 2. process generation module, 3. excipient modification module and 4. validation module.

First, the concentration adjustment module generates a concentration of each excipient and calculates this into an exact amount with regards to total tablet weight and API amount. Second, the process generation module is designed to generate a manufacturing process of arranged methods as tablet production instruction. Third, the excipient modification module generates a list of proposed excipients and modifies those which cause invalid validation. Two strategies are used for modification of excipients: 1. adding another excipient and 2. substituting a suspicious excipient. The system selects a strategy based on the role of the excipient causing invalid validation. Together, the purpose of the first three modules is to generate a reasonable tablet formulation and instruction, whereas the last, the validation module, is implemented to evaluate quality control of a tablet produced from a suggested formulation and instruction.

The validation module is designed to validate tablet quality in two aspects. The first is to evaluate standard quality control of a suggested generic tablet production and a suggested herbal tablet production, and the second is for generic tablet production only, to validate a pharmaceutical equivalence between a suggested generic tablet production and its original product.

Information required for standard quality control is different dependent on tablet type. For a herbal tablet, information is required on disintegration time and friability, whereas information for a generic tablet also includes dissolution. Standards for each generic tablet are variable. For a herbal tablet in Thailand, disintegration time is specified to be less than 30 min after consumption and below 2% of friability is allowed.

For generic tablet production only, pharmaceutical equivalence is investigated as it is a requirement to qualify a generic version of a tablet product. To compare tablet pharmaceutical equivalence between an original product and a suggested product, difference (f_1) and similarity (f_2) factors are determined by performing the requisite dissolution rate testing on 12 tablets according to the FDA's *Guidance on Dissolution Testing of Immediate Release Solid Oral Dosage Form* (Shargel and

Kanfer, 2005). The difference factor (f_1) is a measurement of the relative error between the generic drug formulation curve and the trade name drug formulation curve, whereas the similarity factor (f_2) is a measurement of the dissolution curve between the generic drug and the trade name drug. If the f_1 values range between 0 and 15 and the f_2 values range between 50 and 100, both dissolution curves are compared. The range of similarity of f_1 and f_2 is set up between 0 and 100. The suggested generic drug tablet is satisfactory unless the curve reaches over the acceptable range. The difference factor and the similarity factor can be calculated from following equations respectively (Shargel and Kanfer, 2005).

$$f_1 = \left\{ \frac{\left[\sum \left| R_t - T_t \right|\right]}{\left[\sum R_t\right]} 100 \right\}$$

$$f_2 = 50 \log \left\{ \left[1 + \frac{I}{n} \sum w_t \left(R_t - T_t \right)^2 \right]^{-0.5} 100 \right\}$$

where f is a fit factor, R_t is a reference assay at time t (per cent dissolved), T_t is a test assay at time t (per cent dissolved), n is a number of sample points, w_t is a weight at time t (optional) and Σ is a summation of t from 1 to n.

8.3 OXPIRT process

OXPIRT has a certain work flow to generate a qualified tablet formulation and instruction. A structure of working processes is illustrated in Figure 8.4.

8.3.1 Required information

Before working with OXPIRT, a user must gather information from both preformulation study and patent reviewing. As working processes and validation necessity for generic tablet production and herbal tablet production are slightly different, the information required is accordingly differently. Table 8.3 shows the information required for generic and herbal tablet production.

In cases where the information provided does not include a list of excipients, OXPIRT executes the excipient modification module to generate a list using the given information on API properties by considering

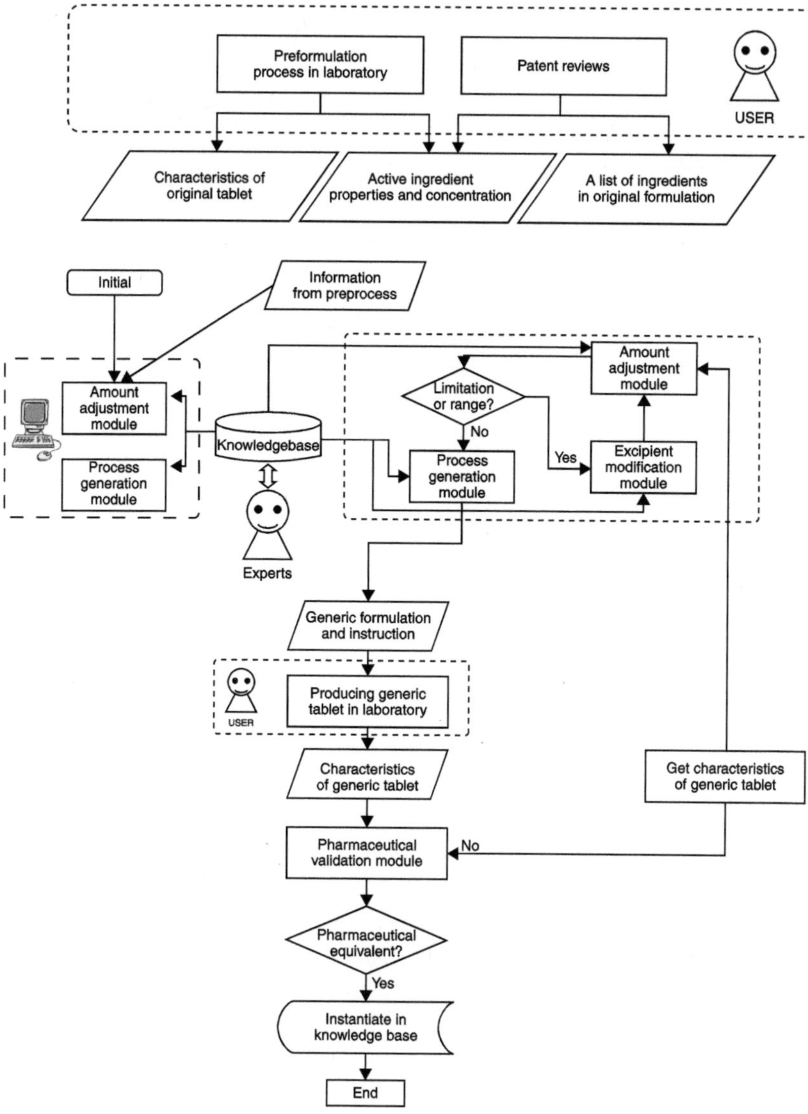

Figure 8.4 A structure of working processes of OXPIRT

compatibility and efficacy. When provided with a complete list of excipients, OXPIRT begins to generate a tablet formulation using the concentration adjustment module. A set of production rules for setting concentration is executed for each excipient by matching conditions from given information. OXPIRT continues to assign a concentration for each excipient and calculate its weight from a total weight of a tablet. The

Table 8.3 **Information required for OXPIRT for generic tablet and herbal tablet production**

	Information	Generic tablet production	Herbal tablet production
API properties	Name	Yes	Yes
	Amount	Yes	Yes
	Solubility	Yes	Yes
	Flowability	Yes	Yes
	Compactibility	Yes	Yes
	Temperature stability	Yes	Yes
	Moisture stability	Yes	Yes
Tablet characteristics	Total weight	Yes	Yes
	Disintegration time	Yes	No
	Hardness	Yes	No
	Dissolution profile	Yes	No
List of excipient names		Optional	Optional

manufacturing process is generated after examining characteristics of ingredients. With the complete result, a tablet formulation and instruction is displayed to the user. Once the user acquires the result for a generic tablet production, he/she is required to produce tablets following OXPIRT to obtain the properties and characteristics of the tablet for evaluating a standard quality control and pharmaceutical equivalence. Those properties and characteristics are a dissolution profile (%) at 5, 10, 15, 30, 45, and 60 min, an average dissolution and a disintegration time. With these data, the evaluation module conducts an approval of tablet quality and returns a validation result. If all criteria are within an acceptable range, OXPIRT displays a validation confirmation to a user. Otherwise, a failure notification is shown and OXPIRT uses the data as additional information for generating an improved result of the tablet formulation and instruction onward until an acceptable validation result is given.

8.3.2 Evaluation

To evaluate OXPIRT at work, four original formulations are selected as generic tablet examples based on two factors which relate to active ingredient (API) information. The first factor is solubility of active ingredient, which

Published by Woodhead Publishing Limited, 2013

Table 8.4 **Four drug representatives highlighting two factors related to active API information**

		Dose and ratio of API	
		1b. API>25%	2b. API<25%
Solubility of API	1a. Very soluble, Freely soluble, or Soluble	Metformin hydrochloride	Hydroxyzine hydrochloride
	2a. Sparingly soluble, Slightly soluble, Very slightly soluble, or Practically insoluble	Paracetamol	Atorvastatin calcium

can be of two types: 1a. better than soluble API and 2a. worse than sparingly soluble API. This factor indicates that the worse the solubility of the API, the more challenging will be selection of excipient, to improve dissolution of the API and overall performance. API with better solubility generally cause less problems in excipient selection and amount adjusting. The second factor is percentage amount of API per manufactured tablet, which can be of two types based on a criterion of content uniformity: 1b. API less than 25% and 2b. API more than 25%. Less than 25% API per tablet signifies difficulty in blending to a homogeneous mixture as large amounts of each excipient are combined. With more than 25% API per tablet, it is hard to identify appropriate amounts of excipients as the window for amount adjustment is too narrow. Combination of these two factors can generate four different groups of drugs, hence four selected representatives are shown in Table 8.4.

Metformin hydrochloride

From preformulation study and its original patent, we obtain information on original metformin hydrochloride as given in Figure 8.5.

Information	Value		
Solubility	Freely soluble		
Flowability	Poor		
Fracture surface	Rough		
Temperature stability	Stable		
Moisture stability	Stable		
API weight	500 mg		
Tablet weight	530 mg		
Hardness	9 kg		
Disintegration time	336 s		
Dissolution profile (%) at 5/10/15/30/45/60 min	53.51/56.92/61.10/85.06/85.59/89.60		
Ingredients I known amount I known function	Metformin hydrochloride	500 mg	API
	Povidone K30	-	Binder and diluent
	Magnesium stearate	-	Lubricant

Figure 8.5 **Information on metformin hydrochloride product from preformulation study and its original patent**

Table 8.5 **Rules used for adjustment concentration of generic metformin hydrochloride production**

Rule	Detail of rule
I	IF <solubility of API is very soluble or freely soluble or soluble> THEN <set the concentration of lubricant at maximum concentration>
II	IF <diluent exists> THEN <fill diluent until obtain the total tablet amount>
III	IF <flowability of API is poor or very poor or extremely poor> AND <fracture surface is rough> AND <temperature stability is stable> AND <moisture stability is stable> AND <API concentration is more than 10%> THEN < set the process type as Wet granulation >

Using the information as shown in Figure 8.5, OXPIRT performs an adjustment for a concentration of excipients. A set of production rules matching the information is executed to compute an exact weight of each excipient. A list of relevant rules is given in Table 8.5.

In detail, OXPIRT inferred a concentration of unknown amount ingredients and later performed a weight calculation based on the assigned concentration and tablet weight. In this case, the two ingredients concerned were magnesium stearate and povidone K30. First, magnesium stearate was involved in Rule I shown in Table 8.5. With the rule, a concentration of magnesium stearate was inferred to maximum as 1% (assigned in PTPO) and it was computed to weight 5.3 mg. Then based on Rule II, the diluent amount was computed by the total weight minus the available left space from the already set ingredients (i.e. 530 – (500 + 5.3) = 24.7 mg). Finally, a set of instructions was generated based on Rule III in Table 8.5. With these calculations, OXPIRT returned the generic reformulation of metformin hydrochloride as shown in Figure 8.6.

Ingredient	Function	Weight
Metformin hydrochloride	API	500.00 mg
Povidone K30	Binder and diluent	24.70 mg
Magnesium stearate	Lubricant	5.30 mg

Manufacturing process	Wet granulation
Instruction	1. Dry mixing metformin hydrochloride, povidone K30 2. Wet mixing mixture with water until wet 3. Communition with sieve no.14 4. Drying 5. Communition with sieve no.18 6. Dry mixing mixture and magnesium stearate 7. Compression

Figure 8.6 **OXPIRT result for an atorvastatin calcium generic product**

Dissolution profile (%)		
min	**Original**	**Generic**
5	53.51	42.75
10	56.92	58.53
15	61.10	69.37
30	85.06	91.72
45	85.59	92.62
60	89.63	90.79
avg	**71.97**	**74.30**

Disintegration time (s)	
Original	**Generic**
336	326
Pharmaceutical equivalence	
F_1	**F_2**
8.21	59.62
=(0–15) Pass	**=(50–100) Pass**

Figure 8.7 **Pharmaceutical equivalence result between the original and the generic atorvastatin calcium**

A result from OXPIRT is required to be produced in a laboratory to examine tablet properties for standard quality control. Figures 8.7 and 8.8 show, respectively, dissolution profile and graph comparing the original and the generic version gained from Figure 8.6, and the result shows pharmaceutical equivalence as the difference (f_1) and similarity (f_2) factors are within acceptable ranges.

Hydroxyzine hydrochloride

Information on original hydroxyzine hydrochloride is given in Figure 8.9.

The IF-THEN rules related to information in Figure 8.9 are listed in Table 8.6.

OXPIRT inferred a concentration of excipients and later performed a weight calculation based on the assigned concentration and tablet weight. In this case, five ingredients, crosscarmellose sodium,

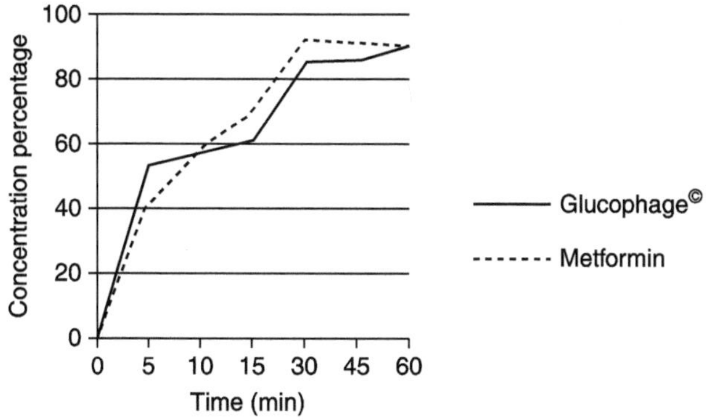

Figure 8.8 **Dissolution profile graph of Glucophage® tablet (original) and generic metformin hydrochloride tablet**

<table>
<tr><th>Information</th><th colspan="3">Value</th></tr>
<tr><td>Solubility</td><td colspan="3">Very soluble</td></tr>
<tr><td>Flowability</td><td colspan="3">Poor</td></tr>
<tr><td>Fracture surface</td><td colspan="3">Rough</td></tr>
<tr><td>Temperature stability</td><td colspan="3">Stable</td></tr>
<tr><td>Moisture stability</td><td colspan="3">Stable</td></tr>
<tr><td>API weight</td><td colspan="3">10 mg</td></tr>
<tr><td>Tablet weight</td><td colspan="3">65 mg</td></tr>
<tr><td>Hardness</td><td colspan="3">2.3 kg</td></tr>
<tr><td>Disintegration time</td><td colspan="3">180 s</td></tr>
<tr><td>Dissolution profile (%) at 5/10/15/30/45/60 min</td><td colspan="3">25.40/52.75/71.25/96.99/101.66/101.06</td></tr>
<tr><td rowspan="6">Ingredients | known amount | known function</td><td>Hydroxyzine hydrochloride</td><td>20 mg</td><td>API</td></tr>
<tr><td>Croscarmellose sodium</td><td>-</td><td>Disintegrant</td></tr>
<tr><td>Microcrystalline cellulose</td><td>-</td><td>Binder</td></tr>
<tr><td>Lactose</td><td>-</td><td>Diluent</td></tr>
<tr><td>Colloidal silicon dioxide</td><td>-</td><td>Lubricant</td></tr>
<tr><td>Magnesium stearate</td><td>-</td><td>Lubricant</td></tr>
</table>

Figure 8.9 Information on hydroxyzine hydrochloride product from preformulation study and its original patent

Table 8.6 Rules used for adjustment concentration of generic hydroxyzine hydrochloride production

Rule	Detail of rule
I	IF <hardness of the original is between 2.0 and 5.0 kg> AND <type of binder is hardest> THEN <set the concentration of binders at medium concentration>
II	IF <solubility of API is very soluble or freely soluble or soluble> AND <there is more than one lubricant > THEN <set the concentration of lubricant at minimum concentration>
III	IF <disintegration time of the original is less than or equal to 180 s> AND <type of disintegrant is super-disintegrant> THEN <set the concentration of disintegrants at maximum concentration>
IV	IF <diluent exists> THEN <fill diluent until obtain the total tablet amount>
V	IF <flowability of API is poor or very poor or extremely poor> AND <fracture surface is rough> AND <temperature stability is stable> AND <moisture stability is stable> AND <API concentration is more than 10%> THEN < set the process type as Wet granulation >

microcrystalline cellulose, colloidal silicon dioxide, magnesium stearate and lactose were considered. First, crosscarmellose sodium was involved in Rule III shown in Table 8.6. With the rule, a concentration of crosscarmellose sodium was inferred to maximum as 5% and it was computed to weight 3.25 mg. Second, microcrystalline cellulose was

Published by Woodhead Publishing Limited, 2013

involved in Rule I shown in Table 8.6. With the rule, a concentration of microcrystalline cellulose was inferred to maximum as 10% and it was computed to weight 6.5 mg. Third, colloidal silicon dioxide and magnesium stearate were involved in Rule II shown in Table 8.6. With the rule, a concentration of colloidal silicon dioxide was inferred to minimum as 0.1% and it was computed to weight 0.07 mg, and a concentration of magnesium stearate was inferred to minimum as 0.2% and it was computed to weight 0.13 mg. Fourth, the diluent amount is computed based on Rule IV by the total weight minus the available remaining space from the already set ingredients (i.e. $65 - (10 + 3.25 + 6.5 + 0.07 + 0.13) = 45.05$ mg). Last, the process type is set to wet granulation following Rule V. With all weight computed, OXPIRT returns a result as given in Figure 8.10.

A result of OXPIRT is required to be produced in laboratory to examine tablet properties for standard quality control. Figures 8.11 and 8.12 show, respectively, a dissolution profile and graph comparing the original and the generic version gained from Figure 8.10 and the result

Ingredient	Function	Weight
Hydroxyzine hydrochloride	API	10.00 mg
Croscarmellose sodium	Disintegrant	3.25 mg
Microcrystalline cellulose	Binder	6.50 mg
Lactose	Diluent	45.05 mg
Colloidal silicon dioxide	Lubricant	0.07 mg
Magnesium stearate	Lubricant	0.13 mg

Manufacturing process	Wet granulation
Instruction	1. Dry mixing hydroxyzine hydrochloride, croscarmellose sodium, microcrystalline cellulose and lactose 2. Wet mixing mixture with water until wet 3. Communition with sieve no.14 4. Drying 5. Communition with sieve no.18 6. Dry mixing mixture, colloidal silicon dioxide and magnesium stearate 7. Compression

Figure 8.10 OXPIRT result for a hydroxyzine hydrochloride generic product.

	Dissolution profile (%)	
Min	Original	Generic
5	25.40	28.24
10	52.75	54.71
15	71.25	81.77
30	96.99	93.77
45	101.66	100.65
60	101.06	103.30
avg	71.97	74.30

Disintegration time (s)	
Original	Generic
180	200
Pharmaceutical equivalence	
F_1	F_2
8.21	59.62
=(0–15) Pass	=(50–100) Pass

Figure 8.11 Pharmaceutical equivalence result between the original and the generic hydroxyzine hydrochloride

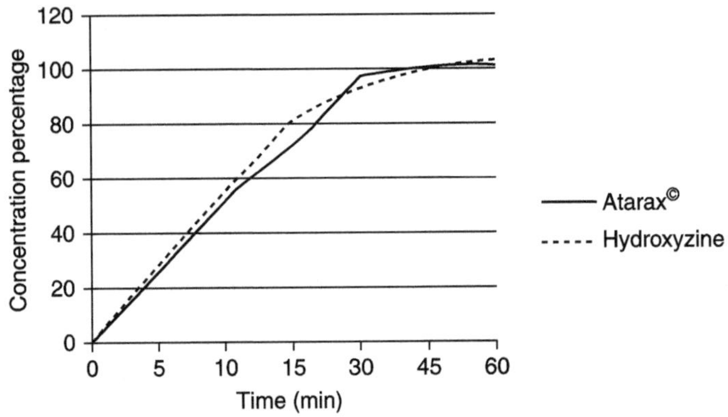

Figure 8.12 Dissolution profile of original Atarax® tablet and generic hydroxyzine hydrochloride tablet

Information	Value		
Solubility	Sparingly soluble		
Flowability	Poor		
Fracture surface	Rough		
Temperature stability	Stable		
Moisture stability	Stable		
API weight	500 mg		
Tablet weight	630 mg		
Hardness	8.3 kg		
Disintegration time	28 s		
Dissolution profile (%) at 5/10/15/30/45/60 min	81.31/89.27/94.22/98.76/98.12/101.98		
Ingredients I known amount I known function	Paracetamol	500 mg	API
	Microcrystalline cellulose	-	Binder
	Corn starch	-	Diluent
	Sodium starch glycolate	-	Disintegrant
	Magnesium stearate	-	Lubricant

Figure 8.13 Information on a paracetamol product from preformulation study and its original patent

shows pharmaceutical equivalence as difference (f_1) and similarity (f_2) factors are within acceptable ranges.

Paracetamol

As usual, information required for input gained from preformulation study and patent reviewing is fundamental to begin the system. The information on original paracetamol is shown in Figure 8.13.

The IF-THEN rules related to information in Figure 8.14 are listed in Table 8.7.

Published by Woodhead Publishing Limited, 2013

Ingredient	Function	Weight
Paracetamol	API	500.00 mg
Microcrystalline cellulose	Binder	94.50 mg
Corn starch	Diluent	2.70 mg
Sodium starch glycolate	Disintegrant	31.50 mg
Magnesium stearate	Lubricant	0.13 mg

Manufacturing process	Wet granulation
Instruction	1. Dry mixing metformin hydrochloride, sodium starch glycolate, microcrystalline cellulose, and corn starch 2. Wet mixing mixture with water until wet 3. Communition with sieve no.14 4. Drying 5. Communition with sieve no.18 6. Dry mixing mixture and magnesium stearate

Figure 8.14 OXPIRT result for a paracetamol generic product

Table 8.7 Rules used for adjustment concentration of the generic paracetamol production

Rule	Detail of rule
I	IF <hardness of the original is more than 5.0 kg> AND <type of binder is hardest> THEN <set the concentration of binders at maximum concentration>
II	IF <disintegration time of the original is less than or equal to 180 s> AND <type of disintegrant is super-disintegrant> THEN <set the concentration of disintegrants at maximum concentration>
III	IF <solubility of API is sparingly soluble or slightly soluble or very slightly soluble or practically insoluble> THEN <set the concentration of lubricant at minimum concentration>
IV	IF <diluent exists> THEN <fill diluent until obtain the total tablet amount>
V	IF <flowability of API is poor or very poor or extremely poor> AND <fracture surface is rough> AND <temperature stability is stable> AND <moisture stability is stable> AND <API concentration is more than 10%> THEN < set the process type as Wet granulation >

OXPIRT inferred a concentration of excipients and later performed a weight calculation based on the assigned concentration and tablet weight. In this case, four ingredients, microcrystalline cellulose, corn starch, sodium starch glycolate, and magnesium stearate, were considered. First, microcrystalline cellulose was involved in Rule I shown in Table 8.7.

With the rule, a concentration of microcrystalline cellulose was inferred to maximum as 15% and it was computed to weight 94.50 mg. Second, sodium starch glycolate was involved in Rule II shown in Table 8.7. With the rule, a concentration of sodium starch glycolate was inferred to maximum as 5% and it was computed to weight 31.50 mg. Third, magnesium stearate is involved in Rule III shown in Table 8.7. With the rule, a concentration of magnesium stearate was inferred to minimum as 0.2% and it was computed to weight 0.13 mg. Fourth, the diluent amount is computed based on Rule IV by the total weight minus the available remaining space from the already set ingredients (i.e. 630 – (500 + 94.5 + 31.5 + 0.13) = 2.7 mg). Last, the process type is set to wet granulation following Rule V. With all weight computed, OXPIRT returns a result as given in Figure 8.14.

A result of OXPIRT is required to be produced in the laboratory to examine tablet properties for standard quality control. Figures 8.15 and 8.16 show, respectively, dissolution profile and graph comparing the original and the generic version gained from Figure 8.14 and the result shows pharmaceutical equivalence as difference (f_1) and similarity (f_2) factors are within acceptable ranges.

Atorvastatin calcium

From preformulation study and its original patent, we obtain information on atorvastatin calcium as shown in Figure 8.17.

With the information in Figure 8.17, OXPIRT performs an adjustment for a concentration of excipients. A set of production rules that match in this case are executed to compute an exact weight of each excipient. A list of relevant rules is given in Table 8.8.

With such rules, we obtain certain weights for ingredients. The ingredients and their amounts are sent to the process generation module to complete a production guideline result with a production instruction.

	Dissolution profile (%)	
Min	**Original**	**Generic**
5	81.31	73.01
10	89.27	82.05
15	94.22	84.75
30	98.76	87.25
45	98.12	91.22
60	101.98	90.50
avg	**93.94**	**84.80**

Disintegration time (s)	
Original	**Generic**
28	33
Pharmaceutical equivalence	
F_1	**F_2**
9.74	53.03
=(0–15) Pass	**=(50–100) Pass**

Figure 8.15 Pharmaceutical equivalence result between the original and the generic paracetamol

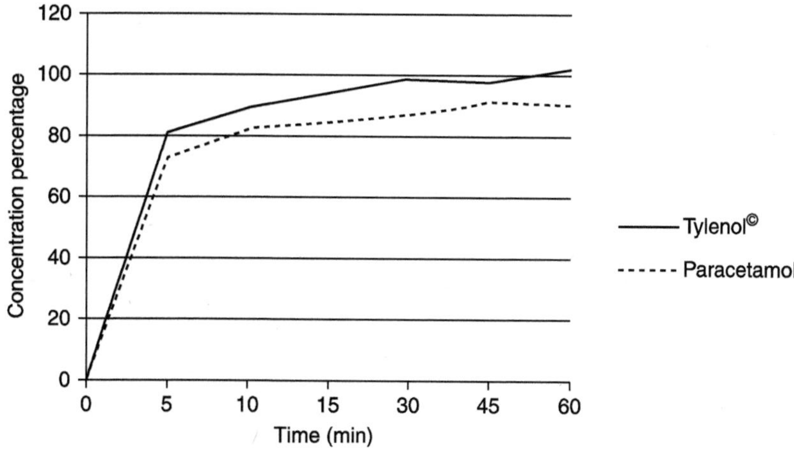

Figure 8.16 Dissolution profile of original Tylenol® tablet and generic paracetamol tablet

Information	Value		
Solubility	Very slight soluble		
Flowability	Fair		
Fracture stability	Rough		
Temperature stability	Stable		
Moisture stability	Stable		
API weight	20 mg		
Tablet weight	300 mg		
Hardness	5.2 kg		
Disintegration time	50 s		
Dissolution profile (%) at min 5/10/15/30/45/60	91.08/98.37/101.07/101.28/101.20		
Ingredients I Known amount I Known function	Atorvastatin calcium	20 mg	API
	Calcium carbonate	-	Buffering agent
	Croscarmellose sodium	-	Disintegrant
	Microcrystalline cellulose	-	Binder
	Lactose	-	Diluent
	Magnesium stearate	-	Lubricant
	Polysorbate 80	-	Solubiliser

Figure 8.17 Information on an atorvastatin calcium product from preformulation study and its original patent

Table 8.8 **Rules used for adjustment concentration of the generic atorvastatin calcium production**

Rule	Detail of rule
I	IF <buffering agent exists> THEN <set the concentration of buffering agent at normal concentration>
II	IF <disintegration time of the original is less than or equal to 180 s> AND <type of disintegrant is super-disintegrant> THEN <set the concentration of disintegrant at maximum concentration>
III	IF <hardness of the original is more than 5 kg> AND <type of binder is hardest> THEN <set the concentration of binders at maximum concentration>
IV	IF <solubility of API is sparingly soluble or slightly soluble or very slightly soluble or practically insoluble > THEN <set the concentration of lubricant at minimum concentration>
V	IF <solubility of API is sparingly soluble, slightly soluble, very slightly soluble, or practically insoluble> THEN <set the concentration of solubilizer at maximum>
VI	IF <diluent exists> THEN <fill diluent until obtain the total tablet amount>
VII	IF < API concentration is less than 10%> THEN < set the process type as Wet granulation >

Ingredient	Function	Weight
Atorvastatin calcium	API	20.00 mg
Calcium carbonate	Buffering agent	60.00 mg
Croscarmellose sodium	Disintegrant	15.00 mg
Microcrystalline cellulose	Binder	45.00 mg
Magnesium stearate	Lubricant	0.60 mg
Polysorbate 80	Solubilizer	12.00 mg
Lactose	Diluent	147.40 mg

Manufacturing process	Wet granulation
Instruction	1. Wet mixing API and solubilizer 2. Dry mixing the mixture from 1 with disintegrant, binder, buffering agent and diluent 3. Wet mixing the mixture from 2 with water until wet 4. Communition with sieve no.14 5. Drying 6. Communition with sieve no.18 7. Compression

Figure 8.18 **OXPIRT result for an atorvastatin calcium generic product**

A result from OXPIRT for an atorvastatin calcium generic product is shown in Figure 8.18.

A result of OXPIRT is required to be produced in the laboratory to examine tablet properties for standard quality control. The result shown in Figure 8.18 gives an examination result as shown in Figure 8.19.

Published by Woodhead Publishing Limited, 2013

Dissolution profile (%)		
Min	Original	Generic
5	91.08	54.05
10	98.37	61.75
15	101.04	64.25
30	101.07	65.22
45	101.28	65.50
60	101.20	66.38
avg	**99.01**	**62.86**

Disintegration time (s)	
Original	Generic
50	193
Pharmaceutical equivalence	
F_1	F_2
36.51	23.75
=(0–15) Fail	=(50–100) Fail

Figure 8.19 Pharmaceutical equivalence result between the original and generic atorvastatin calcium

The information must be manually input into the validation module to automatically approve a suggestion. Unless any criteria are unacceptable, OXPIRT will terminate the suggestion process and store the accepted suggestion to instantly result further on. Otherwise, the information will be used to improve the result. The result shown in Figure 8.19 is, unfortunately, not satisfactory because of an unacceptable rate of disintegration time. In detail, the average dissolution profile of the generic version is over the acceptable rate of ±10%. Moreover, the disintegration time of generic product also needs improvement as it exceeds 10% of the disintegration time of the original product. To improve the suggestion, another set of rules is applied within the excipient modification module. The relevant rules for this case are listed in Table 8.9. After the rules for improvement are activated, the generic production result is given as shown in Figure 8.20.

Table 8.9 Rules used for improving a production suggestion of generic atorvastatin calcium production

Rule	Detail of rule
I	IF <dissolution profile is over an acceptable range> AND <solubilizer is at maximum> AND <wetting agent does not exist> THEN <add wetting agent excipient with half the amount of existing solubilizer and decrease the amount of the existing solubilizer to half>
II	IF <disintegration is over an acceptable range > AND <disintegrant is at maximun> AND <type of disintegrant is super-disintegrant> AND <another excipient has a possible role as disintegrant> THEN <set a concentration of the excipient that has a possible role as disintegrant to perform the role of disintegrant function>

List of ingredients	Function	Weight
Atorvastatin calcium	Active ingredient	20.00 mg.
Calcium carbonate	Buffering agent	60.00 mg.
Croscarmellose sodium	Disintegrant	15.00 mg.
Microcrystalline cellulose	Binder	**75.00 mg.**
Magnesium stearate	Lubricant	0.60 mg.
Polysorbate 80	Solubilizer	**6.00 mg.**
Sodium lauryl sulfate	**Wetting agent**	**6.00 mg.**
Lactose	Diluent	**117.40 mg.**

Manufacturing process	Wet granulation
Instruction	1. Wet mixing API and solubilizer 2. Dry mixing the mixture from 1 with disinitegrant, binder, buffering agent and diluent. 3. Wet mixing the mixture from 2 with water until wet. 4. Communition with sieve no.14 5. Drying 6. Communition with sieve no.18 **7. Dry mixing mixture and magnesium stearate** 8. Compression

Figure 8.20 Improved OXPIRT result for an atorvastatin calcium generic product

With the result in Figure 8.20, the changes are an addition of 6 mg wetting agent and the solubilizer amount is reduced to half as according to the first rule in Table 8.9. Moreover, the amount of binder is increased to 75 mg and an the diluent is reduced to 117.40 mg from the second rule in Table 8.9. Using the new substance, the instruction is generated again. The improved result is produced in the laboratory once more to examine tablet properties for standard quality control and the pharmaceutical equivalence result between the original and the improved generic atorvastatin calcium are shown in Figure 8.21, while the dissolution profiles of original Lipitor® tablet and the generic atorvastatin tablet from the last result are acceptably similar, as shown in Figure 8.22.

Dissolution profile (%)		
Min	Original	Generic
5	91.08	89.81
10	98.37	100.86
15	101.04	102.91
30	101.07	102.86
45	101.28	103.06
60	101.20	103.45
avg	**99.01**	**100.49**

Disintegration time (s)	
Original	Generic
50	46
Pharmaceutical equivalence	
F_1	F_2
1.93	84.29
=(0–15) Acceptable	=(50–100) Acceptable

Figure 8.21 Pharmaceutical equivalence result between the original and generic atorvastatin calcium (improved result)

Published by Woodhead Publishing Limited, 2013

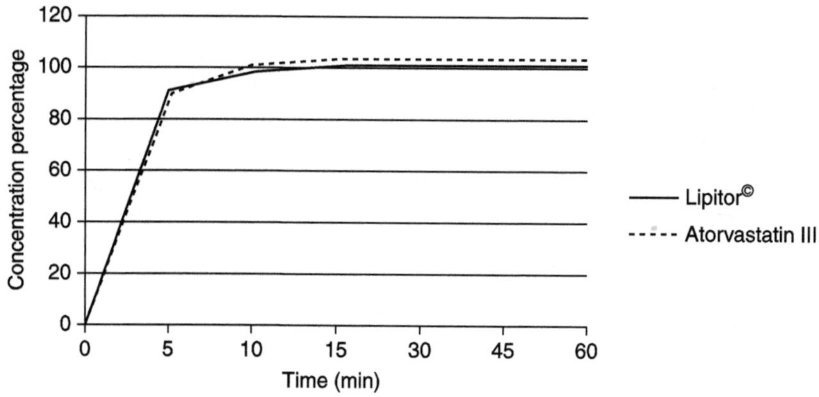

Figure 8.22 Dissolution profile of original Lipitor® tablet and generic atorvastatin tablet

8.4 Conclusion and future work

In this chapter, we presented a framework of a pharmaceutical support system for both generic tablet and herbal tablet reformulation and production. An ontology is exploited to represent domain knowledge of excipients and tablet formulation from documents, literature and patent reviews. Production rules represent operation knowledge from experience of experts and generic drug tablet formulation experiments. The system consists of four modules which are the amount adjustment module, the excipient modification module, the process generation module and the pharmaceutical validation module. The first three modules assist a user in generating generic drug production. The pharmaceutical validation module facilitates the user to validate pharmaceutical equivalence between the generic products following the suggestion of the system and the original products.

Based on our evaluation result, the system has potential in terms of successful reformulation of four random sampling originals. Three in particular showed pharmaceutical equivalence to their original products from the first recommendation.

In the future, we plan to develop a user-friendly interface for users to directly input their excipient information and condition rule into the knowledge base. Moreover, we plan to improve the system for supporting herbal tablet production, which is a traditional product in the pharmaceutical markets of a number of countries. Lastly, we plan to adapt our system and ontology to other dosage forms such as capsule, liquid and powder.

8.5 References

Augsbuger LL and Hoag SW. *Pharmaceutical Dosage Forms: Tablets Rational Design and Formulation.* (2008): Informa Healthcare.

Bateman SD, Verlin J, Russo M, Guillot M and Laughlim SM. The development and validation of a capsule formulation knowledge-based system. *Pharmaceutical Technology* (1996) 20, 174–84.

Christian S. (2010). 'Knowledge sources, patent protection, and commercialization of pharmaceutical innovations.' *Research Policy* 39(6), 810–21.

Davies J, Studer R and Warren P. *Semantic Web Technologies Trends and Research in ontology-based systems.* (2006): John Wiley & Sons Ltd.

Friedman-Hill E. *JESS in Action.* (2003): Maning Publications Co.

Kozaki K, Kitamura Y, Ikeda M and Mizoguchi R. *Hozo: An Environment for Building/Using Ontologies Based on a Fundamental Consideration of 'Role' and 'Relationship'.* In the 13th International Conference Knowledge Engineering and Knowledge Management (EKAW2002) (2002) Siguenza, Spain. 213–18.

Lacy LW. *OWL: Representing Information Using the Web Ontology Language.* (2004): Trafford Publishing.

Morales FJ and van Boekel MAJS. (1997) 'A study on advanced Maillard reaction in heated casein/sugar solutions: Fluorescence accumulation.' *International Dairy Journal* 7(11), 675–83.

Nopphadol Chalortham, et al. *'Ontology Development for Pharmaceutical Tablet Production Expert System'.* in Electrical Engineering/Electronics, Computer, Telecommunications and Information Technology, 2008. (ECTI-CON 2008) 5th International Conference, 2008.

Nopphadol Chalortham, Phuriwat Leesawat, Taneth Ruangrajitpakorn and Thepchai Supnithi. 'A Framework of Ontology-Based Tablet Production Supporting System for a Drug Reformulation' *IEICE Transactions on Information and Systems* E94-D No.3, 448–55, 2011.

Rowe RC. Film coating formulation using an expert system. *Pharmaceutical Technology* (1998) 10, 72–82.

Rowe RC and Sheskey PJ. *Handbook of Pharmaceutical Excipients.* (2005) 5edn.: APhA Publications.

Shargel L and Kanfer I. *Generic Drug Product Development: Solid Oral Dosage Forms.* (2005): Marcel Dekker, Inc.

Sirisinsuk Y and Katechroen A. *Annual Report of Drug System Situation in 2009* (2009).

Wood M. *Lab Equipment Digest* (1991), 17–19.

Published by Woodhead Publishing Limited, 2013

9

Optimisation of compression parameters with AI-based mathematical models

Aleš Belič and Igor Škrjanc, University of Ljubljana, Slovenia, Damjana Zupančič-Božič and Franc Vrečer, Novo Mesto, Slovenia

DOI: 10.1533/9781908818508.229

Abstract: This chapter describes a study of the influence of particle size and the settings of tableting parameters on tablet capping tendency. Artificial neural network (ANN) and fuzzy models were used for modelling the effect of particle size and tableting machine settings on the capping coefficient. The basic principles of the tableting process are described, followed by a description of principal components analysis, then ANN and fuzzy models. Finally, a real tableting case is presented. The suitability of routinely measured quantities for prediction of the tablet quality was tested. Results showed that model-based expert systems developed on the contemporary routinely measured quantities can significantly improve manual trial-and-error procedures; however, they cannot replace them. The results also suggest that where it is not possible to obtain a sufficient number of measurements to uniquely identify the model, it is beneficial to use several modelling techniques to estimate the quality of model prediction.

Key words: tableting, optimisation of machine settings, artificial neural networks, fuzzy models, principal component analysis.

9.1 Introduction

Although tablets are now one of the most common drug formulations, the processes involved in compression and compaction are still being researched, with optimisation of production being a major research goal. In spite of the high technology level of tablet production, tableting parameter optimisation in industry is still relatively basic. In most cases the optimisation is performed manually, by applying experiences from the past tableting batches. This manual optimisation by trial-and-error is quite lengthy and, therefore, not very cost effective. There are several tableting process parameters that must be included in optimisation which make optimisation a high-dimensional problem. The physics of tableting is also quite complex, which results in a non-linear, high-dimensional criterion function with possibly multiple local minima. The manual optimisation procedure is therefore slow to converge to some optimal tableting machine settings, especially as the particle compression also exhibits some random phenomena. As each input material batch has specific properties, the characteristics of which can vary within specific intervals, that may influence the tableting process and tablet quality, the optimisation procedure must be applied to each new batch. Typical tableting parameters that can be set directly are tableting speed, compression force and pre-compression force, whereas input material characteristics vary between batches. The tablet quality is usually described via tablet mass variability, crushing strength variability, capping coefficient, etc. A high quality compression process must produce tablets with low capping coefficient, low mass and crushing strength variability at compression speeds as high as possible. These requests often contradict each other; therefore, it is difficult to find optimal tableting machine settings to fulfil all requests. In this chapter we present a mathematical model-based optimisation procedure as one possible solution to this problem. The presented optimisation procedure was developed with the aim of assisting the conventional manual procedure by aggregating the knowledge from past batches into a non-linear black-box model which would indicate the most promising regions of tableting machine settings with respect to the new input material batch characteristics, and would therefore shorten the optimisation procedure of tableting setting at the production scale.

Published by Woodhead Publishing Limited, 2013

9.2 Compression process

The tablet is the most common pharmaceutical dosage form; it is produced by compression of a powder mixture containing the active ingredient and auxiliary materials (excipients) into a solid dosage form. The process of tableting consists of three stages: 1. the powder mixture fills the die; 2. compaction, when the powder is compressed inside the die by two punches, the next stage is particle deformation (plastic, elastic deformation and/or particle fragmentation), so forming bonds among the particles; and 3. ejection, when the tablet is ejected from the die. The most desirable method of tablet production is direct compression, which includes tableting of the powder mixture without any prior particle agglomeration. This is a technologically and economically optimal procedure if the formulation characteristics (especially the compressibility and flowability of the mixture of active ingredient and excipients) allow this method. If a high percentage of active ingredient is used in the formulation, the compressibility of the formulation can be poor as active ingredients usually have poor flowability and compressibility. In such cases dry or wet granulation is often needed to achieve suitable tablet characteristics. The flowability and compressibility properties of the powder mixture can, together with other characteristics, significantly affect the quality of the tablet, in terms of tablet crushing strength, the standard deviations of the tablet mass and hardness, the capping tendency, etc. Today, tableting is performed on modern, rotary tableting machines, which require optimised formulation and process settings for their high-capacity performance and high tablet quality.

In dry granulation, the particles are agglomerated into compacts using a physical load; these are then crushed and sieved prior to tableting in order to get the desired particle size distribution. There are two methods of dry granulation: 1. slugging (compacts are made using a tableting machine) and 2. roller compaction (compacts are made by compacting powder between two rollers on a roller compactor). The particle size distribution is normally shifted towards larger particles, leading to improved powder flowability and compressibility with a diminished capping tendency [1–3].

If the intensity of the elastic relaxation during the decompression phase overcomes the strength of the interparticulate bonding formed during compression, it can lead to separation of the upper part of the tablet from the tablet body (known as capping), which is a serious problem affecting the tablet's mechanical strength and its quality [4]. Mass and crushing strength may be affected as well.

Many studies have been performed studying the relationship between the powder's mechanical characteristics, the cohesion, the deformation mechanisms and the elastic recovery of the tablet [5–16]; however, generally only powders with up to two different materials under laboratory conditions were evaluated in these studies. Because real pharmaceutical formulations are usually complex, practical experience shows that it is not possible to apply a model developed in laboratory-scale studies (e.g. [17–20]) for large-scale production situations in the pharmaceutical industry. The mechanical properties of powder mixtures with a large number of components are too complex to be described in a transparent mathematical model based on theory, thus the mathematical models developed in [6–16] are often not precise enough for the purpose of adjusting the parameters of a tableting machine to inter-batch differences.

9.3 Principal component analysis

Principal component analysis (PCA) [21] is used to transform the original set of variables into new, uncorrelated variables, called the principal components, that are linear combinations of the original variables. The principal components lie along the directions of maximum variances of the original data set. PCA is also known as eigenvector analysis, eigenvector decomposition, Karhunen-Loeve expansion or SVD decomposition. The main purpose of PCA is to represent the samples in a reduced coordinate system, where only the directions of the eigenvectors with most significant variances are taken into account. In the first step the original raw data matrix $\mathbf{Z}^0 \in \mathbb{R}^{m \times n}$ of n samples (columns) and m variables (rows) is normalised to a matrix $\mathbf{Z}$ with zero mean as follows:

$$Z = (Z^0 - bI_n)$$

where $I_n = [1, 1, 1, \ldots, 1] \in \mathbb{R}^n$, $b \in \mathbb{R}^m$ stands for the mean of each variable (row) and is defined as

$$b = \frac{1}{n} Z^0 I_n^T$$

Then the covariance matrix $\boldsymbol{R} \in \mathbb{R}^{m \times m}$, which is symmetrical and positive definite is calculated and transformed into the form $R = ZZ^T = PDP^T$,

Published by Woodhead Publishing Limited, 2013

where $P \in \mathbb{R}^{m\times m}$ stands for the matrix of eigenvectors which are written in decreasing order of eigenvalues ($\lambda_1, \lambda_2, \ldots, \lambda_m$) which are the diagonal elements of the eigenvalue matrix $D \in \mathbb{R}^{m\times m}$ ($D = \mathrm{diag}[\lambda_1, \lambda_2, \ldots, \lambda_m]$). Defining the symmetrical, positive definite matrix D as a product of the matrix and its transpose $D = S^{\mathrm{T}}S$, this means that PCA practically transforms the normalised data matrix Z into a product of two matrices, one of which contains the information about the samples (($S \in \mathbb{R}^{n\times p}$) and the other about variables ($P \in \mathbb{R}^{p\times p}$). The matrix S_p contains the scores of the n measurements on p principal components (the scores are the projections of the samples on the principal components) and the other gives the information about the variables (P_p). The decomposition results in orthogonal matrix S and orthonormal matrix P and the residual matrix $\tilde{Z}$. This means that the normalised matrix Z is decomposed as follows:

$$Z = S_p P_p^{\mathrm{T}} + \tilde{Z} = S_p P_p^{\mathrm{T}} + \tilde{S}\tilde{P}^{\mathrm{T}} = [S_p, \tilde{S}]\,[P_p, \tilde{P}]^{\mathrm{T}} = SP^{\mathrm{T}}$$

where the columns of P_p are actually eigenvectors of the correlation matrix R associated with the p largest eigenvectors, and the columns of $\tilde{P}$ are the remaining eigenvectors ($m - p$). Because the trace of the matrix corresponds to the sum of all eigenvalues of the same matrix, the criterion of proper selection of p is given as:

$$\frac{\mathrm{trace}(P_p S_p^{\mathrm{T}} S_p P_p^{\mathrm{T}})}{\mathrm{trace}(PS^{\mathrm{T}} SP^{\mathrm{T}})} \geq \in$$

where $\in$ is a selected threshold. The typical value of this threshold is equal to 0.95. The columns of matrix S_p are now called the scores of the original variables in the transformed coordinate system and are denoted as $s_j = [s_{1j}, s_{2j}, \ldots, s_{nj}]^{\mathrm{T}}$ where $j = 1, 2, \ldots, p$. The value of p also denotes the dimensionality of the analysed data, and the remaining components represent the measurement noise.

9.4 Artificial neural networks and fuzzy models

In cases where physical relations are very complex and not entirely understood, artificial intelligence methods can be used for modelling the relations. Although the efficiency of the methods is limited with data quality and may be primarily used for interpolation purposes, they can be successfully used in complex control engineering problems. As in tableting, the useful range of process variables can be estimated and, as the process variables' space can be efficiently experimentally covered, the ANN and fuzzy models can be efficiently applied.

9.4.1 Artificial neural networks

ANN [22] are general-purpose non-linear models with the ability to describe any non-linearity with desired precision. However, their flexibility can also be a drawback as they can also approximate the measuring imprecision, when not applied carefully. ANN characteristics depend on their structure and the training algorithm. The basis of the ANN is a natural neuron-like structure, usually with several inputs (x) and one output (y). The input signals are multiplied with the corresponding weights (w) and added to the neuron bias (b). The sum is then used as an argument for the transfer functions that is usually some non-linear function ($f(.)$) (step function, continuous sigmoidal function, Gaussian function, . . .), depending on the shape of the non-linearity that should be described with the ANN.

$$y = f(wx + b)$$

As the ANN developed, several network structures have been developed. The structure of the ANN defines the connections between the neurons in the network and thus defines the network properties. Some of the network structures are: perceptrons, Kohonnen networks, Hopfield networks, recurrent networks, feed-forward networks, and many more. Let us look closer at feed-forward networks, which have been used in our studies.

Feed-forward neural network

Feed-forward ANN [22] consist of several layers of neurons. The first layer is connected to inputs. All the inputs are connected to all the neurons of the first layer, and all the outputs of the layers are connected to all the neurons of the next layer. The last layer outputs are the outputs of the network. The number of neurons of the last layer is equal to the number of outputs. See Figure 9.1 for a schematic representation of the feed-forward network.

The output of the network is calculated in a step-wise procedure where the outputs of each layer are consecutively calculated from input to output. For the network with layers the equation would be:

$$y = y^c = f^c(W^c(f^{c-1}(W^{c-1}(f^{c-2}(. . .(W^1 x + b^1). . .)) + b^{c-1})) + b^c)$$

Published by Woodhead Publishing Limited, 2013

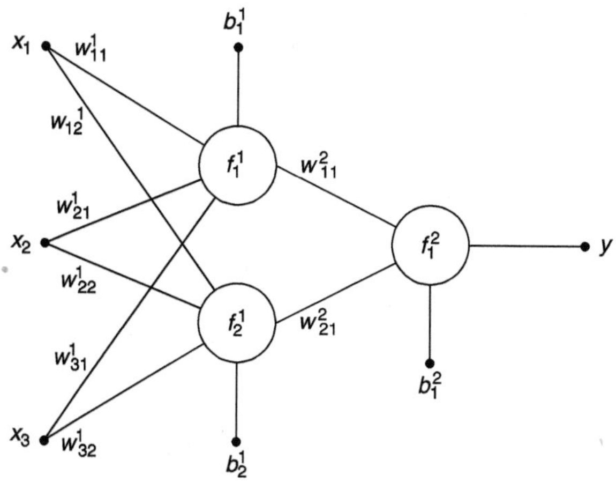

Figure 9.1 **Graphical representation of a simple feed-forward network with three inputs and one input, two layers with two neurons in the first layer and one neuron in the output layer: *x* – inputs, *w* – weights, *b* – biases, *f* – transfer functions, *y* – output**

However, before the network can describe a particular non-linear relation, weights and biases of all the layers must be identified from the data. Most common training algorithms for feed-forward networks are numerous variations of the back-propagation algorithm.

The back-propagation training algorithm

Let us consider a system with one output; however, the procedures are similar for a multi-output network. The algorithm starts with randomly distributed values of weights and biases. In the first step, the outputs of the network y_k are calculated for all the input vectors x_k, $k = 1, 2, \ldots, n$. As there are observations of the system, the input column-vectors can be arranged in a matrix and the output can be arranged in a row-vector:

$$X = [x_1, x_2, \ldots, x_n], \quad y = [y_1, y_2, \ldots, y_n]$$

The layer outputs for all c layers are then calculated as:

$$Y^i = f^i(W^i Y^{i-1} + b)^i, \qquad i = 1,2, \ldots, c$$
$$Y^0 = X$$
$$y = y^c$$

Next, the difference function ($\ddot{F}(X)$) between the network outputs and the target outputs is estimated,

$$\ddot{F}(X) = E[e^T e] = E[(t - y)^T (t - y)]$$

Now the weights and the biases have to be adapted to reduce the difference

$$w^i_{ml}(j+1) = w^i_{ml}(j) - \alpha \frac{\partial \ddot{F}}{\partial w^i_{ml}}$$

$$b^i_m(j+1) = b^i_m(j) - \alpha \frac{\partial \ddot{F}}{\partial b^i_m}$$

where i stands for the layer, j stands for training iteration step, m is consecutive number of a neuron in i-th layer and l is consecutive number of a neuron in the $i+1$-st layer and α is a learning factor that defines the change of parameter values in iterations. Considering the network structure, the two partial derivatives can be rearranged by using the argument a into the m-th neuron transfer function of the i-th layer n^i_m:

$$a^i_m = \sum_{l=1}^{L^{i-1}} w^i_{ml} y^{i-1}_l + b^i_m$$

where L^i is the number of neurons in the i-th layer. The partial derivatives can now be transformed into indirect partial derivatives:

$$\frac{\partial \ddot{F}}{\partial w^i_{ml}} = \frac{\partial \ddot{F}}{\partial a^i_m} \frac{\partial a^i_m}{\partial w^i_{ml}}$$

$$\frac{\partial \ddot{F}}{\partial b^i_m} = \frac{\partial \ddot{F}}{\partial a^i_m} \frac{\partial a^i_m}{\partial b^i_m}$$

which can be further simplified, as partial derivatives of the transfer function arguments are calculated as:

$$\frac{\partial a^i_m}{\partial w^i_{ml}} = y^{i-1}_l, \quad \frac{\partial a^i_m}{\partial b^i_m} = 1$$

If we define the sensitivity of the transfer function s as:

$$s^i_m = \frac{\partial \ddot{F}}{\partial a^i_m}$$

the partial derivatives can be rewritten as:

$$\frac{\partial \ddot{F}}{\partial w^i_{ml}} = s^i_m y^{i-1}_l, \quad \frac{\partial \ddot{F}}{\partial b^i_m} = s^i_m$$

and finally, the rule for updating the weights and biases in training iterations in matrix form can be written as:

$$W^i(j+1) = W^i(j) - \alpha s^i (Y^{i-1})^T$$

$$b^i(j+1) = b^i(j) - \alpha s^i$$

where

$$s^i = \left[\frac{\partial \hat{F}}{\partial a_1^i}, \frac{\partial \hat{F}}{\partial a_2^i}, \ldots, \frac{\partial \hat{F}}{\partial a_{L^i}^i}\right]^T$$

In the final step, the sensitivity of the layer should be rewritten in order to eliminate the transfer function arguments from the equation. This can be done by introducing the matrix of partial derivatives of the function arguments over the previous layer transfer function arguments:

$$\frac{\partial a^{i+1}}{\partial a^i} = \begin{bmatrix} \frac{\partial a_1^{i+1}}{\partial a_1^i} & \frac{\partial a_1^{i+1}}{\partial a_2^i} & \cdots & \frac{\partial a_1^{i+1}}{\partial a_{L^i}^i} \\ \frac{\partial a_2^{i+1}}{\partial a_1^i} & \frac{\partial a_2^{i+1}}{\partial a_2^i} & \cdots & \frac{\partial a_1^{i+1}}{\partial a_{L^i}^i} \\ \vdots & \vdots & \ddots & \vdots \\ \frac{\partial a_{L^{i+1}}^{i+1}}{\partial a_1^i} & \frac{\partial a_{L^{i+1}}^{i+1}}{\partial a_2^i} & \cdots & \frac{\partial a_{L^{i+1}}^{i+1}}{\partial a_{L^i}^i} \end{bmatrix}$$

Each element of the matrix can be further rewritten:

$$\frac{\partial a_l^{i+1}}{\partial a_m^i} = \frac{\partial\left(\sum_{o=1}^{L^i} w_{ol}^{i+1} y_o^i + b_o^{i+1}\right)}{\partial a_m^i} = w_{ml}^{i+1} \frac{\partial y_m^i}{\partial a_m^i} = w_{ml}^{i+1} \frac{\partial f^i(a_m^i)}{\partial a_m^i}$$

Thus the matrix can be rewritten as:

$$\frac{\partial a^{i+1}}{\partial a^i} = W^{i+1} \dot{F}^i(a^i)$$

where $\dot{F}^i(a^i)$ is a diagonal matrix of transfer function derivatives of the -th layer. Hence, the sensitivity becomes:

$$s^i = \frac{\partial \hat{F}}{\partial a^i} = \left(\frac{\partial a^{i+1}}{\partial a^i}\right)^T \frac{\partial \hat{F}}{\partial a^{i+1}} = \dot{F}^i(a^i)(W^{i+1})^T \frac{\partial \hat{F}}{\partial a^{i+1}} = \dot{F}^i(a^i)(W^{i+1})^T s^{i+1}$$

The sensitivity is, therefore, calculated from the last layer to the first, hence the name error back-propagation. The final algorithm looks like:

$$Y^0 = X$$

$$Y^{i+1} = f^{i+1}(W^{i+1}Y^i + b^{i+1}), \qquad i = 1, 2, \ldots, c$$

$$y = y^c$$

$$s^c = -2\dot{F}^c(a^c)(t - y)$$

$$s^i = \dot{F}^i(c^i)(W^{i+1})^T s^{i+1}, \qquad i = c - 1, c - 2, \ldots, 1$$

$$W^i(j+1) = W^i(j) - \alpha s^i (Y^{i-1})^T$$

$$b^i(j+1) = b^i(j) - \alpha s^i$$

The loop runs until changes of weights and biases drop under a prescribed limit that depends on the data quality. A problematic issue in the algorithm presents the learning factor α. The method for calculation of α is what defines the efficiency of the training algorithms. Probably the most efficient training algorithm to date is the Levenberg-Marquadt algorithm, an adaptation of Gauss-Newton's optimisation method [23]. Let p represent the vector of parameters to set with optimisation procedure and let j represent the iteration. The rule for adapting the parameters can be written as:

$$p(j+1) = p(j) - A^{-1}(j)g(j)$$

where $A(j) = \nabla^2 F(p(j))$, which is Hessian matrix, and $g(j) = \nabla F(p(j))$ denoting gradient function. Since $F(p)$ is a norm function that can produce only non-negative values, it can be written as $F(p) = \Sigma^n_{i=1} e^2_i(p)$, where n denotes the number of the system observations. The components of the function F gradient are then written as:

$$\left[\nabla F\left(p(j)\right)\right]_k = \frac{\partial F(p)}{\partial p_k} = 2\sum_{i=1}^{n} e_i(p)\frac{\partial e_i(p)}{\partial p_k}$$

or in a matrix form:

$$\nabla F(p) = 2J(p)e(p)$$

where J stands for Jacobian matrix of partial derivatives of the functions e over the components of the parameter vector p. Now let us apply the same definition of $F(p)$ for calculation of the Hessian:

$$\left[\nabla^2 F(p)\right]_{kl} = \frac{\partial^2 F(p)}{\partial p_k \partial p_l} = 2\sum_{i=1}^{n}\left\{\frac{\partial e_i(p)}{\partial p_k}\frac{\partial e_i(p)}{\partial p_l} + e_i(p)\frac{\partial^2 e_i(p)}{\partial p_k \partial p_l}\right\}$$
$$= 2J^T(p)J(p) + 2S(p)$$

where $S(p) = \Sigma^{n}_{i=1} e_i(p)\nabla^2 e_i(p)$ and is small compared with the rest of the term when approaching optimum; therefore, it can be neglected. The rule for updating the optimised parameter values is thus transformed into:

$$p(j+1) = p(j) - [J^{T}(p(j))J(p(j))]^{-1}J^{T}(p(j))e(p(j))$$

which is a form of Gauss-Newton algorithm. However, the problems arise with inversion of $J^{T}J$ which may become singular. To avoid this, a Levenberg-Marquadt variation is used. Let us define matrices $H = J^{T}J$ and $G = H + \mu I$, where μ is some positive number such that $\lambda_i + \mu > 0$ for all eigenvalues λ_i of matrix H, as the product of matrix G and any eigenvector z_i of matrix H yields $Gz_i = [H + \mu I]z_i = Hz_i + \mu z_i = \lambda z_i + \mu z_i = (\lambda_i + \mu)z_i$, we can see that both matrices have the same eigenvectors; however, in any iteration the value of μ that prevents singularity of the Hessian matrix can be found. Therefore, the Levenberg-Marquadt algorithm can be written as:

$$p(j+1) = p(j) - [J^{T}(p(j))J(p(j)) + \mu(j)I]^{-1} J^{T}(p(j))e(p(j))$$

The Jacobian J is calculated with the back-propagation algorithm and the algorithm applied for setting the weights and biases of the neural network is written as:

$$W^{i}(j+1) = W^{i}(j) - [(J^{i})^{T}J^{i} + \mu(j)I]^{-1} (J^{i})^{T}(y(j) - t)(Y^{i-1})^{T}$$

$$b^{i}(j+1) = b^{i}(j) - [(J^{i})^{T}J^{i} + \mu(j)I]^{-1}(J^{i})^{T}(y(j) - t)$$

9.4.2 Fuzzy models

The bases of fuzzy models are fuzzy sets [24]. Fuzzy sets represent a generalisation of traditional, crisp sets, where an element is either a member of the set or not. In fuzzy sets an element is not necessarily a full member of any set. In fact, it can be a partial member of a number of sets, while the sum of all the partial membership functions values should be 1. Such a notion is similar to human reasoning, where not all things have sharp borders. For instance, a person's membership of the sets 'young' and 'old' of (linguistic) variable age depends on the age and the background of the person who is asked to perform the sorting. When describing a population response to an age-sorting problem, this cannot be realistically performed by crisp sets. In more complicated cases where a relation is described by more than one variable and each variable consists of several fuzzy sets, complex algorithms are necessary for identification of fuzzy models.

Fuzzy c-means clustering

When trying to find the fuzzy model of a relationship between the input and output data of a certain system, first the input matrix **X** must be combined of key independent variables of the system. In cases where a dynamical system is modelled, the independent variables must be sorted by the time of observation and the delayed versions of the variables must also be included in **X**. The main objective of clustering is to partition the data set **X** into *c* sub-sets, which are called clusters. The fuzzy partition of the set **X** is a family of fuzzy sub-sets $\{A_i; 1 \le i \le c\}$. The fuzzy sub-sets are defined by their membership functions, which are implicitly defined in the fuzzy partition matrix $U = [\mu_{ik}] \in \mathbb{R}^{cxn}$, where n is the number of observations of the system. The i-th row of matrix **U** contains values of the membership function of the i-th fuzzy sub-set A_i of data set **X**. The partition matrix satisfies the following conditions: the membership degrees are real numbers from the interval $\mu_{ik} \in [0,1]$, $1 \le i \le c$, $1 \le k \le n$; the total membership of each variable in all the clusters equals one $\Sigma^{c}_{i=1}\mu_{ik} = 1, 1 \le k \le n$; none of the fuzzy clusters is empty nor contains all the data $1 \le \Sigma^{n}_{k=1}\mu_{ik} \le n$, $1 \le i \le c$. This means that the fuzzy partition matrix U belongs to the fuzzy partition set which is defined as:

$$M = \left\{ U \in \mathbb{R}^{cxn} \middle| \mu_{ik} \in [0,1], \forall i,k; \sum_{i=1}^{c} \mu_{ik} = 1, \forall k; 1 < \sum_{k=1}^{n} \mu_{ik} < n, \forall i \right\}$$

The fuzzy partition matrix is obtained by applying the fuzzy c-means algorithm based on the Mahalanobis distance norm. The algorithm is based on minimisation of the fuzzy c-means functional given as:

$$J(X,U,V) = \sum_{i=1}^{c} \sum_{k=1}^{n} \mu_{ik}^{m} \, d_{ik}^{2}$$

where *U* is the fuzzy partition matrix of **X**, and **V** is the vector of cluster prototypes (centres) $V = [v_1, v_2, \ldots, v_c]$, $v_i \in \mathbb{R}^p$ c, which have to be estimated, and

$$d^2_{ik} = (x_k - v_i)^T \, C^{-1} (x_k - v_i)$$

is the inner-product distance norm, where

$$C = \frac{1}{n} \sum_{k=1}^{n} (x_k - \bar{x})(x_k - \bar{x})^T$$

and $\bar{x}$ denotes the mean of the data. This allows the detection of hyper-ellipsoidal clusters in the distribution of the data. If the data are distributed along the non-linear hyper-surface, the algorithm will find the clusters that are local linear approximations of this hyper-surface. The cluster overlapping is defined by the parameter $m \in [1, \infty]$.

The number of clusters is defined using the cluster validity measure or by iterative merging or insertion of the clusters. The overlapping factor or the fuzziness parameter m influences the fuzziness of the resulting partition; from the hard $(m=1)$ to the partition which is completely fuzzy $(m=\infty)$. In our approach the standard value $m=2$ is used.

For the given data set **X**, the number of clusters c, the chosen weighting exponent $m > 1$ and the algorithm termination tolerance $\in_{end} > 0$ the algorithm of fuzzy c-means clustering is the following:

- Initialisation of fuzzy partition matrix $U \in M$ (randomly) and calculation of the norm-inducing matrix **C** which equals:

$$C = \frac{1}{n}\sum_{k=1}^{n}(x_k - \bar{x})(x_k - \bar{x})^T, \ \bar{x} = \frac{1}{n}X^T I_n, \ I_n = [1,1,1, ..., 1]^T \in \mathbb{R}^n, \ r = 0$$

- Repeat

  $r = r + 1$

  – Computation of cluster centres

$$- \ v_i^{(r)} = \frac{\sum_{k=1}^{n}(\mu_{ik}^{(r)})^m x_k}{\sum_{k=1}^{n}(\mu_{ik}^{(r)})^m}, 1 < i < c$$

- Computation of the distance from the cluster centres

$$- \ d_{ik}^2 = (x_k - v_i^{(r)})^T C^{-1}(x_k - v_i^{(r)}), \quad 1 < i < c, \quad 1 < k < n$$

  – Update of the partition matrix:

$$if \ d_{ik} > 0, \ \mu_{ik}^{(r)} = \frac{1}{\sum_{j=1}^{c}\left(\frac{d_{ik}}{d_{jk}}\right)^{\frac{2}{m-1}}}$$

- Until $\| U^{(r)} - U^{(r-1)} \| < \in_{end}$.

Fuzzy model in Takagi-Sugeno form

The fuzzy model, in Takagi-Sugeno (TS) form [25], approximates the non-linear system by smoothly interpolating affine local models. Each local model contributes to the global model in a fuzzy sub-set of the space characterised by a membership function. We assume a set of input vectors $X = [x_1, x_1, \ldots, x_n]^T$ and a set of corresponding outputs which is defined as $Y = [y_1, y_2, \ldots y_n]^T$. A typical fuzzy model [25] is given in the form of rules:

$$R_i: \text{if } x_k \text{ is } A_i \text{ then } \hat{y}_k = \phi_i(x_k), \quad i = 1, \ldots, c$$

The vector x_k denotes the input or variables in premise, and the variable $\hat{y}_k$ is the output of the model at time instant k. The premise vector x_k is connected to one of the fuzzy sets $(A_1, \ldots, A_c)$ and each fuzzy set $A_i (i = 1, \ldots, c)$ is associated with a real-valued function $\mu_{Ai}(x_k)$ or μ_{ik}: $\mathbb{R} \rightarrow [0,1]$ that produces the membership grade of the variable x_k with respect to the fuzzy set Ai. The functions $\phi(.)$ can be arbitrary smooth functions in general, although linear or affine functions are normally used. The model output is now described in closed form as follows:

$$\hat{y}_k = \frac{\sum_{i=1}^{c} \mu_{ik} \phi_i(x_k)}{\sum_{i=1}^{c} \mu_{ik}}$$

To simplify the equation, a partition of unity is considered where the functions $\beta_i(x_k)$, defined by:

$$\beta_i(x_k) = \frac{\mu_{ik}}{\sum_{i=1}^{c} \mu_{ik}}, \; i = 1, \ldots, c$$

give information about fulfilment of the respective fuzzy rule in the normalised form. It is obvious that $\sum_{i=1}^{c} \beta_i(x_k) = 1$ irrespective of x_k as long as the denominator of $\beta_i(x_k)$ is not equal to zero (this can be easily prevented by stretching the membership functions over the whole potential area of x_k). Combining the above equations we arrive at the following equation:

$$\hat{y}_k = \sum_{i=1}^{c} \beta_i(x_k) \phi_i(x_k), \; k = 1, \ldots, n$$

Very often, the output value is defined as a linear combination of consequence states

$$\phi_i(x_k) = x_k \theta_i, \; i = 1, \ldots, c, \; \theta_i^T = [\theta_{i1}, \theta_{i2}, \ldots, \theta_{ip}]$$

The vector of fuzzified input variables at time instant k is written as

$$\psi_k = [\beta_1(x_k) x_k, \ldots, \beta_c(x_k) x_k], \; k = 1, \ldots, n$$

and then the fuzzified data matrix follows as:

$$\Psi^T = [\psi_1^T, \psi_2^T, \ldots, \psi_n^T]$$

Published by Woodhead Publishing Limited, 2013

If the matrix of the coefficients for the whole set of rules is written as $\Theta^T = [\theta^T{}_1, \theta^T{}_2, \ldots, \theta^T{}_n]$, then the output equation can be rewritten in the matrix form

$$\hat{y}_k = \psi_k \Theta$$

and the compact form which describes the relation from the whole set of data becomes

$$\hat{Y} = \Psi\Theta$$

where $\hat{Y}$ stands for the vector of model outputs $\hat{y}_k$ where $k = 1, \ldots, n$ ($\ddot{Y} = [\hat{y}_1, \hat{y}_2, \ldots, \hat{y}_n]^T$). The fuzzy model in the presented form is referred to as the affine TS model and can be used to approximate any arbitrary function with any desired degree of accuracy [26–28]. The generality can be proven with the Stone-Weierstrass theorem [29], which suggests that any continuous function can be approximated by a fuzzy basis function expansion [30].

Identification of affine TS fuzzy model parameters

Estimation of the fuzzy model parameters will be done using the least square error approach. The measurements satisfy the non-linear equation of the system

$$y_k = g(x_k), \qquad k = 1, \ldots, n$$

According to the Stone-Weierstrass theorem, for any given real continuous function g on a compact set $U^c \subset \mathbb{R}^p$ and arbitrary $\delta > 0$, there exists a fuzzy system f such that

$$\max_{x_k \in X} |f(x_k) - g(x_k)| < \delta, \forall k$$

This implies the approximation of any given real continuous function with a fuzzy function from class $\mathcal{F}^p$. However, it has to be pointed out that lower values of δ imply higher values of c that satisfy the above equation. In the case of the approximation, the error between the measured values and the fuzzy function outputs can be defined as

$$e_k = y_k - f(x_k) = y_k - \hat{y}_k, \qquad k = 1, \ldots, n$$

where y_k stands for the measured output and $\hat{y}_k$ for the model output at time instant k. To estimate the optimal parameters of the proposed fuzzy function (Θ), minimisation of the sum of square errors over the whole input set of data is performed:

$$E = \sum_{k=1}^{n} e_k^2 = (Y - \hat{Y})^T (Y - \hat{Y}) = (Y - \Psi\Theta)^T (Y - \Psi\Theta)$$

The parameter Θ is obtained as:

$$\frac{\partial E}{\partial \Theta} = 0$$

and becomes

$$\Theta = (\Psi^T\Psi)^{-1}\Psi^T Y$$

The idea of an approximation can be interpreted as the most representative fuzzy function to describe the domain of outputs Y as a function of inputs X. This problem can also be viewed as a problem of data reduction, which often appears in identification problems with large data sets.

9.5 Improved compression process optimisation procedure

As explained above, currently, mainly manual tableting optimisation procedures are in industrial use, which in cases of substances with poor compressibility and flowability characteristics can prove to be rather demanding. A procedure starts with some initial setting of the machine, which can be an optimal setting for the previous batch of the same powder mixture or is deduced from past experiences with similar mixtures. If the quality of the tablets is within some tolerance band the settings are fixed and the procedure is finished; however, if the tablet quality is outside the prescribed limits, some changes to the settings must be introduced. In cases where no prior knowledge exists, the parameters must be varied around the initial settings values and then their influence on tablet quality is observed. Therefore, for each set of settings a short run of the machine must be performed and the tablets must be analysed for mechanical quality, which is a lengthy procedure that cannot be performed on-line. On the other hand, for machines which are capable of producing several hundred thousand tablets per minute, a short run results in several thousands of tablets that must be destroyed if the quality does not comply with the standards. Testing a set of settings is, therefore, quite lengthy and expensive. If initial settings are far from the region of optimal settings, it can take a lot of trials before some acceptable settings are found. In order to shorten the procedure, records of past trials can be collected and a model can be designed, describing the quality parameters

Published by Woodhead Publishing Limited, 2013

with respect to machine settings and batch characteristics. The idea is to use the information from commonly measured properties of the batch and tablet quality descriptors to build the model. Next, the model is used to determine the suitable region for tableting machine settings with respect to the powder mixture batch properties. Within the region a few machine settings are tested and the best are used for production.

The first step in building a model is analysis of the model input data. Two goals must be achieved with the analysis: identification of important inputs, and estimation of data distribution throughout the input space. In order to build a reliable model, input data should be equally spread throughout the input data space. PCA is the most common tool for analysis of the input data distribution. The input data distribution is directly influenced by experimental design, which must be set up to cover the input data space areas of interest. However, when data are obtained from experiments that are not designed specifically for the modelling, it is necessary to evaluate the distribution of the input data in order to correctly set the limits for valid values of model inputs, as fuzzy models and ANN have poor extrapolation capabilities. Low numbers of significant principal components (cumulatively accounting for at least 95% of total input variance) with respect to the number of inputs, suggest poor input data distribution and, consequently, very limited sub-space of valid model input values. If such distribution is caused by physical limits of the technology, this has no effect on model efficiency as the inputs outside the sub-space that was covered with experiments have no practical significance. However, if the limited coverage of the input space is not subject to some physical limitations of the process, any model designed on such data sets should be used with caution. As the presented method is designed to operate on commonly measured variables of the tableting process, at least the data for initial model design should be obtained with some pilot study designed specifically for the model development, while the model improvements can be performed on the data obtained with the manual tableting optimisation procedures. In the long run, such a procedure is more cost and time effective, as suitable tableting machine settings for each new batch can be found more quickly.

9.6 Testing feasibility of the improved optimisation procedure

The method for optimising the tableting process using a mathematical model (ANN and fuzzy) was created and tested on a high-capacity Killian

T300/40 tableting machine, with a formulation including a 75% loading of the active ingredient from the group of macrolide antibiotics [31–33]. The formulation had poor flow and compressibility characteristics and a strong tendency to exhibit capping. A dry granulation of this formulation led to a larger particle size, improved powder flowability, better compressibility properties and a significantly lower capping tendency [22].

9.6.1 Production of model tablets

In order to study the influence of dry granulation compared with direct tableting on tablet quality, three types of powder mixtures for tableting were prepared:

1. Powder for direct compression without prior granulation step (Type: 'direct' – 1 sample, see Table 9.1),
2. Granulate prepared by slugging (dry granulation on a tableting machine), using different setting parameters of tableting speed and compression force (Type: 'slugging' – 4 samples – see Table 9.1),
3. Granulate prepared by dry granulation on a roller compactor using different parameters of compacting speed and force (Type: 'roller' – 4 samples – see Table 9.1).

The qualitative and quantitative compositions of all the powder mixtures were the same, and the milling and sieving of the compacts were performed on the same equipment using a 1.5 mm sieve. The nine samples were compressed into tablets on a Killian® T300/40 (IMA, Germany) tableting machine equipped with round, concave punches (Ø = 13 mm,

Table 9.1 Process parameters for dry granulation on a tableting machine (slugging) and on a roller compactor (roller)

Slugging			Roller		
Label	Speed (1000 tbl/h)	Compression pressure (bar)	Label	Speed (rev/min)	Compression pressure (bar)
S26/21	26	21	R12/60	12	60
S100/21	100	21	R20/60	20	60
S26/14	26	14	S16/85	16	85
S100/14	100	14	S20/85	20	85

Table 9.2 Values of the process parameters

Main compression force (kN)	Pre-compression force (kN)	Tableting machine speed (1000 tbl/h)
7	5	26
14	7.5	40
18	9	67.5
21		100

R = 26 mm) using different combinations of parameter settings: main compression force, pre-compression force and tableting speed (Table 9.2). The tablet mass was 0.550 g.

Each powder mixture was compressed at different combinations of setting parameters during the compression trial. We produced 76 types of tablets, and a sample of 10 tablets was evaluated from each sample type. If all the process-parameter settings (see Table 9.1) were to be used on all the powder types, there would have been a total of 432 tablet types. However, making 432 tablet types would require too much work, and thus the 76 types that were the most interesting for industrial procedures were selected.

The tablets were evaluated in terms of mass variability, crushing strength variability and a capping coefficient (CC). The CC was evaluated during testing of the tablet crushing strength. The tablet was considered to have a capping tendency if the upper part of the tablet completely fell apart from the tablet body during testing of crushing strength or if typical relief (a significant step form) appeared on the fractured surface of the tablet, which would indicate that there is a large probability that the tablet would break during subsequent steps in production. The CC was calculated as a fraction of the tablets with a capping tendency compared to all the evaluated tablets.

The CC of each tablet type was analysed with respect to the following experimental values: the main compression force, the pre-compression force, the tableting speed, the Carr index and the particle size distribution of the powder (which is related to the powder type). The Carr index is a well-established index for describing the compressibility of powders [12]. Each powder type was also characterised with a particle size distribution based on a sieve analysis using the following sieve ranges: 0–0.045 mm (d1), 0.045–0.071 mm (d2), 0.071–0.125 mm (d3), 0.125–0.25 mm (d4),

0.25–0.5 mm (d5), 0.5–0.71 mm (d6), 0.71–1.0 mm (d7) and 1.0–1.25 mm (d8). Each powder type was characterised by the proportion of particles belonging to each particle size group.

9.6.2 Identifying the dimensionality of the input data set

Using PCA, the input data distribution was tested. The dimensionality of input data reveals the randomness of experimental design. To produce a reliable model, experimental design must cover the interesting design parameters space as evenly as possible. At the same time, the number of most important principal components defines the dimension of the sub-space that was sufficiently covered with the experiments. The estimated dimension of the sub-space also defines the approximate number of independent input variables that can be used as model inputs. If a much higher number of model inputs is selected, the model is valid for a very limited area of the design space. In our case, the input space was defined by the tableting machine settings (compression force, pre-compression force and speed), and the particle size composition of the powder (d1–d8) resulting in 11-dimensional input space. PCA was performed on input data and 95% of the total input data variability can be described with only two principal components (see Figure 9.2).

This suggests that we can afford to use models with only a few inputs to obtain good prediction by the model for the whole range of interesting values of input values. Observing Figure 9.1, it makes sense to use up to three or four of the most significant principal components as inputs, or a similar number of selected original inputs. Using principal components is more beneficial for model training as they are linearly independent; however, calculation of original input values from the principal components is an underdetermined problem and may produce large computational errors. In cases where a number of original inputs can be selected that is close enough to the identified dimension of the sub-space and still provides good model prediction, this solution has an advantage over the principal components as model inputs. In our case a selection of original inputs provided only marginally worse prediction than principal components as model inputs, therefore the original inputs were selected as model inputs.

A separate PCA of the particle size distribution of the used powder mixtures suggested that there is only one significant principal component. Hence, a median of particle size distribution was used as a descriptor of powder composition.

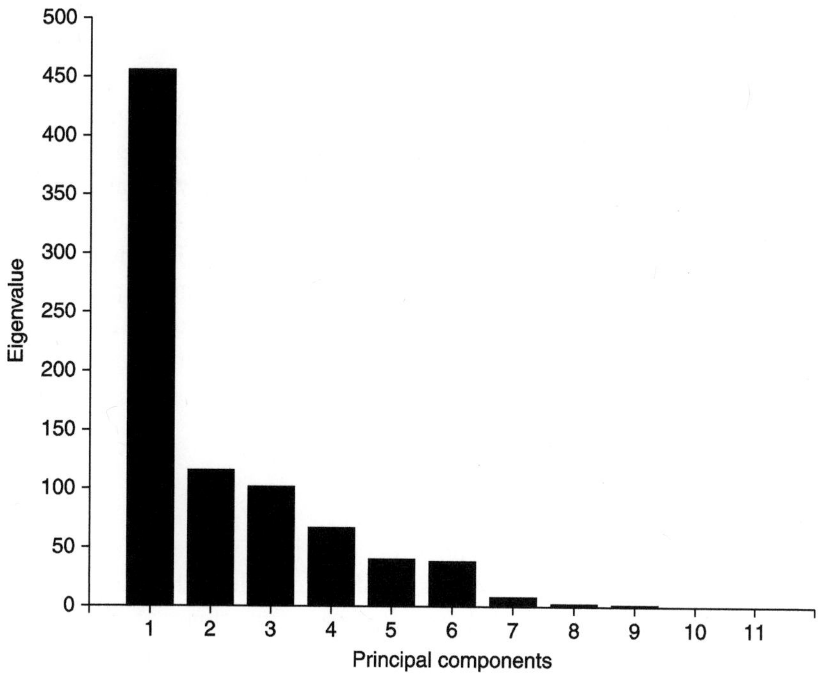

Figure 9.2 Principal components of the input space

9.6.3 Training and validation procedures

The training procedures were unique for each type of the model; however, validation of both models was performed in a similar way. Validation was performed with a variant of the leave-one-out procedure, where 16 data points were left for the validation and 60 points were randomly selected for the training. After several repetitions of the training and validation procedures on the same training-validation data set, a new data set was created by randomly selecting another 60 points for the training and 16 points for the validation data set. The procedure of randomly selecting the training-validation sets was repeated several times. The model prediction was validated by applying the R^2 measure [34].

$$R^2 = \frac{1 - \sum (T_s - T)^2}{\sum (T_s - T)^2 - \sum (T_s - \bar{T})}$$

The models achieved R^2 values between 0.87 and 0.66.

Artificial neural networks

To model the system's characteristics, a feed-forward ANN [24] was used. The neural network consisted of two or three neurons with a tangens sigmoid transfer function on the first layer and one neuron with a linear transfer function on the output layer. The ANN was trained with the Levenberg-Marquadt algorithm. The network was trained several hundred times to analyse the stability of the result. The number of neurons in the first layer was selected according to the model prediction value. The starting structure was one neuron and then the neurons were added as long as each new neuron caused significant improvement of the R^2 value.

Fuzzy model

In this study a TS-type fuzzy model was used [25], wherein an arbitrary function of the input variables is used to calculate the output. For simplicity of interpretation, however, linear functions of the input variables are often selected. Thus, the TS model of a system with two inputs and, where each input is divided between the two fuzzy sets, fuzzy sets, $x_1 \in X_{11}$, X_{12} and, $x_2 \in X_{21}$, X_{22} is described as:

$$\text{IF}(x_1 \in X_{11}) \cap (x_2 \in X_{21}) \text{ THEN } y_1 = k_{11}x_1 + k_{12}x_2 + n_1$$

$$\text{IF}(x_1 \in X_{11}) \cap (x_2 \in X_{22}) \text{ THEN } y_2 = k_{21}x_1 + k_{22}x_2 + n_2$$

$$\text{IF}(x_1 \in X_{12}) \cap (x_2 \in X_{21}) \text{ THEN } y_3 = k_{31}x_1 + k_{32}x_2 + n_3$$

$$\text{IF}(x_1 \in X_{12}) \cap (x_2 \in X_{22}) \text{ THEN } y_4 = k_{41}x_1 + k_{42}x_2 + n_4$$

Each logical statement defines a region of input space and the corresponding output function. Each input variable is first fuzzified, by calculating the memberships of the fuzzy sets that describe the particular input variable. Next, the output of each statement is calculated, and then the outputs are aggregated by calculating the weighted sum of the outputs, the weights being the corresponding results of the premises.

$$CC = (\mu_1 y_1 + \mu_2 y_2 + \mu_3 y_3 + \mu_4 y_4)/(\mu_1 + \mu_2 + \mu_3 + \mu_4)$$

where μ_i represents the result of a premise statement:

$$\mu_1 = (x_1 \in X_{11}) \cap (x_2 \in X_{21}) = \min(x_1 \in X_{11}, x_2 \in X_{21})$$

$$\mu_2 = (x_1 \in X_{11}) \cap (x_2 \in X_{22}) = \min(x_1 \in X_{11}, x_2 \in X_{22})$$

$$\mu_3 = (x_1 \in X_{12}) \cap (x_2 \in X_{21}) = \min(x_1 \in X_{12}, x_2 \in X_{21})$$

$$\mu_4 = (x_1 \in X_{12}) \cap (x_2 \in X_{22}) = \min(x_1 \in X_{12}, x_2 \in X_{22})$$

The number of input variables was selected with respect to R^2 measure. The initial structure of the model had all four possible input variables as inputs (particle size distribution, compression force, pre-compression force, tableting speed). Next, the input that had the least effect on R^2 was removed. All inputs that had insignificant influence on R^2 were removed. Each input was fuzzified by two linguistic variables that had piece-wise linear membership functions.

Modelling of CC

For the ANN, two inputs were identified as the most important for good model prediction: the median of the particle size distribution of the powder, and the compression force. Therefore, the final ANN had two inputs that were connected to the two neurons of the first layer and the two neurons were connected to the output neuron. The output of the output neuron was the predicted CC. In Figure 9.4(a) the identified CC relation with respect to the compression force and the particle size distribution is shown.

For the fuzzy model, the same two inputs were identified as for the ANN. The identified membership functions are shown in Figure 9.3.

In Figure 9.4(b) the identified relation for the fuzzy model is presented.

Modelling of crushing strength variability

For the ANN, three inputs were identified as the most important for good model prediction: the median of the particle size distribution of the powder, the compression force and the pre-compression force. The final ANN had three inputs that were connected to the three neurons of the first layer and the three neurons were connected to the output neuron. The output of the output neuron was the predicted crushing strength variability. In Figure 9.6 the identified relation with respect to the particle size distribution, the compression force and the pre-compression force is shown.

For the fuzzy model, the same three inputs were identified as for the ANN. The identified membership functions are shown in Figure 9.5. The predicted relation is shown in Figure 9.6.

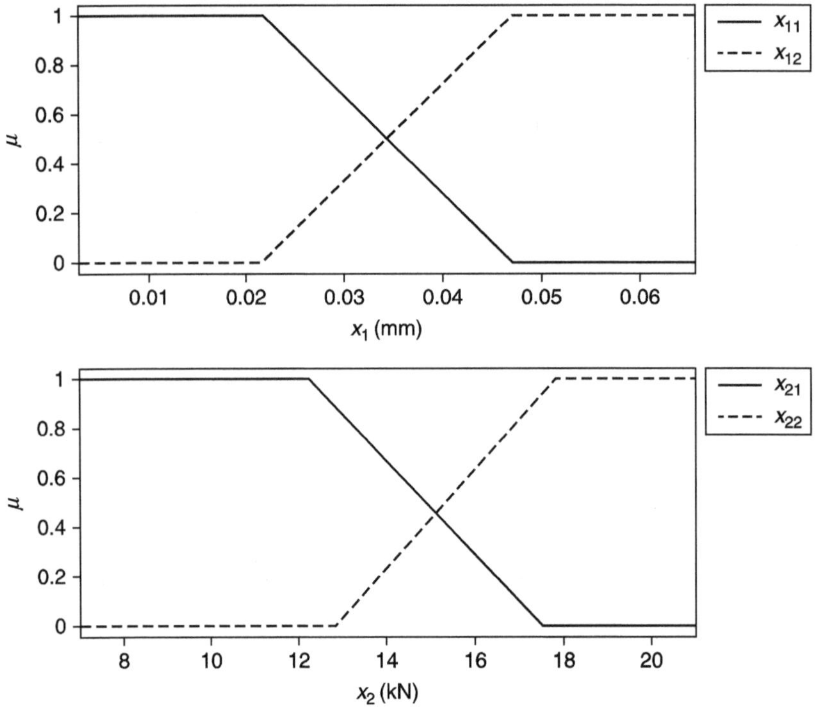

Figure 9.3 Membership functions for CC prediction: μ – grade of membership, x_1 – particle size distribution median, x_2 – compression force, X_{11},X_{12} – linguistic variables fine and coarse particle size distribution, X_{21},X_{22} – linguistic variables low and high compression force

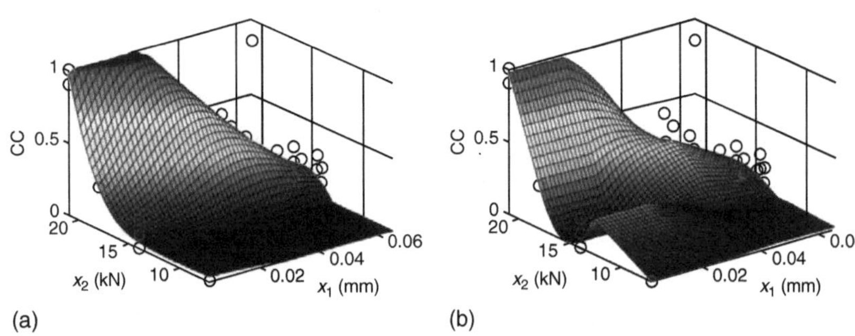

Figure 9.4 Identified effects of particle size distribution median (x_1) compression force (x_2) on CC: (a) ANN model, (b) fuzzy model. Surface represents the identified relation, circles represent measured effects

Published by Woodhead Publishing Limited, 2013

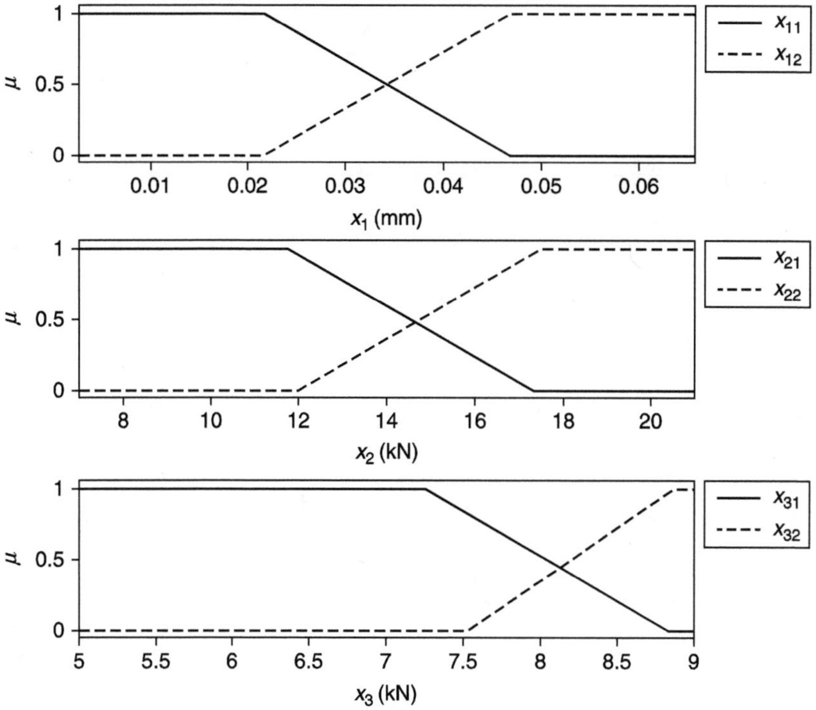

Figure 9.5 **Membership functions for σF_c prediction: μ – grade of membership, x_1 – particle size distribution median, x_2 – compression force, x_3 – pre-compression force, X_{11},X_{12} – linguistic variables fine and coarse particle size distribution, X_{21},X_{22} – linguistic variables low and high compression force, X_{31},X_{32} – linguistic variables low and high pre-compression force**

Modelling of mass variability

For the ANN, four inputs were identified as the most important for good model prediction: the median of the particle size distribution of the powder, the compression force, the pre-compression force and tableting speed. The final ANN had four inputs that were connected to the two neurons of the first layer and the two neurons were connected to the output neuron. The output of the output neuron was the predicted mass variability. In Figure 9.8 the identified relation with respect to the particle size distribution, the compression force, the pre-compression force and tableting speed is shown.

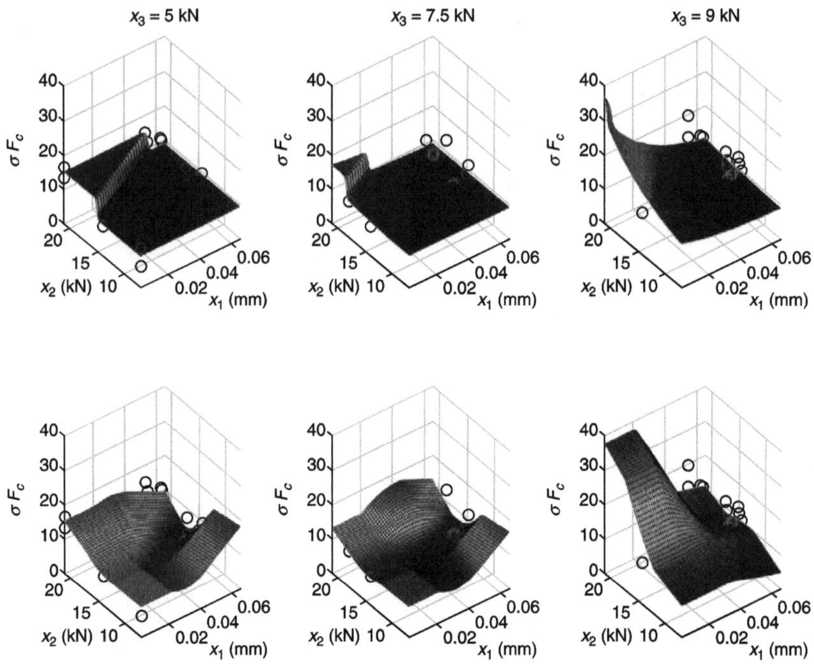

Figure 9.6 Identified effects of particle size distribution median (x_1), compression force (x_2), and pre-compression force (x_3) on crushing strength variability (σF_c): first line – ANN model, second line – fuzzy model, columns represent a single value of x_3. Surface represents the identified relation, circles represent measured effects

For the fuzzy model, the same four inputs were identified as for the ANN. The identified membership functions are shown in Figure 9.7. The predicted relation is shown in Figure 9.9.

9.6.4 *Finding optimal tableting parameters*

Once the model has been developed and validated, it can be used for optimisation procedures. The goal of the optimisation procedure is to get optimal tableting machine settings for a given powder. The powder with the same characteristics as the tableting mixture prepared for direct tableting (without prior granulation) was chosen for the test. The first step of optimisation procedure is to define the optimisation goal. In our

Published by Woodhead Publishing Limited, 2013

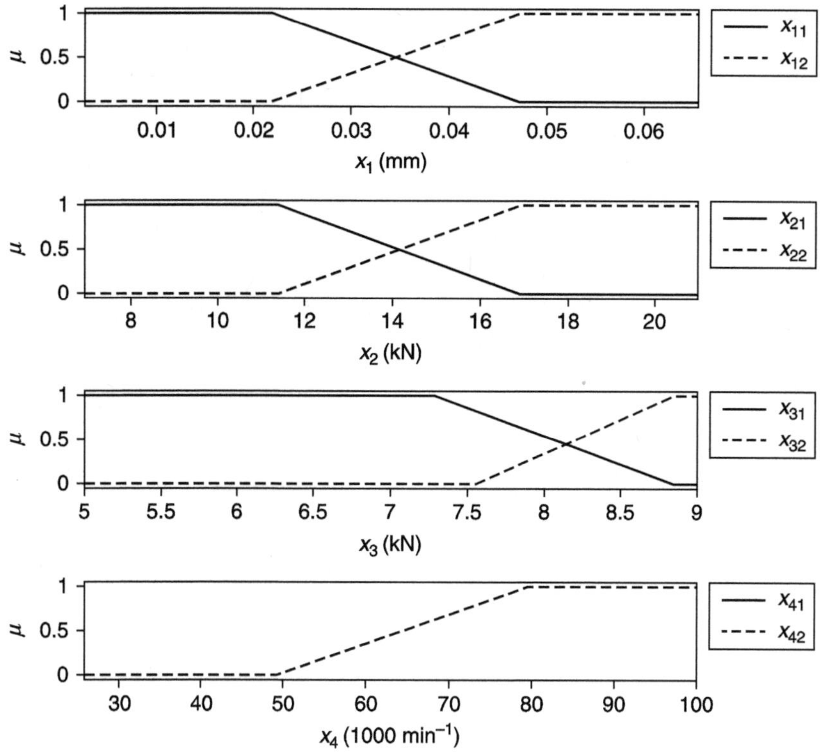

Figure 9.7 **Membership functions for σ_m prediction: μ – grade of membership, x_1 – particle size distribution median, x_2 – compression force, x_3 – pre-compression force, x_4 – tableting speed, X_{11},X_{12} – linguistic variables fine and coarse particle size distribution, X_{21},X_{22} – linguistic variables low and high compression force, X_{31},X_{32} – linguistic variables low and high pre-compression force, X_{41},X_{42} – linguistic variables low and high tableting speed**

case, it would be optimal to have no tablets with capping tendency (CC) and no variability of crushing strength (σF_c) or mass (σ_m), while the tableting machine would operate at the highest possible speed (v_t). The mathematical description of the criterion would, therefore, look like:

$$J = CC + \sigma F_c + \sigma_m + \frac{1}{v_t}$$

and the goal would be to find the minimum of the function. However, as the values of the variables included in the criterion have quite different

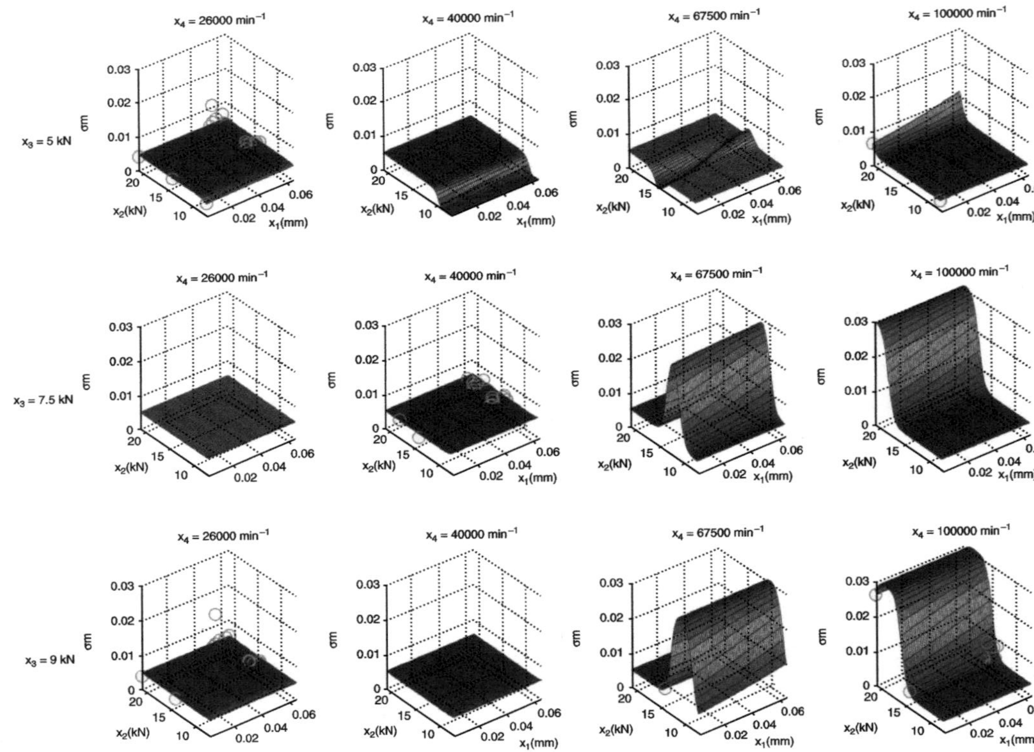

Figure 9.8 ANN identification of effects of particle size distribution median (x_1), compression force (x_2), pre-compression force (x_3), and tableting speed (x_4) on mass variability (σm): lines represent a single value of x_3, columns represent a single value of x_4. Surface represents the identified relation, circles represent measured effects

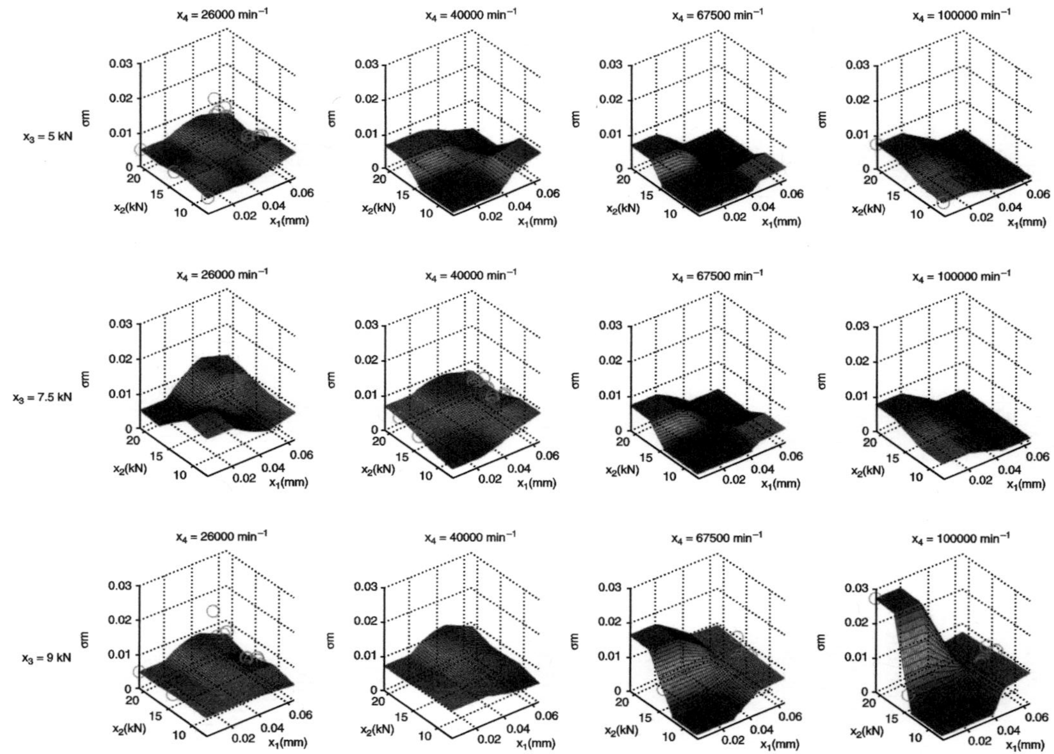

Figure 9.9 Fuzzy identification of effects of particle size distribution median (x_1), compression force (x_2), pre-compression force (x_3), and tableting speed (x_4) on mass variability (σm): lines represent a single value of x_3, columns represent a single value of x_4. Surface represents the identified relation, circles represent measured effects

ranges of values, each variable must be scaled in order to achieve the desirable effect. In cases where the ideal solution $J = 0$ can be achieved the scaling is irrelevant; however, in real cases $J = 0$ can never be achieved, as contradictory situations might occur where reduction of one variable's value would cause elevation of the other variable's value. In such cases the scaling of variables defines the optimum of the criterion and must be carefully chosen. In our case the variables were scaled with their maximal value as was measured in the experiments, ensuring equal effects of all the variables on the criterion. The simplex method [23], as implemented in Matlab's *fmeansearch* function, was used to find the minimum of the function. Regardless of the model type, the optimal setting for the tableting machine for the raw powder was identified at compression force of 8.7 kN, pre-compression force of 6.4 kN and tableting speed of 100 000 tablets per minute. Another suitable solution was found for compression force of 19.6 kN, pre-compression force of 5.0 kN and tableting speed of 100 000.

9.7 Conclusions

The proposed model-assisted tableting machine setting, as described in this chapter, has some advances over the classical, completely manual approach.

Fuzzy models are not very often used in the field of pharmaceutical technology; however, they have some significant advantages over ANN. Most importantly, it is possible to use other knowledge than just the measured data for their identification, which reduces the need for large quantities of data when identifying non-linear relations. The fuzzy model can be built on the basis of piece-wise linear models that are often used in pharmacy. Thus, we also obtain better model transparency, which is very important for the understanding of complex non-linear relations.

By observing relatively large differences between the surfaces predicted by the two models, it is clear that any numerical estimations of the prediction quality, such as R^2, are not entirely unbiased. Although R^2 is relatively high for both models (0.87 for ANN, and 0.82 for the fuzzy model), suggesting high quality of the models' predictions, the comparison of the surfaces identified with the two models resulted in large differences in areas where measurements were sparse. This suggests that in cases where it is not possible to obtain a sufficient number of measurements to uniquely identify the model, it is beneficial to use several modelling techniques to identify the quality of model prediction. In input space areas

Published by Woodhead Publishing Limited, 2013

that are too sparsely covered with the measured points, the characteristics of the used model prevail over the characteristics of the modelled system.

Although the surface of the identified relation is not equal for both models and, therefore, completely automated setting of the tableting machine, with respect to a powder batch, is not possible, the model represents valuable information for the operator about useful ranges of machine settings with respect to the physical properties of the powder. Using a model is also more cost effective than a trial-and-error approach. Optimisation of the tableting machine's settings by trial and error produces a relatively large number of faulty tablets and is very time consuming, especially when the starting settings of the machine were poorly guessed, and the procedure has to be repeated for characteristics of each new powder batch. In an industrial environment with a PAT system [5] implemented, development of the model would have to be divided into two stages. First, the data generation for building the model would be organised as a dedicated experiment that should cover the area of interest described by the machine's setting parameters and the properties of the powder. For the modelling, the machine's settings must be systematically chosen to cover the whole area of interesting values and tested for several batches. Next, the model would be validated and further developed with data from large-scale production. Production monitoring data typically contribute relatively dense data points from the near-optimal areas of the experimental space that were not included at the beginning in the experimental plan. Experiments for modelling purposes are more expensive than those for optimisation with trial and error; however, the model can be used for the prediction of optimal settings for new batches, which substantially shortens the time for optimising the tableting machine with respect to a new batch and reduces the number of faulty tablets and shortens the machine set up times which contribute to a production optimisation. In any case, the models that will be built on the contemporary routinely measured quantities will most likely never be precise enough for completely automated adaptation of the machine settings as a compensation for batch-to-batch differences, but they can serve as a significant improvement to the trial-and-error procedure.

9.8 References

[1] Soares L, González Ortega G, Petrovick P and Schmidt P. 2005 Dry Granulation and Compression of Spray-Dried Plant Extracts. *AAPS PharmSciTech* 6(3), E359–66.

[2] von Eggelkraut-Gottanka S, Abed S, Müller W and Schmidt P. 2002 Roller Compaction and Tabletting of St. John's Wort Plant Dry Extract Using a Gap Width and Force Controlled Roller Compactor. I. Granulation and Tabletting of Eight Different Extract Batches. *Pharmaceutical Development and Technology* 7(4), 433–45.

[3] Kochhar S, Rubinstein M and Barnes D. 1995 The Effect of Slugging and Recompression on Pharmaceutical Excipients. *International Journal of Pharmaceutics* 115(1), 35–43.

[4] Picker K. 2001 Time Dependence of Elastic Recovery for Characterization of Tableting Materials. *Pharmaceutical Development and Technology* 6(1), 61–70.

[5] Informa. *PAT – Quality by design and process improvement*, Amsterdam, 2007.

[6] Sebhatu T, Ahlneck C and Alderborn G. 1997 The Effect of Moisture Content on the Compression and Bond-Formation Properties of Amorphous Lactose Particles. *International Journal of Pharmaceutics* 146(1), 101–14.

[7] Rios M. 2006 Developments in Powder Flow Testing. Pharmaceutical Technology 30(2), 38–49.

[8] Sorensen A, Sonnergaard J and Hovgaard L. 2006 Bulk Characterization of Pharmaceutical Powders by Low-Pressure Compression II: Effect of Method Settings and Particle Size. *Pharmaceutical Development and Technology* 11(2), 235–41.

[9] Zhang Y, Law Y and Chakrabarti S. 2003 Physical Properties and Compact Analysis of Commonly Used Direct Compression Binders. *AAPS PharmSciTech* 4(4), E62.

[10] Gohel M and Jogani P. 2002 Functionality Testing of a Multifunctional Directly Compressible Adjuvant Containing Lactose, Polyvinylpyrrolidone and Croscarmellose Sodium. *Pharmaceutical Technology* 26(3), 64–82.

[11] Sucker H. 1982 Test Methods for Granulates. *Pharmazeutische Industrie* 44(3), 312–6.

[12] Li Q, Rudolph V, Weigl B and Earl A. 2004 Interparticle van der Waals Force in Powder Flowability and Compactibility. *International Journal of Pharmaceutics* 280(1–2), 77–93.

[13] Parrott E 1990. Compression. In Liberman H, Lachman L and Schwartz J, editors. *Pharmaceutical Dosage Forms: Tablets, 2nd ed.*, New York: Marcel Dekker, pp. 201–43.

[14] Nystrom C, Alderborn G, Duberg M and Karehill P. 1993 Bonding Surface-Area and Bonding Mechanism – 2 Important Factors for the Understanding of Powder Compactibility. *Drug Development and Industrial Pharmacy* 19(17–8), 2143–96.

[15] Luangtana-Anan M and Fell J. 1990 Bonding Mechanisms in Tabletting. *International Journal of Pharmaceutics* 60(3), 197–202.

[16] Sonnergaard J. 2006 Quantification of the Compactibility of Pharmaceutical Powders. *European Journal of Pharmaceutics and Biopharmaceutics* 63(3), 270–7.

[17] Wu C, Ruddy O, Bentham A, Hancock B, Best S and Elliott J. 2005 Modelling the Mechanical Behaviour of Pharmaceutical Powders During Compaction. *Powder Technology* 152(1–3), 107–17.

Published by Woodhead Publishing Limited, 2013

[18] Ilkka J and Paronen P. 1993 Prediction of the Compression Behaviour of Powder Mixtures by the Heckel Equation. *International Journal of Pharmaceutics* 94(1–3), 181–7.
[19] Carstensen J, Geoffroy J and Dellamonica C. 1990 Compression Characteristics of Binary-Mixtures. *Powder Technology* 62(2), 119–24.
[20] Busignies V, Leclerc B, Porion P, Evesque P, Couarraze G and Tchoreloff P. 2006 Compaction Behaviour and New Predictive Approach to the Compressibility of Binary Mixtures of Pharmaceutical Excipients. *European Journal of Pharmaceutics and Biopharmaceutics* 64(1), 66–74.
[21] Jackson JE. 1991 *A User Guide to Principal Components*. New York: John Wiley & Sons, inc.
[22] Hagan M, Demuth H and Beale M. 1996 *Neural Network Design. 1st ed.*, Boston: Thomson Learning.
[23] Fletcher R. 1969 *Optimization*. London: Academic Press.
[24] Zadeh LA. 1965 Fuzzy sets. *Information and Control* 8(3), 338–53.
[25] Takagi T and Sugeno M. 1985 Fuzzy identification of systems and its applications to modelling and control. *IEEE Transactions on Systems, Man, and Cybernetics* 15, 116–32.
[26] Kosko B. 1994 Fuzzy systems as universal approximators. *IEEE Transactions on Computers* 43(11), 1329–33.
[27] Ying Gc Y. 1997 Necessary conditions for some typical fuzzy systems as universal approximators. *Automatica* 33, 1333–8.
[28] Wang LX and Mendel JM. 1992 Fuzzy basis functions, universal approximation, and orthogonal least-squares learning. *IEEE Transactions on Neural Networks* 3(5), 807–14.
[29] Goldberg RR. 1976 *Methods of Real Analysis. 2nd Ed.*, New York: John Wiley and Sons.
[30] Lin CH. 1997 Siso nonlinear system identification using a fuzzy-neural hybrid system. *International Journal of Neural Systems* 8(3), 325–37.
[31] Zupancic-Bozic D, Dreu R and Vrecer F. 2008 Influence of Dry Granulation on Compactibility and Capping Tendency of Macrolide Antibiotic Formulation. *International Journal of Pharmaceutics* 357(1–2), 44–54.
[32] Belič A, Škrjanc I, Zupančič-Božič D, Karba R and Vrečer F. 2009 Minimisation of the capping tendency by tableting process optimisation with the application of artificial neural networks and fuzzy models. *European Journal of Pharmaceutics and Biopharmaceutics* 73(1), 172–8.
[33] Belič A, Škrjanc I, Zupančič-Božič D and Vrečer F. 2009 Tableting process optimisation with the application of fuzzy models. *International Journal of Pharmaceutics* 389(1–2), 86–93.
[34] Draper NR and Smith H. 1998 *Applied Regression Analysis. 3rd Ed.*, New York: John Wiley and Sons.

Index

Published by Woodhead Publishing Limited, 2013